Two week loan

Please return on or before t
date stamped below.
Charges are made for la

PRINCIPLES OF MOLECULAR PATHOLOGY

PRINCIPLES
OF MOLECULAR
PATHOLOGY

By

ANTHONY A. KILLEEN, MB, BCh, PhD

Department of Laboratory Medicine and Pathology,
University of Minnesota, Minneapolis, MN

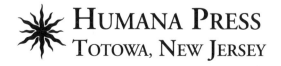
HUMANA PRESS
TOTOWA, NEW JERSEY

© 2004 Humana Press Inc.
999 Riverview Drive, Suite 208
Totowa, New Jersey 07512

www.humanapress.com

Production Editor: Tracy Catanese.
Cover Illustrations: Figures 23 and 25A–D from Chapter 4, "Methods in Molecular Pathology"; Figure 5 from Chapter 3, "Mutation"; and Figure 9 from Chapter 2, "Genetic Inheritance."

Cover design by Patricia F. Cleary.

This publication is printed on acid-free paper. ∞
ANSI Z39.48-1984 (American National Standards Institute) Permanence of Paper for Printed Library Materials.

For additional copies, pricing for bulk purchases, and/or information about other Humana titles, contact Humana at the above address or at any of the following numbers: Tel.: 973-256-1699; Fax: 973-256-8341; E-mail: humana@humanapr.com or visit our website: http://www.humanapress.com

Printed in the United States of America.   10   9   8   7   6   5   4   3   2   1

1-59259-431-X (e-book)

Library of Congress Cataloging-in-Publication Data

Killeen, Anthony A.
    Principles of molecular pathology / by Anthony A. Killeen.
       p. cm.
    Includes bibliographical references and index.
    ISBN 1-58829-085-9 (alk. paper)
       1. Pathology, Molecular. 2. Genetic disorders. I. Title.

 RB113.K47 2003
 616.07'56--dc21

                                                                        2003041737

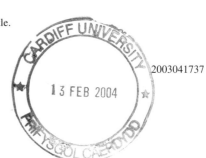

DEDICATION

In memoriam parentium, Professor James Francis and Joyce Killeen.

PREFACE

Principles of Molecular Pathology provides a comprehensive, but concise introduction to this rapidly growing subject. It will be useful to a wide readership including residents and fellows in laboratory medicine and pathology, practicing pathologists who have not had a formal exposure to this relatively new field, and our medical and scientific colleagues in related laboratory and clinical disciplines.

Only a few years ago, experts debated whether molecular pathology was a bona fide academic discipline, or merely the application of new laboratory techniques that would find their roles in existing areas of the clinical laboratories. Now it is clear that this field is far more than just a set of novel techniques. Molecular pathology has a grand theme, and that theme is the study of genetic mutations, both inherited and acquired, and their effects on the structure and function of the cell. Within this theme, molecular pathology brings together concepts from molecular biology, genetics, and traditional pathology to provide new insights into human diseases, new ways of classifying certain types of diseases, and the technologies to provide new diagnostic and prognostic information. There is no doubt that the practice of laboratory medicine and pathology will be significantly altered by the principles and laboratory methods of molecular pathology.

The topics in *Principles of Molecular Pathology* were chosen to provide a broad overview of the field. Basic concepts of human molecular biology and genetics are followed by a description of the most commonly used analytical methods. This background is followed by a discussion of the acquired genetic abnormalities that underlie human malignancies. Chapters on pharmacogenetics and identity testing emphasize the growing importance of these areas in clinical practice. The application of molecular methods to the detection of microbial pathogens has assumed an essential role in clinical laboratory practice, and this important area is illustrated using common viral infections as examples.

I hope that *Principles of Molecular Pathology* will stimulate interest in this exciting field. I welcome comments from readers at akilleen@akilleen.com.

Acknowledgments

First and foremost, I thank my wife, Randee, for her love and support, and for her patience during the course of my writing this book. It would never have been completed without the time she afforded me to write. Our children, Olivia and Trevor, were a constant source of energy and enthusiasm during this project.

I acknowledge with gratitude the excellent support of my colleagues at the University of Minnesota and my former colleagues at the University of Michigan. Several have read and commented on chapters, including Matt Bower, Charlotte Brown, Michelle Dolan, Betsy Hirsch, Mark Linder, Elizabeth Petty, and Rima Tinawi-Aljundi. I thank them sincerely for their suggestions.

Anthony A. Killeen

CONTENTS

1 Basic Concepts in Molecular Pathology

BASIC TERMINOLOGY

Human diseases that have a genetic basis, whether hereditary or acquired, arise from changes in the sequence or pattern of expression of genes. A gene, which is the unit of heredity, is a piece of DNA that encodes a protein or RNA. The position at which a given gene is found on a chromosome is known as its locus. Sequence variants of a gene are known as alleles, and the most common functional allele at a locus is known as the wild-type allele. Changes in the sequence of DNA are known as mutations. In genetic use, the term mutation does not necessarily mean that the effect of the change in sequence is deleterious to the organism. By definition, a sequence change that is present in at least 1% of the population is known as a polymorphism.

In the haploid cell, the human genome is composed of approximately 3×10^9 bp of DNA, the sequence of which has largely been determined through the efforts of the public and commercial human genome projects *(1,2)*. Most of the genome is located in the nucleus, but mitochondria also contain a small genome that is approximately 16.5 kb in length. The set of genes that is expressed in a cell determines the structure and functions of the cell.

STRUCTURE OF NUCLEIC ACIDS

Both DNA and RNA are polymers composed of repeating units of sugars (deoxyribose or ribose, respectively) with attached bases. The sugars are joined by phosphodiester linkages between the 3′ carbon of one sugar and the 5′ carbon of the next sugar in the polymer (Fig. 1). A strand of DNA or RNA therefore has polarity: the end with the terminal 5′-carbon is known as the 5′ end, and the other end of the strand, which has an unlinked 3′-hydroxyl group, is

From: *Principles of Molecular Pathology*
Edited by: A. A. Killeen © Humana Press Inc., Totowa, NJ

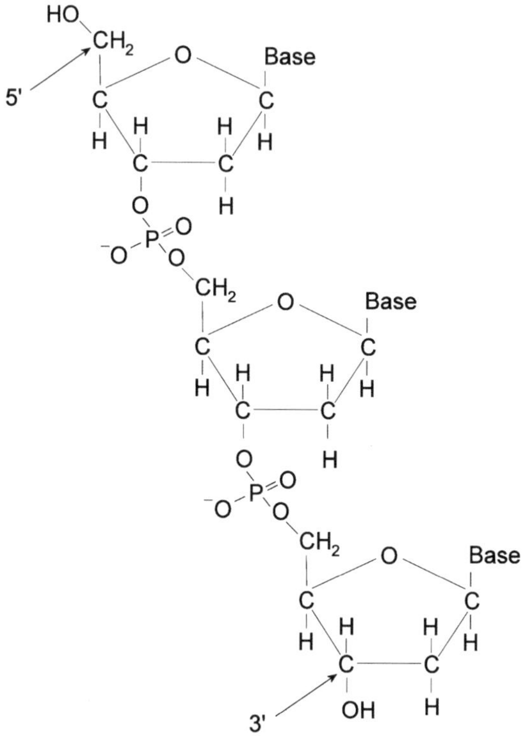

Fig. 1. Structure of a strand of nucleic acid (DNA shown). The strand is composed of a polymer of sugar residues joined by phosphate linkages between the 3′-carbon of one sugar and the 5′-carbon of the next sugar. Each sugar is attached to a base. The 5′ and 3′ ends of the polymer are shown by arrows.

known as the 3′ end. Ribose and deoxyribose differ at the 2′-carbon, which has a hydroxyl group in ribose (Fig. 2). Both DNA and RNA are composed of purine and pyrimidine bases (Fig. 3). The standard base composition differs between DNA and RNA: in DNA the bases adenine (A), cytidine (C), guanine (G), and thymidine (T) are present. In RNA, uracil (U) is present in place of thymidine. The structures of these are shown in Figs. 4 and 5. In addition to these standard bases, other bases are found in DNA and RNA. The most frequent modification is methylation of cytidine at carbon 5, giving rise to 5-methylcytidine.

A strand of DNA forms interstrand hydrogen bonds with another DNA strand of complementary sequence. In this arrangement, A forms a base pair with T on the complementary strand, and C forms

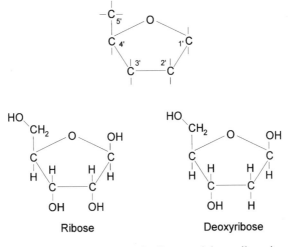

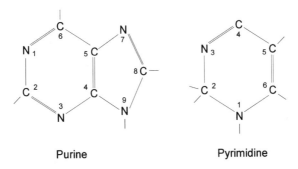

Fig. 2. The numbering of carbon atoms in ribose and deoxyribose in nucleic acids is shown at the top. The structures of ribose and deoxyribose differ at the 2′-carbon, which is linked to a hydroxyl group in ribose. In DNA and RNA, the bases are joined at the 1′ carbon.

Purine

Pyrimidine

Fig. 3. Basic structure and numbering of carbon atoms in purine and pyrimidine.

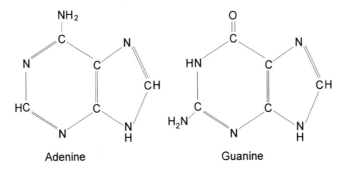

Adenine

Guanine

Fig. 4. Structures of the purines adenine and guanine.

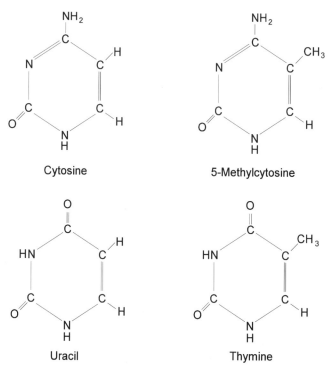

Fig. 5. Structures of the pyrimidines cytosine, 5-methylcytosine, uracil, and thymine.

a base pair with G. Two hydrogen bonds can form between A and T, whereas three bonds can form between C and G. Bonding of the latter base pair is therefore stronger than the former. In addition, the two complementary strands of DNA are oriented in opposite directions and adopt a double-helix structure.

RNA generally exists as single-stranded molecules; however, intrastrand base pairing can form, giving rise to molecules with complex three-dimensional structures. An RNA strand can also form a double helical molecule with another RNA strand of complementary sequence, or with a DNA strand of complementary sequence.

The ability of complementary strands of nucleic acid to bind to each other is the most important property of DNA and RNA in laboratory genetic analysis. It is because of this property that in vitro hybridization of nucleic acids can be used for applications as

diverse as polymerase chain reaction, Southern blotting, and fluorescence *in situ* hybridization (FISH).

TYPES OF DNA

Single-Copy Sequences

Based on the number of copies of a particular sequence in the
genome, DNA sequences can be classified as single copy or as
repetitive. Most genes exist in single copies in the haploid genome,
whereas repetitive DNA sequences are present in multiple copies.
These copies may be adjacent to each other in a head-to-tail
arrangement, or they may be dispersed across different chromosomes. The former are referred to as satellite DNA, and the latter are
known as interspersed repeats.

Genes account for less than 5% of total DNA, but they represent
the most important fraction of the genome for cell structure and
function. Genes encode proteins that are responsible for the biological functions of a cell. Different cells express different sets of the
total repertoire of genes, giving rise to distinct structural and functional characteristics that distinguish one tissue from another. It is
estimated that there are approx 26,000 genes in the human genome,
but that because of alternative splicing, these can give rise to at least
twice as many distinct proteins *(1,2)*. At least 35% of human genes
undergo alternative splicing, giving rise to multiple proteins from
these genes *(3)*. From analysis of sequence information and comparison with genes of known function, the biological function of
proteins or RNAs encoded by most genes identified through large-
scale sequencing projects is known or predicted. However, the function of a large fraction—as much as 40%—of identified genes is
entirely unknown *(2)*.

Repetitive DNA

Repetitive DNA accounts for at least 50% of the human genome
(1). Several classes of repetitive DNA exist (Table 1). The bulk of
repetitive DNA is accounted for by sequences derived from trans-
posable elements, i.e., sequences that are capable of being copied
and inserted into another region of the genome. Among these repetitive elements are short interspersed elements (SINEs), such as
Alu, and long interspersed elements (LINEs), such as LINE1 (L1).

Table 1
Classes of Repetitive DNA[a]

Class	Example
Interspersed repeats	Short interspersed elements (SINEs)
	Long interspersed elements (LINEs)
Retroposed genes	Processed pseudogenes
Simple sequence repeats (SSRs)	Mono-, di-, and trinucleotide repeats
Segmental duplications	HLA class I genes
Tandemly repeated blocks	Centromeres, telomeres, and short arms of acrocentric chromosomes

[a] Based on ref. *1*.

Both SINEs and LINEs have several subclasses. Alu repeats are approx 100–300 bp in length and are present in 1.5 million copies, representing 13% of the genome. LINE elements, of which there are about 850,000 copies, are approximately 6 kb in length, and represent 21% of the human genome *(1)*. Functional LINEs are capable of autonomous retrotransposition by a process that uses RNA polymerase II to produce the LINE mRNA. This encodes a reverse transcriptase and other proteins needed for reverse transcription and reinsertion of the LINE sequence at a new position in the genome. Reverse transcription usually fails to generate a complete cDNA, and so most LINEs are incomplete, with an average length of 900 bp *(1)*. Both Alu and L1 elements have been implicated in human diseases by inactivating genes through insertion and by involvement in misalignment and crossing over during meiosis, leading to duplication and deletion of genes. These effects are discussed in Chapter 3.

Processed pseudogenes arise by an alternative mechanism. These pseudogenes lack the introns found in their normal counterparts. They are believed to arise by reverse transcription of mRNA transcripts of functional genes, followed by integration into a chromosome. The mechanism whereby a mRNA transcript is reverse transcribed is unclear. As previously mentioned, the L1 repeats may be capable of inserting DNA into the genome. The location of insertion of a processed pseudogene in the genome is usually not related to the location of the normal gene. In contrast, nonprocessed pseudogenes located in duplicated segments of DNA are situated close to their normal counterpart and retain the normal organizational structure including the introns. For example, *psiPTEN*, which is located on chromosome 9p, is a processed pseudogene derived from the tumor suppressor gene, *PTEN,* which is located on 10q *(4)*. By contrast, the steroid 21-hydroxylase pseudogene, *CYP21P,* is located approximately 30 kb from the functional gene, *CYP21,* in a duplicated region on chromosome 6p *(5)*.

Simple sequence repeats (SSRs) involve short segments of DNA that are repeated in a head-to-tail fashion. The length of the repeat can be as little as a single nucleotide, or a few base pairs in length. These can be situated in genes or in noncoding regions of the genome. SSRs are of medical interest because there are several examples of diseases, such as the unstable trinucleotide repeat diseases, that are caused by instability of the repeat, i.e., the number of copies changes between generations. If situated in a gene, these changes can alter the level of gene expression or the sequence of the encoded protein. Examples of these are discussed in Chapters 3 and 5. SSRs are also of use in identity testing because some are highly polymorphic and can be used for identification of samples in paternity testing, forensic testing, and bone marrow engraftment monitoring (*see* Chap. 10).

Segmental duplications involve regions of DNA of 1 kb to >200 kb. These account for approximately 5% of the human genome *(1,6)*. Duplication can occur through misalignment and unequal crossing-over during meiosis, leading to a duplication of the segment in a tandem arrangement. However, many duplicated segments have also been found on different chromosomes, indicating that some other mechanism, which is not understood, is involved in their origin *(6)*. An example is provided by the adrenal leukodystrophy gene, *ABCD1,* on the X chromosome (OMIM 300100). This gene is involved in entry of very long chain fatty acids into peroxisomes for catabolism. The disorder has variable phenotypic expression that includes elevated levels of very long chain fatty acids, adrenal insufficiency, and neurological decline *(7)*. Portions of this gene, including exons 7–10, have been duplicated and inserted in the pericentromeric region of chromosomes 2, 10, 16, and 22 *(8)*. Segmental duplications are frequently observed in the pericentromeric and subtelomeric regions of chromosomes and are particularly common in the Y chromosome *(1)*.

TYPES OF RNA

Based on their function, several types of RNA exist. Messenger RNA (mRNA) is used to transfer genetic information, in the form of nucleotide sequence, from genes to ribosomes, where the genetic sequence is used to determine the sequence of amino acids in a polypeptide. Ribosomal RNA (rRNA) is the major component of ribosomes, the structures on which polypeptides are synthesized. rRNA comprises most RNA within a cell. Transfer RNA (tRNA) functions as an adaptor that links the sequence of nucleotides in mRNA to the sequence of amino acids in a polypeptide.

Chromosomes

Humans have 22 pairs of autosomes and a pair of sex chromosomes, X/X in females and X/Y in males. Members of a pair of chromosomes are known as homologs. For each pair of homologous chromosomes, one member is inherited from the father, and the other from the mother. The Y chromosome, which is the only chromosome that is not essential for life, has genes determining that the fetus develops a male phenotype. It is transmitted from father to son.

Chromosomes are numbered and grouped according to their relative sizes and the positions of the centromeres. A chromosome is composed of DNA, histone proteins, and nonhistone proteins. Euchromatin refers to regions of a chromosome in which the chromatin is relatively open. Most transcribed genes are located in euchromatin. Heterochromatin refers to chromatin that is more tightly packed and in which few genes are transcribed.

The ends of chromosomes are known as telomeres. These structures contain multiple copies of a repetitive sequence, TTAGGG. Replication at the end of a linear DNA molecule involves loss of some sequence and so telomeres tend to shorten with successive cell divisions. Telomerase, an enzyme that can add the telomere sequence to the end of a chromosome, is responsible for maintenance of telomere length in normally dividing cells. It is reactivated in most malignancies; this is discussed further in Chapter 6. The subtelomeric regions of chromosomes tend to be rich in genes and have a composition that includes large duplicated segments of DNA varying in length between individuals *(9,10)*. Various chromosomal abnormalities involving subtelomeric sequences have been implicated as a relatively common etiology of moderate-to-severe mental retardation (11).

Following DNA replication, which occurs prior to cell division, each chromosome is present in two copies known as sister chromatids. The structures at which these are joined are the centromeres, also known as primary constrictions. Centromeres are sites of attachment of the microtubule spindle apparatus that is involved in the correct segregation of chromosomes to the two daughter cells during cell division. Chromosomes may be classified as metacentric if the centromere is roughly in the middle of the chromosome, sub-metacentric if the centromere is between the middle and one end of the chromosome, or acrocentric if the centromere is almost at one end of the chromosome.

Centromeres contains repetitive DNA sequences known as α-satellites that are composed of repeats of 171-bp units (12). These repeat structures are arranged into higher order repeats that can span several million base pairs. Probes for specific α-satellites can be used to enumerate and identify chromosomes or fragments of chromosomes in cytogenetic studies using FISH.

RECOMBINATION DURING MEIOSIS

During meiosis, homologous chromosomes pair and exchange segments of DNA. This process is known as recombination. The chromosomes resulting from recombination contain novel combinations of sequences from paternal and maternal chromosomes. The number of recombination events along a particular chromosome depends on the length of the chromosome and on the presence of hot spots of recombination. Recombination rates in females are higher than those in males.

If two loci are closely linked, it is unlikely that a recombination event will occur between them, and so alleles at closely linked loci will usually be inherited together. Alleles that are on the same chromosome are said to be syntenic. The further apart the loci, the more likely it is that a recombination event during meiosis will occur between the two loci, but the possibility of multiple recombination events also increases as the distance between two loci increases. Alleles of distantly separated loci may therefore remain syntenic if an even number of recombination events occurs between the loci.

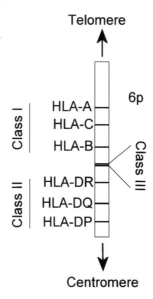

Fig. 6. Arrangement of genes in the HLA region on 6p.

The recombination rate between loci is used to measure genetic distance in centiMorgans (cM). An observed recombination rate of 0.01 (1%) between two loci is expressed as a genetic distance between the loci of 1 cM. This generally corresponds to a physical distance of approx 1 million base pairs of DNA.

HAPLOTYPES AND LINKAGE DISEQUILIBRIUM

When several genes or genetic markers are closely spaced on a chromosome, they tend to be inherited together as a group, and such a group of genetic markers on a chromosome is known as a haplotype. For example, the HLA loci encode highly polymorphic genes that are located in a region of approx 3.6 million bp on the short arm of chromosome 6. This region of the genome is known as the major histocompatibility complex (MHC); the MHC includes class I and class II HLA genes, several genes that encode components of the complement system, and several other genes such as tumor necrosis factor and steroid 21-hydroxylase (Fig. 6). An MHC haplotype includes several million base pairs of DNA, as exemplified by the frequent Caucasian haplotype HLA-A3, -B8, -DRB1*0301, which spans over 2 million bp *(13)*. Identification of MHC haplotypes is of importance when searching for a potential donor for organ or bone marrow transplantation. Siblings have a 1-in-4 probability of having inherited the same MHC haplotypes from their parents and are therefore the most likely potential donors of an MHC-identical match.

When several alleles exist at independent polymorphic loci, the frequencies of expected combinations of alleles in the population is given by the product of the allele frequencies. For example, if locus A has two alleles, A_1 and A_2, with frequencies of 0.3 and 0.7, and locus B also has two alleles, B_1 and B_2, with frequencies of 0.6 and 0.4, then the expected frequencies of combinations of alleles are A_1/B_1 0.18 (i.e., 0.3×0.6); A_1/B_2 0.12; A_2/B_1 0.42; and A_2/B_2 0.28. If these findings were observed in a population, then the markers would be referred to as being in linkage equilibrium. When markers on a chromosome are not randomly associated with each other, they are said to be in linkage disequilibrium. For example, a deletion that includes both the steroid 21-hydroxylase gene *(CYP21)* and the adjacent complement *4B* gene is frequently seen on a haplotype that includes the HLA markers A3, B47, and DR7 *(14)*. This haplotype is associated with congenital adrenal hyperplasia because of deficiency of steroid 21-hydroxylase, an autosomal recessive inborn error of metabolism. Similarly, hereditary hemochromatosis resulting from a mutation, C282Y, in the *HFE* gene, is in linkage disequilibrium with the *HLA-A3* gene.

Linkage disequilibrium may indicate a founder effect. For example, the C282Y mutation in *HFE* arose in a chromosome that also contained the *HLA-A3* allele, and this combination of alleles at these two loci has been transmitted to the descendents of the individual in whom this mutation occurred. Because the *HFE* locus and the *HLA-A* locus are in relatively close proximity, the *HFE* mutation is still in linkage disequilibrium with the *HLA-A3* allele. Over many generations, recombinations between *HFE* and *HLA-A* would be expected to bring the *HFE* mutation into chromosomes with different *HLA-A* alleles. The extent of linkage disequilibrium between a founder mutation and other closely spaced genetic markers is therefore a function of the age of the mutation as well as the distance between the loci in question. For example, based on haplotype analysis, it has been estimated that the C282Y mutation in *HFE* arose approximately 60–70 generations ago *(15)*.

Several examples of linkage disequilibrium involving disease-causing genes provide insight into the structure of human populations. The C282Y mutation in *HFE* is found in 10% of the Caucasian population of northern European (Celtic) ancestry, which means that 1 in 10 people of this group are descendents of a single founder individual. In the United States alone, these number approx 20 million people. Similarly, 5–8% of the Caucasian population have the factor V Leiden mutation, which predisposes to thrombophilia. Haplotype analysis of markers in and around the factor V gene in these people demonstrates that these are also descendents of a single founder individual *(16)*.

BASIC GENE STRUCTURE AND FUNCTION
Promoter and Enhancer Elements

The 5' region of genes contains DNA sequences known as promoters that bind transcription factors. These in turn are involved in the recruitment of RNA polymerase II, which transcribes the sequence in a gene into an mRNA. Most messenger RNAs that encode proteins are synthesized by RNA polymerase II. Ribosomal RNAs are transcribed by RNA polymerase I, whereas transfer RNAs are transcribed by RNA polymerase III. Some promoter elements are common to many genes, and others are essentially unique to a particular gene. Enhancers increase the rate of transcription of a gene, but whereas promoters are situated within close proximity to the point at which transcription begins, enhancers may be located several kilobases distant either upstream or downstream of the gene, or even within the gene. Distantly situated enhancers may be brought closer to a gene by looping of DNA. Unlike promoters, enhancers can function irrespective of their orientation relative to the gene.

One of the most common promoter elements is the TATA box, located approximately 25–35 bp upstream of the RNA transcription initiation site. The consensus sequence of this element is TATAAAA. The TATA box binds TATA-binding protein (TBP), a component of a multiprotein complex known as transcription factor IID (TFIID). The TATA box appears to function primarily to identify the transcription initiation site.

Whereas TFIID functions as a member of the core set of transcriptional factors, other transcription factors function to stimulate transcription of a more limited set of target genes to achieve a specific biological effect. For example, a particular group of transcription factors, collectively known as nuclear factor-κB (NF-κB), or Rel, is involved in mediation of a very wide range of cellular inflammatory responses. NF-κB transcription factors bind as dimers to a 10-bp promoter sequence, leading to stimulation of transcription. This transcription factor was initially identified in regulating expression of the κ-light chain in B-cells, but further studies revealed that expression of a very large number of genes is stimulated by NF-κB. These genes encode members of various classes of proteins that are involved in the inflammatory response such as cytokines, HLA molecules, tumor necrosis factor, cellular adhesion molecules, acute-phase proteins, and growth factors *(17)*.

Pseudogenes

Pseudogenes contain sequences that are derived from functional genes, but they contain mutations that render them nonfunctional. They are generally believed to be remnants of formerly functional genes that have acquired mutations during evolution. They are commonly found in regions of the genome that have undergone duplication, and frequently, at least one fully functional copy of the gene still exists in the genome. Examples of pseudogenes occurring in duplicated regions of DNA are found in the α- and β-globin gene clusters, the HLA class I and class II regions, and the steroid 21-hydroxylase region. In all of these examples, at least one functional copy of the gene and a pseudogene are present in duplicated blocks of DNA.

Transcription

RNA transcription begins at the initiation site, which is upstream of the first codon, and continues to the end of the gene. Genes vary considerably in their overall length, but the median length of a gene is 14 kb. The longest human gene is the dystrophin gene, which is mutated in patients with Duchenne's and Becker's muscular dystrophy. This gene is over 2.4 million bp in length. Genes contain exons that encode the sequence of amino acids in proteins. Exons are interrupted by intervening sequences (also known as introns) in the majority of genes. The longest coding region, nearly 81 kb, is found in the titan gene. This gene also has the longest single exon, which is over 17 kb in length. In general, introns tend to be longer than exons.

Over 50% of introns are between 101 bp and 2 kb in length (the median being 1023 bp), whereas the median length of an exon is just 125 bp. The median length of the coding sequence in a gene is 1100 bp, corresponding to a protein of approximately 367 amino acids.

The region between the beginning of the mRNA and the first codon is known as the 5′ untranslated region (5′-UT). The corresponding position between the end of the coding region and the end of the mRNA tail is known as the 3′ untranslated region (3′-UT). The 5′-UT contains sequences that are essential for ribosomal binding and translation of mRNA. The 3′-UT contains sequences that direct mRNA transport and affect stability.

Newly synthesized RNA encoding a typical protein undergoes three alterations during its processing to form a mature mRNA. First, the 5′ end of the RNA is modified by addition of a cap site that confers stability against exonucleases, facilitates export of the mRNA from the nucleus, and allows for binding to ribosomes where translation occurs *(18)*. The cap is composed of 7-methyl-guanosine joined to the mRNA in a 5′-5′ linkage. Second, the introns are spliced out, and third, a tract of approx 200 adenine residues, known as a poly(A) tail, is added to the 3′ end.

Splicing of mRNA involves removal of the introns. More than 98% of introns begin with the dinucleotide GU and end with another dinucleotide, AG. Other, less common, intron boundaries include GC/AG and AU/AC. Because of the inevitable occurrence of any dinucleotide throughout exons and introns, not every GU or AG in a mRNA represents a splice site. In addition to these highly conserved dinucleotides, other neighboring nucleotides form a splice recognition site. The consensus 5′ splice site is AGGURAGU, and the consensus 3′ splice site sequence is YAGRNNN. [The conserved dinucleotides are underlined, R is a purine, Y is a pyrimidine, and N is any nucleotide *(18)*.]

In addition to these markers of the boundaries of an intron, an internal intron sequence known as the branch point sequence (BPS) is required for splicing. During splicing, the 5′ end of the intron is cut, and the free end is joined in a 5′-2′ linkage to a conserved A residue in the consensus branch site CURAY, usually located approx 100 nucleotides upstream from the 3′ end of the intron. The resulting structure is commonly known as a lariat. The 3′ end of the upstream exon then participates in a nucleophilic attack on the 3′ end of the intron, displacing the intron and resulting in a fusion between the upstream and downstream exons. Splicing takes place on a structure known as the spliceosome. This is composed of 5 small nuclear ribonucleoprotein (snRNP) complexes (U1, U2, U4, U5, and U6) and other additional proteins. Mutations that disrupt normal splice sites or create new splice sites in exons or introns are commonly seen in human diseases; they are generally known as splice mutations and are discussed in Chapter 3.

Alternative splicing of introns can generate multiple proteins from a single gene, resulting in encoding of more than one protein from a single DNA sequence. This mechanism enables a genome of only 30,000–40,000 genes to encode many more distinct proteins. Alternative splicing can involve different mechanisms, for example, skipping of an exon, retention of an intron, and use of alternative splice sites that result in a longer or shorter exon, as well as and change of the translational reading frame *(19)*. The mechanisms that govern alternative splicing are poorly understood, but it is estimated that at least 35% of genes exhibit alternative splicing *(3)*.

CDKN2A

One of the most striking examples of the effect of alternative splicing on the protein produced from a gene is provided by the cyclin-dependent kinase inhibitor 2A *(CDKN2A)* locus, which is also known as *p16* or *INK4a,* and is situated on chromosome 9p21. Germline mutations in this gene are associated with some cases of familial melanoma (*see* Chap. 7). The p16 protein, which functions as a tumor suppressor gene, is encoded by three exons, designated 1α, 2, and 3. The same locus also encodes a second tumor suppressor gene, $p14^{ARF}$, which uses an alternative first exon, 1β, and a portion of exon 2 of *p16/INK4a* (Fig. 7) *(20)*. The portion of exon 2 is translated in an alternative reading frame, so the two proteins have no amino acids in common. The remainder of exon 2 (and exon 3) provide 3′ untranslated sequences for $p14^{ARF}$.

Another example of generation of multiple distinct proteins from a single region of DNA is provided by the UDP-glucuronosyltransferase 1A locus *(UGT1A).* Multiple isoforms of this enzyme exist that have different substrate affinities. The enzyme is deficient in

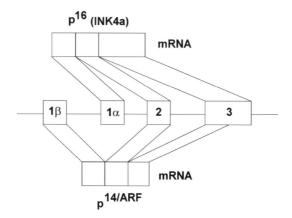

Fig. 7. Coding of two distinct proteins, p16 and p14, from a single region of DNA. Exons 1β, 1α, 2, and 3 are shown in the center of the figure. p16 and p14 use different first exons, and share a common 2nd exon and part of a common 3rd exon (but in different reading frames). The resulting proteins are entirely different in their amino acid sequences, but both function as tumor suppressor genes.

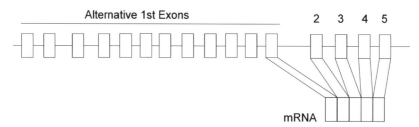

Fig. 8. The UGT1A gene is composed of 12 alternative 1st exons and a single set of exons 2–5. If transcription begins at one of the more upstream alternative first exons, the transcript is spliced so that only one first exon is present.

patients with inherited defects in bilirubin conjugation, namely, Gilbert's syndrome and Crigler-Najjar syndrome, types I and II. Twelve distinct exon 1 sequences are present at the *UGT1A* locus, each with its own promoter elements for binding RNA polymerase II. These are designated exons 1.1–1.12. The 3′ end of each of these exons contains an intron 5′-splice recognition sequence. A single set of exons 2–5 encodes the rest of the protein. Depending on which promoter is used, a different first exon becomes the first exon, and the other possible first exons are removed by splicing (Fig. 8).

Polyadenylation

The poly(A) tail is not encoded in DNA but is added at the 3′ end of the mRNA by a multimeric complex known as poly(A) polymerase. Before the poly(A) tail can be added, the nascent RNA molecule must be cleaved. A conserved polyadenylation signal, AAUAAA, located approx 11–30 nucleotides upstream of the poly(A) addition site, is required for termination of RNA polymerase activity and for polyadenylation *(21)*. Many genes have multiple polyadenylation signals, and the pattern of usage may vary between tissues *(22)*. In addition to the polyadenylation signal, a sequence rich in GU or U residues, located 10–30 nucleotides downstream of the cleavage site, is present in many transcripts prior to polyadenylation *(23)*. Mutation of the polyadenylation signal can result in continuation of transcription of the gene to the next available polyadenylation signal, resulting in production of a mutant protein *(24)*. The poly(A) tail is believed to stabilize the RNA and to facilitate its translation.

RNA Editing

Occasionally, the sequence of a messenger RNA transcript differs from the sequence in the coding regions of the gene. The process that gives rise to such alterations, which involves changes to single bases, is known as RNA editing *(25)*. The first described example of this phenomenon in humans involves the transcript of the *APOB* gene. In the liver, apolipoprotein B is produced as a 500-kDa protein known as apoB-100, whereas in the small intestine it is produced as a 250-kDa protein known as apoB-48. Both proteins are encoded by the same *APOB* gene. In the small intestine, the transcript is edited so that a glutamine codon, CAA, is changed to a stop codon, UAA, leading to translation of a much smaller protein (Fig. 9) *(26)*. This change is catalyzed by a multisubunit enzyme with cytidine deaminase activity known as APOBEC-1 *(27)*. In another example of RNA editing, two adenine residues in transcripts of the glutamate receptor B-subunit gene are deaminated to form inosine (which is read as guanine during translation), leading to changes in the encoded amino acids *(28)*. The enzyme responsible for this deamination, which is known as ADAR2, requires formation of a double-stranded RNA by base pairing between the exon containing the adenine base that is to undergo deamination and a complemen-

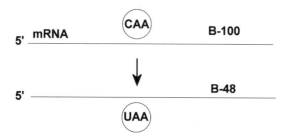

Fig. 9. Editing of the *APOB* mRNA transcript causes a glutamine codon (CAA) to be converted to a stop codon (UAA). This shortens the encoded protein.

tary sequence in the downstream intron. These examples of RNA editing involve codon changes by deamination of a single base. This appears to be the major mechanism of this type of RNA editing.

Although the extent of editing of RNA transcripts in humans is largely unknown, one disease, an autosomal recessive form of immunodeficiency associated with increased levels of IgM and decreased levels of other immunoglobulins (hyper-IgM syndrome, type 2) is known to be associated with mutations in a gene encoding a cytidine deaminase known as activation-induced cytidine deaminase (AID) *(29)*.

Translation

Following its processing, the mRNA molecule is exported from the nucleus through pores in the nuclear membrane into the cytoplasm. In the cytoplasm the mRNA binds to ribosomes where protein translation occurs. The ribosomes are complex structures composed of RNA and proteins. In eukaryotic cells, the ribosomal subunits are 60S and 40S and contain RNAs of 28S, 18S, 5.8S, and 5S. In prokaryotic cells, the subunits are 50S and 30S and contain RNAs of 23S, 16S, and 5S. Recent evidence suggests that some protein translation may occur in the nucleus itself. Mitochondria also have ribosomes that are used for translation of mitochondrial genes. The structure of these is of interest because they are similar in size to prokaryotic ribosomes, supporting the idea that mitochondria are of eubacterial origin *(30)*.

During translation, the genetic code in mRNA is read three nucleotides at a time to determine the corresponding amino acids to be incorporated into the polypeptide being synthesized. A triplet of

Table 2
The Genetic Code

	U	C	A	G
U	UUU Phe	UCU Ser	UAU Tyr	UGC Cys
	UUC Phe	UCC Ser	UAC Tyr	UGU Cys
	UUA Leu	UCA Ser	UAA Stop	UGA Stop
	UUG Leu	UCG Ser	UAG Stop	UGG Trp
C	CUU Leu	CCU Pro	CAU His	CGU Arg
	CUC Leu	CCC Pro	CAC His	CGC Arg
	CUA Leu	CCA Pro	CAA His	CGA Arg
	CUG Leu	CCG Pro	CAG Gln	CGG Arg
A	AUU Ile	ACU Thr	AAU Asn	AGU Ser
	AUC Ile	ACC Thr	AAC Asn	AGC Ser
	AUA Ile	ACA Thr	AAA Lys	AGA Arg
	AUG Met	ACG Thr	AAG Lys	AGG Arg
G	GUU Val	GCU Ala	GAU Asp	GGU Gly
	GUC Val	GCC Ala	GAC Asp	GGC Gly
	GUA Val	GCA Ala	GAA Glu	GGA Gly
	GUG Val	GCG Ala	GAG Glu	GGG Gly

bases that encodes a particular amino acid is known as a codon. The bases in a codon form complementary base pairs with tRNA molecules that are linked to their specific amino acids. Each tRNA molecule carries 1 of the 20 amino acids found in proteins. The tRNA molecules are therefore the adaptors between nucleic acids and peptides. Attachment of the appropriate amino acid to the 3′ end of the tRNA molecule is catalyzed by enzymes known as aminoacyl tRNA synthases. Each of these enzymes adds the correct amino acid to a tRNA.

Because there are only four nucleotides in mRNA, a combination of three bases is the minimum number required to code for the 20 amino acids that are found in proteins. In fact, three bases are sufficient to code for up to 64 (4^3) unique amino acids or stop codons, so the genetic code has redundancy, with some amino acids being encoded by more than one codon. The genetic code is shown in Table 2.

Changes in the Reading Frame

Because of the mechanism whereby bases are read in groups of three, deletion or insertion of a number of bases that is not a multiple of 3 will change the reading frame. This is known as a frame shift mutation. Mutations of this kind generally have highly dele-terious effects on protein structure and function because they lead to a change in amino acid sequence as a result of the change in reading frame. This occurs in addition to whatever changes result directly from the deletion or insertion of base pairs. Commonly, after a frame shift mutation, the new reading frame includes a premature stop codon that leads to premature termination of pro-tein synthesis.

Control of Gene Expression at Translation

In most situations, gene expression is controlled at the level of gene transcription, which is governed by the structure of chro-matin, and by transcriptional factors that bind to promoters and enhancers, thereby regulating the binding of RNA polymerase II. Expression of some genes is also regulated at the level of transla-tion. An example of this is provided by the iron binding proteins, ferritin and transferrin.

The level of iron in a cell is closely regulated so as to balance the needs of the cell for iron and the dangers associated with toxicity of this metal. Ferritin mRNA contains several iron response elements (IREs) in its 5′-UT region *(31)*. These IRE sequences are bound by iron regulatory proteins (IRPs, or IRE-binding proteins). Binding of IRP to the IREs impedes translation of ferritin mRNA. When iron levels rise, the IRPs bind the metal, leading to their dissociation from the mRNA, thus allowing the ferritin mRNA to be translated. Sequestration of iron in ferritin reduces the toxicity of the metal.

IREs are also present in the 3′-UT of transferrin receptor (TfR) mRNA *(31)*. Binding of IRPs stabilizes this mRNA against degrada-tion by nucleases. In the presence of low iron concentrations, this prolongs the half-life of TfR mRNA, allowing for synthesis of more of this receptor, which, in turn, allows iron entry into cells. When iron levels rise, the IRPs dissociate from TfR mRNA, resulting in a shorter half-life of these transcripts and production of lower amounts of the receptor. This reduces further iron entry into cells.

Degradation of Proteins in the Proteasome

Controlled termination of protein activity is essential to maintain cellular homeostasis. Extracellular proteins are generally removed by pinocytosis or by receptor-mediated endocytosis, leading to degradation in lysosomes. Intracellular proteins are generally removed by the proteasome, a complex that hydrolyzes proteins.

Proteins that are to be degraded in the proteasome are first coupled with ubiquitin, a 76-amino acid polypeptide. Ubiquitin is activated in an ATP-dependent reaction by formation of a thiolester bond between the C-terminus of ubiquitin and a cysteine residue in E1, a ubiquitin-activating enzyme. The activated ubiquitin is then transferred to a cysteine residue in a ubiquitin-conjugating enzyme (Ubc), and from there it is transferred to the target protein either directly or through another Ubc. Ubc enzymes are also known as E2 enzymes. The protein that is to be ubiquinated in this process is complexed with a ubiquitin protein ligase, also known as E3 enzymes. Linkage of ubiquitin is at lysine residues in the target protein, and a chain of ubiquitin molecules can be formed by successive additions of ubiquitin to previously linked units.

Disturbances in the ubiquitin-proteasome pathway have been implicated in several disease states. For example, p53, a critical regulator of cell cycle progression, is normally inactivated by this pathway. p53 can halt cell cycle progression at G1 or induce apoptosis and thus is a major defense against uncontrolled cell proliferation (discussed in Chapter 6). In infections with strains of human papillomavirus (HPV), the viral E6 protein targets p53 for destruction, thereby eliminating this important protein and impairing the normal regulation of cell growth.

CONTROL OF GENE EXPRESSION BY EPIGENETIC EFFECTS

The term *epigenetics* has been defined as "heritable changes in gene expression that occur without a change in DNA sequence" *(32)*. Examples of physiologic epigenetic effects include inactivation of one X chromosome in female cells and genomic imprinting. Epigenetic effects that lead to silencing of some tumor suppressor genes are an important factor in the development of some cancers (*see* Chap. 6). The molecular bases of epigenetic effects that regulate gene expression involve changes that include methylation of DNA and structural alternations to chromatin including covalent modification of histone proteins. Far from being an inert scaffolding for DNA, the histone proteins are emerging as a dynamic support that plays an integral role in the regulation of gene transcription.

Methylation of DNA

Methylation of cytosine residues is the most common epigenetic modification of DNA. In many eukaryotic species, methylation of cytosine residues is a mechanism of regulation of gene transcription. Many genes contain "CpG islands" in their 5′ promoter regions. These are regulatory elements that contain multiple copies of the dinucleotide 5′-CG-3′. The "p" in CpG represents the phosphate group between the nucleosides.

Methylation is of significance in human pathology for two reasons. First, methylation of CpG islands generally leads to decreased levels of transcription of the gene. Several examples of tumor suppressor genes that are inactivated by methylation are known. Second, spontaneous deamination of 5-methylcytosine leads to the formation of thymine. This is a frequent type of mutation leading to human diseases as a result of changes in the coding region of genes. The frequency of CpG in human DNA is only 5–10% of the expected frequency, and the loss of CpG dinucleotides is believed to be the result of spontaneous deamination of 5-methylcytosines.

Methylation of cytosine residues is catalyzed by DNA methyltransferases (Dnmt). Two classes of these enzymes are recognized: first, maintenance methylase activity is responsible for methylating a hemimethylated CpG group, and second, enzymes that can methylate a completely unmethylated CpG group *de novo*. Maintenance methylation by Dnmt1 is responsible for perpetuating a methylation pattern after DNA replication. Following replication of a methylated CpG group, the cytosine on the old strand is methylated, but the newly synthesized strand is unmethylated. Methylation of the latter strand re-establishes the symmetrical methylation of the cytosines on both strands in daughter cells. In some situations, such as inactivation of an X chromosome and genomic imprinting, the pattern of methylation is maintained throughout life, but in gametes and preimplantation embryos the methylation pattern is reset. Dnmt1 is believed to be responsible for maintenance of the methylation pattern.

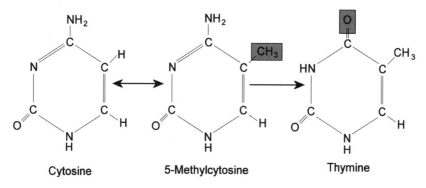

Fig. 10. Mechanism of conversion of C-T. Methylation of cytosine at carbon 5 forms 5-methylcytosine. Spontaneous deamination of 5-methylcytosine leads to formation of thymine.

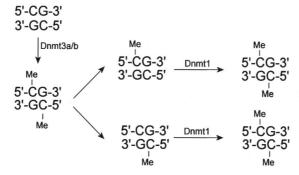

Fig. 11. Different enzymes catalyze formation of 5-methylcytosine. DNA methyltransferases (Dnmt) 3a and 3b are capable of *de novo* methylation of unmethylated DNA. Dnmt1 is capable of completing methylation of previously hemimethylated DNA and functions to maintain a previously established methylation pattern following DNA replication.

De novo methylation is catalyzed by Dnmt3a and Dnmt3b. The latter enzyme is deficient in patients with a rare genetic disease known as immunodeficiency with centromere instability and facial anomalies (ICF, OMIM 242860) *(33)*.

Methylation of DNA can prevent gene transcription by interfering with binding of methylation-sensitive transcription factors to DNA or by recruitment of specific methyl-DNA binding proteins that form complexes with other proteins that alter the structure of histones or chromatin.

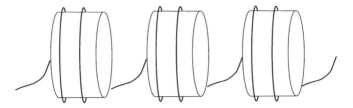

Fig. 12. Structure of the nucleosome. The core consists of an octomer composed of histone proteins H2A, H2B, H3, and H4 (each is present twice). The strand of DNA wraps around this core.

Histones

The major histones in DNA include H1, H2A, H2B, H3, and H4. The histones form an octamer composed of two of each of the core histone proteins, H2A, H2B, H3, and H4. A strand of DNA consisting of 146 bp wraps twice around the histone octamer, forming a nucleosome (Fig. 12). The DNA in contact with the octamer is known as core DNA, whereas the DNA between adjacent nucleosomes is known as linker DNA. Histone H1 binds to the linker DNA.

Histones have a globular domain and a basic tail containing lysine and arginine residues that can undergo several types of covalent modification, including phosphorylation, methylation, and acetylation. Acetylation is catalyzed by histone acetyl transferase (HAT) activity, and acetyl groups are removed by histone deacetylases (HDACs). Histone acetylation is associated with formation of an open chromatin structure and with activation of gene transcription. Histone deacetylation has the opposite effects. Methylation of DNA and histone acetylation are linked processes. Several proteins are known that bind to methylated DNA and recruit other protein complexes, including the histone deacetylases, HDAC1 and HDAC2. Among the proteins that bind to methylated DNA are MeCP2 and four proteins that share a methylated DNA binding domain, MBD1–4.

Deregulation of the normal process of gene transcription by acetylation and deacetylation of histones is emerging as an important aspect of development of certain kinds of malignancies. For example, acute promyelocytic leukemia is characterized by a translocation involving the promyelocytic leukemia *(PML)* gene on chromosome 15 and the retinoic acid receptor α *(RARα)* gene on chromosome 17 *(see* Chap. 8). Under normal circumstances, retinoic acid receptors form dimers that bind to specific gene pro-moter elements. These dimers are capable of recruiting a nuclear co-repressor complex (NCoR) that, in turn, associates with HDAC, leading to deacetylation of local chromatin and repression of tran-scription of target genes. In the presence of retinoic acid, the ligand for the retinoic acid receptors, NCoR, and HDAC dissociate from the receptors and are replaced by histone acetylases that acetylate histones and allow for gene transcription to occur. The PML-RARα complex does not release the NCoR-HDAC complex at physiologi-cal levels of retinoic acid, and so transcription of genes that are involved in further maturation of promyelocytes is blocked. How-ever, pharmacological levels of retinoic acid can cause release of the complex containing HDAC activity and allow histone acetylases to bind, thereby altering the chromatin to allow gene transcription to occur, producing factors that are needed for cell maturation.

Inactivation of the X Chromosome

In cells in a female, one of the two X chromosomes is inactivated. Selection of the chromosome chosen for inactivation begins in early embryonic life and, as cells divide, the pattern of X inactivation is maintained in daughter cells. Tissues in females are therefore mosaic, being composed of some cells in which the paternal X chro-mosome is active and other cells in which the maternal X chromo-some is active. In individuals with abnormal karyotypes in which there are more than two X chromosomes, only one of these is active. X-chromosome inactivation compensates for the fact that females and males have different numbers of X chromosomes. After inacti-vation, each sex has just one functional X chromosome. Abnormali-ties in which more than one X chromosome is active tend to be associated with mental retardation and dysmorphic features.

The mechanisms by which one of the X chromosomes is selected for inactivation, the inactivation mechanism itself, and the mechanism whereby inactivation is maintained from a cell to its daughters are not fully understood. X-chromosome inactivation involves genes in the X inactivation center, *Xic,* which is located at Xq13. Among these is a gene known as the inactive-X specific transcript *(XIST) (34).* This gene is transcribed from the inactive X and processed to form an RNA of approximately 17 kb in length that coats the inactive X chro-mosome, i.e., it functions in *cis.* The *XIST* RNA transcripts are not used for translation but associate with the inactive X chromosome and are essential for its inactivation. The inactive X chromosome is characterized by other changes including extensive methylation of cytosine residues, hypoacetylation of histones, and the accumulation of a histone known as macroH2A *(35)*. It appears as a Barr body at the periphery of the nucleus of certain interphase cells.

In general, the selection of which X chromosome is initially inactivated in a cell line is random. However, skewing of inactivation in favor of either X chromosome can occur. In patients in whom one X chromosome is abnormal, preferential inactivation of the abnormal X chromosome occurs. This leads to fewer symptoms than are seen with more random inactivation and may be a protective mechanism against development of a deleterious phenotype *(36)*. Skewing of the X inactivation pattern of leukocytes has also been reported to occur in 21–31% of healthy women and to increase in frequency with age after 50 yr *(37)*. Importantly, skewed inactivation can unmask an X-linked recessive trait in a heterozygous female. For example, preferential inactivation of an X chromosome carrying a normal factor VIII gene can result in hemophilia A if the active X chromosome carries a mutation *(38)*.

In chromosomal translocations that involve the X chromosome and an autosome, inactivation can spread beyond just the X chromosome regions to the translocated autosomal regions. Inactivation of these leads to functional monosomy for a portion of the autosome. The other chromosomal product of such a translocation may show failure to inactivate regions of the X chromosome, leading to functional disomy for these regions *(39)*. Not all genes on the X chromosome are inactivated. Approximately 10% of genes escape inactivation, and these are nearly all located on Xp.

Because the pattern of X chromosome inactivation is maintained in daughter cells, clonality of tumors in females can be demonstrated as uniformity of inactivation of a particular X chromosome within tumor cells *(40)*.

Pseudoautosomal Region of the Y Chromosome

The Y chromosome is present in a single copy in male cells. However, two regions on the Y chromosome known as the pseudoautosomal regions (PAR1 and PAR2), which are located at the tips of the short and long arms, respectively, have homologous regions on the X chromosomes, and recombination between the X and Y chromosomes occurs at these sites during male meiosis *(41)*. Genes located within the pseudoautosomal region of the X chromosome escape X inactivation.

Imprinting

Imprinting refers to a situation in which some genes are expressed depending on whether they are on the maternal or paternal homolog of a pair of chromosomes. The mechanism of this effect involves silencing of transcription of the gene on one or another homolog, and this effect is believed to involve methylation of the silenced gene. This surprising phenomenon may be revealed when a mutation disrupts the normally expressed gene. In that case, although the homologous gene is structurally intact, it is functionally absent because of imprinting. Imprinting is maintained throughout life, but the pattern is reset during formation of gametes and then re-established. The role of imprinting in several human diseases is discussed further in Chapter 2.

REFERENCES

1. Lander ES, Linton LM, Birren B, et al. Initial sequencing and analysis of the human genome. Nature 2001;409:860–921.
2. Venter JC, Adams MD, Myers EW, et al. The sequence of the human genome. Science 2001;291:1304–51.
3. Croft L, Schandorff S, Clark F, Burrage K, Arctander P, Mattick JS. ISIS, the intron information system, reveals the high frequency of alternative splicing in the human genome. Nat Genet 2000;24:340–1.
4. Dahia PL, FitzGerald MG, Zhang X, et al. A highly conserved processed PTEN pseudogene is located on chromosome band 9p21. Oncogene 1998;16:2403–6.
5. White PC, New MI, Dupont B. Molecular cloning of steroid 21-hydroxylase. Ann NY Acad Sci 1985;458:277–87.
6. Samonte RV, Eichler EE. Segmental duplications and the evolution of the primate genome. Nat Rev Genet 2002;3:65–72.
7. Kemp S, Pujol A, Waterham HR, et al. ABCD1 mutations and the X-linked adrenoleukodystrophy mutation database: role in diagnosis and clinical correlations. Hum Mutat 2001;18:499–515.
8. Eichler EE, Budarf ML, Rocchi M, et al. Interchromosomal duplications of the adrenoleukodystrophy locus: a phenomenon of pericentromeric plasticity. Hum Mol Genet 1997;6:991–1002.
9. Riethman HC, Xiang Z, Paul S, et al. Integration of telomere sequences with the draft human genome sequence. Nature 2001;409:948–51.
10. Mefford HC, Trask BJ. The complex structure and dynamic evolution of human subtelomeres. Nat Rev Genet 2002;3:91–102.
11. Knight SJ, Regan R, Nicod A, et al. Subtle chromosomal rearrangements in children with unexplained mental retardation. Lancet 1999;354:1676–81.

12. Murphy TD, Karpen GH. Centromeres take flight: alpha satellite and the quest for the human centromere. Cell 1998;93:317–20.

13. Meyer D, Thomson G. How selection shapes variation of the human major histo-compatibility complex: a review. Ann Hum Genet 2001;65:1–26.

14. White PC, Speiser PW. Congenital adrenal hyperplasia due to 21-hydroxylase deficiency. Endocr Rev 2000;21:245–91.

15. Ajioka RS, Jorde LB, Gruen JR, et al. Haplotype analysis of hemochromatosis: evaluation of different linkage-disequilibrium approaches and evolution of disease chromosomes. Am J Hum Genet 1997;60:1439–47.

16. Cox MJ, Rees DC, Martinson JJ, Clegg JB. Evidence for a single origin of factor V Leiden. Br J Haematol 1996;92:1022–5.

17. Pahl HL. Activators and target genes of Rel/NF-kappaB transcription factors. Oncogene 1999;18:6853–66.

18. Proudfoot NJ, Furger A, Dye MJ. Integrating mRNA processing with transcription. Cell 2002;108:501–12.

19. Black DL. Protein diversity from alternative splicing: a challenge for bioinformatics and post-genome biology. Cell 2000;103:367–70.

20. Stott FJ, Bates S, James MC, et al. The alternative product from the human CDKN2A locus, p14(ARF), participates in a regulatory feedback loop with p53 and MDM2. EMBO J 1998;17:5001–14.

21. Edwalds-Gilbert G, Veraldi KL, Milcarek C. Alternative poly(A) site selection in complex transcription units: means to an end? Nucleic Acids Res 1997;25:2547–61.

22. Beaudoing E, Gautheret D. Identification of alternate polyadenylation sites and analysis of their tissue distribution using EST data. Genome Res 2001;11:1520–6.

23. Gil A, Proudfoot NJ. A sequence downstream of AAUAAA is required for rabbit beta-globin mRNA 3′-end formation. Nature 1984;312:473–4.

24. Orkin SH, Cheng TC, Antonarakis SE, Kazazian HH Jr. Thalassemia due to a mutation in the cleavage-polyadenylation signal of the human beta-globin gene. EMBO J 1985;4:453–6.

25. Gerber AP, Keller W. RNA editing by base deamination: more enzymes, more targets, new mysteries. Trends Biochem Sci 2001;26:376–84.

26. Chen SH, Habib G, Yang CY, et al. Apolipoprotein B-48 is the product of a messenger RNA with an organ-specific in-frame stop codon. Science 1987;238:363–6.

27. Anant S, Davidson NO. Molecular mechanisms of apolipoprotein B mRNA editing. Curr Opin Lipidol 2001;12:159–65.

28. Seeburg PH, Higuchi M, Sprengel R. RNA editing of brain glutamate receptor channels: mechanism and physiology. Brain Res Brain Res Rev 1998;26:217–29.

29. Revy P, Muto T, Levy Y, et al. Activation-induced cytidine deaminase (AID) deficiency causes the autosomal recessive form of the hyper-IgM syndrome (HIGM2). Cell 2000;102:565–75.

30. Gray MW, Burger G, Lang BF. The origin and early evolution of mitochondria. Genome Biol 2001;2:1018

31. Thomson AM, Rogers JT, Leedman PJ. Iron-regulatory proteins, iron-responsive elements and ferritin mRNA translation. Int J Biochem Cell Biol 1999;31:1139–52.

32. Wolffe AP, Matzke MA. Epigenetics: regulation through repression. Science 1999;286:481–6.

33. Xu GL, Bestor TH, Bourc'his D, et al. Chromosome instability and immunodeficiency syndrome caused by mutations in a DNA methyltransferase gene. Nature 1999;402:187–91.

34. Brown CJ, Lafreniere RG, Powers VE, et al. Localization of the X inactivation centre on the human X chromosome in Xq13. Nature 1991;349:82–4.
35. Avner P, Heard E. X-chromosome inactivation: counting, choice and initiation. Nat Rev Genet 2001;2:59–67.
36. Wolff DJ, Schwartz S, Carrel L. Molecular determination of X inactivation pattern correlates with phenotype in women with a structurally abnormal X chromosome. Genet Med 2000;2:136–41.
37. El Kassar N, Hetet G, Briere J, Grandchamp B. X-chromosome inactivation in healthy females: incidence of excessive lyonization with age and comparison of assays involving DNA methylation and transcript polymorphisms. Clin Chem 1998;44:61–7.
38. Coleman R, Genet SA, Harper JI, Wilkie AO. Interaction of incontinentia pigmenti and factor VIII mutations in a female with biased X inactivation, resulting in haemophilia. J Med Genet 1993;30:497–500.
39. Schmidt M, Du Sart D. Functional disomies of the X chromosome influence the cell selection and hence the X inactivation pattern in females with balanced X-autosome translocations: a review of 122 cases. Am J Med Genet 1992;42:161–9.
40. Pan L, Peng H. Polymerase chain reaction clonality assays based on X-linked genes. In: Killeen AA., ed. Molecular Pathology Protocols. Totowa, NJ: Humana, 2001:73–80.
41. Graves JA, Wakefield MJ, Toder R. The origin and evolution of the pseudoautosomal regions of human sex chromosomes. Hum Mol Genet 1998;7:1991–6.

2 Genetic Inheritance

The patterns of genetic inheritance within families and the behavior of genes at the level of a population are of fundamental importance in the estimating the future risk of genetic diseases within families and in the general population. In this chapter, the common patterns of inheritance and the mechanisms of estimating risks to future offspring in affected families are described. The ability to perform simple bayesian calculations is of increasing importance in the molecular pathology laboratory as genetic testing becomes more widespread.

PATTERNS OF MENDELIAN INHERITANCE IN FAMILIES

The patterns of inheritance and expression of genetic traits in families depends on whether a genetic locus is on an autosome, on a sex chromosome, or in the mitochondrial genome. Any genetic trait, including a disease, may be recessive or dominant depending on the locus and the mutation in question. The inheritance patterns of most diseases can be classified as autosomal or X-linked and as dominant or recessive. Diseases arising from mutations in mitochondrial DNA have a characteristic pattern of inheritance. Knowledge of the principal features of these inheritance patterns is essential for understanding the molecular basis of genetic diseases. Acquired mutations, such as those arising in malignant diseases, can also be described in terms of dominance and recessiveness at a molecular level.

Autosomal Dominant Diseases

In inherited autosomal dominant diseases, the presence of a single mutant allele on one chromosome is sufficient to cause disease. Although the allele on the homologous chromosome is normal, it does not prevent expression of the mutant phenotype. Autosomal dominant diseases affect both males and females in multiple genera-

From: *Principles of Molecular Pathology*
Edited by: A. A. Killeen © Humana Press Inc., Totowa, NJ

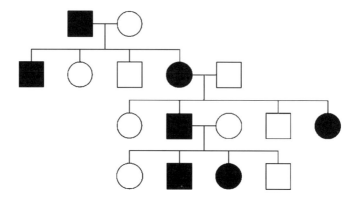

Fig. 1. Autosomal dominant pattern of inheritance. Individuals with the trait are shown in black. Fifty percent of the offspring of an affected individual have the trait. Male-to-male transmission is seen.

tions, and each offspring of a person with an autosomal dominant disease has a 50% chance of inheriting the mutation (Fig. 1). Autosomal dominant disorders can be transmitted from father to son, a feature that distinguishes autosomal dominant from X-linked patterns of inheritance.

Most dominant disorders show a dosage effect so that individuals who are homozygous for a dominant mutation are more severely affected than are individuals who are heterozygous. For example, familial hypercholesterolemia, which is caused by mutations in the low-density lipoprotein receptor gene, shows a marked difference in the severity of hypercholesterolemia and clinical symptoms between heterozygotes and homozygotes. Diseases that have a dose-dependent severity are sometimes referred to as incompletely dominant or semidominant. A notable exception to the influence of mutation dosage is Huntington's disease, which is caused by mutations in the *IT15* gene (*see* Chap. 5). Homozygotes for this disorder are not more severely affected than are heterozygotes *(1)*.

Autosomal Recessive Diseases

In autosomal recessive disorders, the alleles on both homologous chromosomes are mutated. There is therefore no normal allele to provide the missing function encoded by the mutated genes. Most inborn errors of metabolism are caused by autosomal recessive traits. Usually, the heterozygous carriers of autosomal recessive

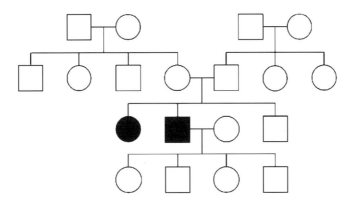

Fig. 2. Autosomal recessive pattern of inheritance. Only a single generation shows affected individuals. Both parents of these individuals are carriers. Other family members may be carriers.

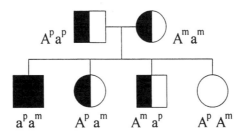

Fig. 3. Transmission of alleles in an autosomal recessive trait. The a allele is recessive to the A allele. The paternal alleles are designated by p and the maternal alleles by m. Both parents are carriers, each having a single a allele. The children show the possible genotypes for offspring of two carrier parents: homozygous affected, two carriers, and a homozygous normal.

traits appear clinically normal, although closer laboratory testing may reveal a biochemical difference from individuals with two functional alleles. Autosomal recessive diseases affect males and females, and often there is no known family history of the disease before the first affected individual comes to medical attention (Fig. 2). Each offspring of the mating of two carriers of an autosomal recessive trait has a 25% risk of being affected, a 50% risk of being a carrier, and a 25% chance of inheriting a normal allele from each parent (Fig. 3). In many autosomal recessive disorders, multiple mutant alleles exist; frequently patients are compound heterozygotes for two distinct mutations.

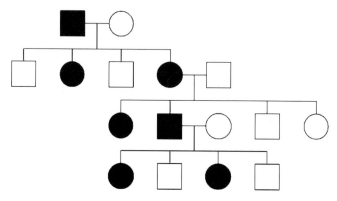

Fig. 4. X-linked dominant pattern of inheritance. Individuals with the trait are shown in black. There is no male-to-male transmission. All the daughters of affected males have the trait, whereas one-half of the offspring of affected females have the trait, regardless of sex.

X-Linked Dominant Diseases

X-linked dominant disorders appear when a dominant mutation is present on the X chromosome. In males, the expression of the disease phenotype is inevitable. In females, although the homologous X chromosome is normal, it is insufficient to prevent the expression of the dominant phenotype (Fig. 4). When analyzing pedigrees, X-linked dominant inheritance can be suspected when there is no male-to-male transmission of a dominant phenotype. Affected females transmit the mutation to 50% of their offspring. Affected males transmit the mutation to all of their female offspring, but not to their male offspring.

X-linked dominance is not a frequent mode of inheritance. A form of hypophosphatemia with rickets (OMIM 307800) is inherited as an X-linked dominant disease. Another X-linked dominant disorder is Rett's syndrome, which is typically characterized by several months of normal infant development, followed by severe neurological decline and acquired microcephaly *(2)*. Most cases of Rett's syndrome are caused by mutations in the *MECP2* gene *(3)*. Nearly all reported cases have been in females, apparently because *de novo* mutations originate predominantly in the paternally derived X chromosome *(4)*. *MECP2* mutations have been reported in infrequently in males with symptoms ranging from severe neonatal encephalopathy to X-linked mental retardation *(5)*.

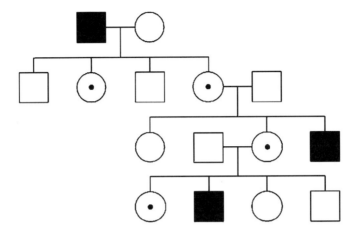

Fig. 5. X-linked recessive pattern of inheritance. Heterozygous females are indicated by circles enclosing a dot. One-half of the sons of heterozygous females express the recessive trait, and one-half of the daughters of heterozygous females are carriers. All the daughters of affected males are carriers. There is no male-to-male transmission.

X-Linked Recessive Diseases

X-linked recessive diseases are generally expressed only in males carrying a mutant X chromosome. Carrier females, who have one normal X chromosome in addition to the mutant chromosome, are generally unaffected, although in unusual situations they may express the phenotype. The absence of affected females and the lack of male-to-male transmission is characteristic of X-linked recessive traits (Fig. 5). Carrier females transmit the mutation to 50% of their offspring. Males who inherit the mutation invariably express the phenotype. Affected males transmit the mutation to all of their female offspring, who are therefore carriers, but not to their male offspring.

It is possible for females to express X-linked recessive traits through several mechanisms. In every somatic cell of a female, one of the two X chromosomes is physiologically inactivated. This X-chromosome inactivation is known as lyonization, after Dr. Mary Lyon, who proposed this concept in 1961. When female cells are viewed with special strains, the inactive X chromosome appears as a condensed piece of chromatin known as a Barr body. The selection of which of the two X chromosomes is inactivated is random, and the process begins in tissues during embryogenesis. Once a particular X chromosome is inactivated, all daughter cells maintain this pattern of X-chromosomal inactivation. Inactivation of genes occurring during lyonization is the result of methylation of large stretches of chromatin that inactivates most, but not all, genes on the X chromosome. If lyonization is skewed such that the normal X chromosome is preferentially inactivated, then an X-linked recessive trait carried on the homologous chromosome may be manifest.

Females can also manifest an X-linked recessive disorder as a result of mating of an affected male with a carrier female. Such a mating will result in 50% of the female offspring being affected because of inheritance of an affected chromosome from each parent. The other 50% will be carriers because of inheritance of an affected chromosome from their father and a normal chromosome from their mother. Finally, females with X-chromosomal abnormalities such as Turner's syndrome (45, X), or microdeletions of X, or some unbalanced translocations, may express an X-linked recessive disease if the remaining X chromosome carries a recessive gene mutation.

Mitochondrial Inheritance

All mitochondria are derived from the oocyte at the time of fertilization and are therefore of maternal origin. Mitochondrial DNA undergoes mutation and accumulates mutations at a faster rate than does nuclear DNA (6). Mutations in mitochondrial DNA usually manifest as multiorgan disease with frequent neuromuscular abnormalities (see Chap. 5). A feature unique to mitochondrial disorders is variable expression of the disease depending on the ratio of normal to mutant mitochondria. This variability in mutation prevalence among mitochondria is termed heteroplasmy. Heteroplasmy depends on the ratio existing at the time of fertilization and on stochastic effects arising from random distribution of normal and mutant mitochondria during mitosis. These give rise to differences in the severity of the phenotype among siblings. Mitochondrial inheritance can be recognized by the exclusive transmission of the phenotype by females (Fig. 6). It is important to note that most proteins expressed in the mitochondria are encoded by nuclear genes. Genetic variation in these follows the usual patterns seen with nuclear genes (see Chap. 5).

Dominance and Recessiveness of Mutations in Tumors

Acquired mutations associated with tumor formation can also be classified as dominant or recessive at a cellular level. For example,

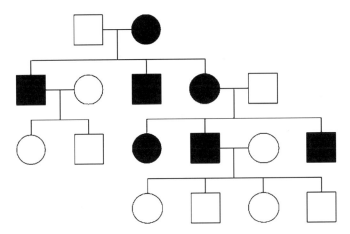

Fig. 6. Mitochondrial pattern of inheritance. The trait is transmitted exclusively by females, and to all of their offspring.

the *BCR-ABL* translocation seen in nearly all cases of chronic myeloid leukemia (CML) functions as a dominant mutation because of activation of the Abelson proto-oncogene. Mutation of a single allele resulting in overexpression of *ABL* leads to CML. Activation of many other oncogenes shows a similar genetic effect in that mutation of one allele is sufficient to manifest the phenotype. In familial cancer syndromes associated with germline oncogene activation, the pattern of inheritance is dominant.

In contrast to activation of oncogenes, tumor suppressor gene function is recessive at a cellular level. Both copies of the tumor suppressor gene must be inactivated for the associated malignant phenotype to develop. For example, retinoblastoma can develop when there is loss of function of both copies of the *RB* gene in the same cell of the developing retina. Having just one copy is sufficient to prevent this phenotype. Paradoxically, although loss of function of a tumor suppressor gene such as *RB* is a recessive trait with regard to tumor development at the molecular level, the inheritance pattern of familial cancers associated with loss of tumor suppressor function may be dominant.

Familial retinoblastoma is usually associated with germline deletions of *RB*. A "second-hit" mutation results in inactivation of the remaining *RB* allele on the homologous chromosome in a retinal cell, leading to tumor formation. Because of the high frequency of such "second hits," the disease can affect multiple generations in a typical autosomal dominant pattern. Other familial cancer syndromes such as breast cancer associated with *BRCA* mutations show a similar pattern of dominance within families but recessiveness at a molecular level.

Mechanisms of Genetic Dominance

A mutation that inactivates a gene on the X or Y chromosome, with the exception of genes located in the pseudoautosomal region of these chromosomes (*see* Chap. 1), might be expected to produce a phenotype in males because of the absence of an alternative allele. However, this explanation for dominant effects of gene mutations does not apply to autosomes, which are present in two copies in both males and females. Why are some mutations dominant whereas others are recessive? A review of the mechanisms of genetic dominance has resulted in the following classification of common reasons for this effect *(7)*.

1. *Reduced gene dosage, also known as haploinsufficiency.* In this situation, loss of a single functional copy of a gene gives rise to disease. Examples of this include some forms of thalassemia, in which loss of a α- or β-globin gene disturbs the normal ratio of α-to-β chains, and DiGeorge's syndrome, caused by loss of *Tbx1,* the dosage of which appears to be critical to normal development of neural crest-derived structures *(8,9)*.

2. *Increased gene dosage.* An example is Charcot-Marie-Tooth disease, which is caused by a duplication of the peripheral myelin protein *(PMP-22)* gene. The reason why the presence of an extra copy of the gene gives rise to disease is not known. It is also of interest in this case that loss of a single copy of the *PMP-22* gene (i.e., haploinsufficiency) gives rise to another neurological disease, hereditary neuropathy with liability to pressure palsies *(HNPP)*.

3. *Changes in the expression of mRNA.* An example of this is provided by the t(14;18) translocation, which brings the *BCL2* gene in proximity to the immunoglobulin heavy chain locus. The latter has strong transcription enhancers that are functional in B-cells and lead to increased production of bcl-2 protein, which is an inhibitor of apoptosis (*see* Chap. 7). This confers a selective growth advantage on cells that harbor this translocation.

4. *Constitutive activation of a protein.* This is seen in, for example, type 2 multiple endocrine neoplasia (MEN2), a group of hereditary cancer syndromes that involve constitutive activation of the *RET* proto-oncogene, a

A **B**

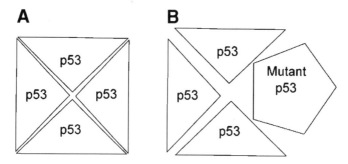

Fig. 7. **(A)** Formation of a p53 tetramer. A single allele, encoding a mutant protein, can disrupt the formation of such a multimer, **(B),** thereby acting as a dominant mutation.

membrane receptor tyrosine kinase. Because of a mutation, the kinase is constitutively active, resulting in transmission of mitogenic signals.

5. *Dominant negative mutations.* When normal protein function requires assembly of several polypeptides, the presence of a population of mutant polypeptides may disrupt normal assembly of a disproportionate fraction of protein complexes. This deleterious effect of mutation of just one polypeptide on the function of such proteins is known as a dominant negative effect. As an example, certain p53 mutations are commonly found in cancer (*see* Chap. 7). p53 functions as a transcriptional activator requiring assembly of a tetramer in order to bind to DNA and stimulate transcription of genes that p53 activates in response to certain cell injuries such as ionizing radiation. Mutations that abolish the ability of p53 to form tetramers prevent this response (Fig. 7). Because of the requirement for formation of tetramers, the presence of a mutant p53 can disrupt the function of wild-type p53 polypeptides. Such mutations are therefore regarded as dominant negative mutations *(10).*

6. *Alterations in structural proteins.* This involves a similar effect as dominant negative mutations but is seen in structural proteins. For example, type I collagen, a major protein constituent of bone, is composed of a trimer consisting of two proα1(I) polypeptides and a proα2(I) procollagen polypeptide. A missense mutation in a proα1(I) gene that results in substitution of a glycine (a frequent amino acid in collagen) by another amino acid leads to assembly of structurally abnormal type I collagen proteins, and these comprise the majority (not just 50%) of all assembled proteins.

7. *Toxic effects of protein alterations.* This is exemplified by the unstable trinucleotide repeat disorders known as polyglutamine diseases . In these disorders, an increase in the number of glutamine residues in the mutant proteins is associated with cellular toxicity. For example, in

Huntington's disease, which is caused by an expansion of a polygluta-mine-encoding region in *IT15,* cytoplasmic and nuclear deposits of pro-teolytic fragments containing the polyglutamine tract are believed to be involved in the pathogenesis of cell death *(11).*

8. *New functions.* In this form of mutation, the mutated protein either has a function not possessed by the wild-type protein, or a new protein is formed. This is commonly seen in translocations associated with malig-nancies. For example, the t(9;22) translocation associated with the Philadelphia chromosome encodes a chimeric protein, bcr-abl, that has a higher level of tyrosine kinase activity and different cellular distribution from the normal protein produced by the *ABL* proto-oncogene.

NONMENDELIAN PATTERNS OF INHERITANCE

In addition to the classic patterns of inheritance, a few unusual types of inheritance pattern are recognized that do not conform to mendelian or multifactorial principles. These include diseases asso-ciated with unstable trinucleotide repeats, imprinting, and uni-parental disomy.

Unstable Trinucleotide Repeat Diseases

Several genetic disorders are characterized by instability of a repetitive sequence consisting of multiple copies of a trinu-cleotide. The instability is characterized by variation in the num-ber of copies of the trinucleotide between generations. When the number of copies of the trinucleotide repeat expands beyond some critical threshold, disease results. Depending on the particu-lar gene, the trinucleotide repeats may be situated in a coding region or in a noncoding region. If the trinucleotide codes for glu-tamine, such diseases are referred to as polyglutamine diseases. The unstable trinucleotide repeat diseases are considered in Chapters 4 and 5.

Imprinting

Imprinting refers to the nonexpression of genes in a manner that is dependent on the parent of origin of the chromosome on which the gene is located. Imprinting violates a fundamental principle of classic mendelian genetics, namely, that genes are equally expressed from both members of a pair of homologous chromo-somes. Genes on an imprinted chromosome, or region of a chromosome, are not expressed depending on whether they were contributed by the mother or by the father. Although the genes on the imprinted chromosome have a normal sequence and are therefore not mutated, they are not capable of being transcribed to form an mRNA and so are functionally absent. The mechanism that leads to imprinting involves methylation of regions of the chromosomes that are imprinted. This is somewhat similar to methylation of one of the two X chromosomes in the somatic cells of normal females, a process referred to as lyonization. However, whereas lyonization involves a random inactivation of an X chromosome, imprinting involves methylation of genes contributed by a specific parent. Depending on the locus, imprinting may involve either the maternal or paternal chromosome.

Several genetic diseases involve imprinted genes. The classic examples of diseases arising from imprinting are Prader-Willi and Angelman syndromes, which involve mutations on chromosome 15q11-q13. Prader-Willi syndrome (PWS; OMIM 176270), which affects approx 1 in 10,000 to 1 in 15,000 newborns, is characterized by hypotonia, short stature, polyphagia, obesity, small hands and feet, hypogonadism, and mild mental retardation. Most cases of PWS are sporadic. In 70% of cases, a cytogenetically visible deletion of 15q11-q13 is present in the paternal chromosome in a region that includes the *SNRPN* gene, which is a candidate gene for this disease. Whether deletion of this gene alone is responsible for the disorder is presently uncertain. The maternal chromosome 15q is imprinted in this region, and therefore subjects with a deletion of this region of the paternal chromosome have no functional copy of the genes that are deleted.

Angelman syndrome (AS; OMIM 105830) is characterized by mental retardation, ataxia, seizures, absence of speech, skin hypopigmentation, sleep disturbance, and spontaneous laughter. The disease has a prevalence of approx 1 in 20,000. Reminiscent of PWS, approx 70% of AS patients have a cytogenetically visible deletion of 15q11-q13 that involves loss of approx 4 Mb of DNA. However, in AS, the deletion is on the maternal chromosome and cannot be compensated for because of imprinting on the homologous region of the paternal chromosome. The specific gene that, when mutated, gives rise to AS is known to be *UBE3A*. This gene encodes a protein, E6-PA, that is involved in transport of other proteins to the proteasome complex in the cytoplasm where protein degradation takes place. The extent of imprinting of *UBE3A* varies between tissues, but imprinting of the paternal allele in the brain is responsible for manifestations of clinical disease. Up to approximately 10% of patients with AS have a mutation in *UBE3A* that inactivates the gene *(12)*. In families with more than one affected individual, mutations in *UBE3A* have been identified in up to 80% of patients. Most of the mutations are truncating. Approximately 7–9% of patients have an imprinting abnormality characterized by a paternal pattern of imprinting on both chromosomes. Some of these patients have defects in a putative imprinting center (IC) that may be responsible for coordinating the switch between maternal and paternal imprinting patterns.

Uniparental Disomy

Both parents contribute equally to the genome of their children, with the exception of the Y chromosome, which is transmitted by fathers to sons, and the mitochondrial genome, which is transmitted exclusively by females. Rarely, individuals have both copies of a chromosome from one parent without the homologous chromosome from the other parent. This phenomenon is termed uniparental disomy (UPD). If UPD includes each member of the pair of chromosomes in a parent, it is termed uniparental heterodisomy. If an individual has two copies of one chromosome from a parent, it is termed uniparental isodisomy.

Several mechanisms might give rise to this phenomenon. At fertilization, an oocyte containing two copies of a chromosome (a result of nondisjunction during meiosis) might fuse with a normal sperm cell containing one copy of the chromosome. The zygote from such a fertilization would be trisomic for the chromosome in question. Re-establishment of a normal chromosome complement would require loss of one the three copies of the chromosome, an event sometimes referred to as "trisomy rescue." Assuming that any of the three chromosomes is equally likely to be lost, in a third of cases the loss will lead to UPD, and because most nondisjunction occurs in female meiosis I, UPD arising by this mechanism will usually be maternal heterodisomy *(13)*. Alternatively, an oocyte may be missing a chromosome, usually as a result of maternal nondisjunction during meiosis I. Fertilization by a normal sperm would yield a zygote that is monosomic for a chromosome. Rescue of this zygote by duplication of the paternal chromosome would lead to paternal uniparental isodisomy. Although these appear to be the most common etiologies of UPD, they are not the only mechanisms. UPD may also arise from mitotic nondisjunction in a conceptus. This can give rise to pure uniparental isodisomy.

The most likely clinical outcome with UPD is that it is asymptomatic. Because uniparental isodisomy leads to homozygosity of genes on that chromosome, it may result in expression of a recessive trait if the involved chromosome carries a recessive mutation. The first patient to be identified with UPD was a child with cystic fibrosis. Her mother was a carrier for the common ΔF508 mutation in *CFTR* and the child was homozygous for this mutation. However, her father did not carry this mutation. Analysis revealed UPD for the maternal chromosome 7 *(14)*.

UPD can also give rise to disease if the chromosome contains imprinted genes because the presence of two copies of an imprinted locus is functionally equivalent to the absence of both copies of the locus. Approximately 25% of patients with Prader-Willi syndrome have maternal UPD in the region of 15q11-q13, and 3–5% of patients with Angelman's syndrome have paternal UPD in this region. Recently, UPD for chromosome 6 has been shown to be associated with transient neonatal diabetes *(15)*.

Recommended Guidelines for Testing for UPD

The American College of Medical Genetics has produced guidelines for laboratory diagnostic testing for UPD *(13)*. These guidelines call for demonstration of UPD by use of polymorphic DNA markers such as microsatellites. At least two fully informative loci should demonstrate absence of inheritance of an allele from one parent for one chromosome, but normal biparental inheritance of markers on other chromosomes. Recommended indications for testing for UPD include prenatal identification of mosaicism for trisomy of chromosomes 6, 7, 11, 14, or 15 or robertsonian translocations involving chromosomes 14 or 15. These chromosomal abnormalities are commonly associated with UPD. Testing is also recommended for patients with features of disorders that are known to be associated with UPD, as shown in Table 1.

Table 1
Diseases Associated with Uniparental Disomy (UPD)[a]

Disease	% with UPD	Chromosome	Parent	OMIM no.
Transient neonatal diabetes mellitus	20	6	Mother	601410
Russell-Silver syndrome	10	7	Mother	180860
Beckwith-Wiedemann syndrome	20	11	Father	130650
upd(14)mat		14	Mother	
upd(14)pat		14	Father	
Prader-Willi syndrome	25	15	Maternal	176270
Angelman's syndrome	3–5	15	Paternal	105830

[a] Features of upd(14)mat and upd(14)pat include short stature, developmental delay, dysmorphic features, and skeletal and joint abnormalities. These disorders are defined by identification of UPD.

Data from ref. 13.

MULTIFACTORIAL INHERITANCE

Most common diseases are not the result of single gene defects. Cancer, heart disease, and diabetes are generally the result of both hereditary and environmental factors. There are examples of single gene disorders that lead to forms of each of these diseases, for example, hereditary retinoblastoma, familial hypercholesterolemia, and maturity onset diabetes of youth (MODY), but these are exceptional forms of disease. Unfortunately, our current state of knowledge of the specific loci and alleles that contribute to most multifactorial disorders is very limited. We have a much better understanding of the molecular pathology of rare, single-gene disorders than we do of the common illnesses that affect large numbers of the population.

Multifactorial disorders tend to aggregate in families, but the risk of first-degree relatives (parents, children, siblings) of an affected patient developing the disease is less than the usual 50 or 25% found in mendelian genetic disorders. As the degree of relationship from an affected patient becomes more remote (e.g., uncles, cousins, second cousins), the prevalence of multifactorial disorders decreases. This has been interpreted as indicating a threshold effect, i.e., the overall genetic risk is influenced by the additive effects of many genes, some of which increase the disease risk, and some of which may lessen the risk. When some critical threshold of genetic and environmental risks is crossed, the disease becomes manifest. There are several predicted consequences of this model *(16):*

1. As the degree of relatedness to an affected family member decreases, the frequency of disease will decline more rapidly than would occur if the disease were caused by a single major locus.
2. The risk of other family members' having a multifactorial disease depends on the degree of severity of the disease in the affected members of the family. If an affected family member has a severe form of the disease, the frequency of other affected individuals will be greater.
3. The risk to other family members also depends on the number of affected individuals. The larger the number of affected individuals, the greater the likelihood that a future sibling will also have the disease.
4. If a disease is normally found with greater frequency in a particular sex, relatives of patients of the less commonly affected sex will have a higher disease frequency than will relatives of patients of the more commonly affected sex. This is another manifestation of the second principle listed above. For a person of the less commonly affected sex to have the disease, the combination of genetic effects is probably more adverse than is required to manifest disease in a person of the sex in which the disease is naturally more prevalent.

Environmental factors are also of importance in multifactorial disease. For example, cigarette smoking, obesity, a high-fat diet, and physical inactivity are associated with increased risk of developing coronary artery disease. From a practical perspective, identification of these is important because environmental risks, unlike genetic risks, are often modifiable.

Traits that are either present or absent are known as qualitative traits. Traits that fall on a continuous scale such as blood pressure, plasma cholesterol, and height are known as quantitative traits, and loci that influence these are known as quantitative trait loci (QTLs). Because a multifactorial trait has both genetic and environmental influences, it is possible by genetic analysis of families to quantify the relative contribution of each to the variance of the trait or phenotype in the population *(16).* The proportion of variance of a phenotype that results from genetic factors is known as the heritability (h^2). Heritability can vary from 0 if genes have no effect on the variance of the trait to 1 if genetic factors are exclusively responsible for variance. As examples, h^2

Table 2
Heritability (h^2) of Lipids[a]

Lipid	h^2 value
Lipoprotein(a)	0.9
LDL and HDL cholesterol	0.5
Triglycerides	0.3

[a] For details, see ref. 23. LDL, low-density lipoprotein; HDL, high-density lipoprotein.

values for different types of plasma lipids are shown in Table 2. The fraction of variance that is not heritable is caused by environmental effects. This is sometimes called environmentability, defined as $1 - h^2$.

GENES IN THE POPULATION

Genetic diseases within families tend to follow the patterns of inheritance outlined above. The relationship between genes and their behavior in a population is governed by other factors, and the Hardy-Weinberg law provides a basis for understanding this behavior.

Hardy-Weinberg Law

At a given locus, if two possible alleles (A and a) can be found and the frequencies of these in a particular population are p and q, then it follows that $p + q = 1$ because no other alleles exist in the population. The possible genotypes that any individual might have are A/A, A/a, a/A, and a/a. The expected frequencies of these genotypes are p^2, pq, qp, and q^2. Because no other genotypes exist,

$$p^2 + 2pq + q^2 = 1 \qquad (1)$$

This simple relationship was independently described by Hardy and Weinberg in 1908. A population in which this formula holds true is said to be in Hardy-Weinberg equilibrium. In such a population, it can be shown that the ratio of the three genotypes will remain constant from one generation to the next. Although it is known as the Hardy-Weinberg law, it is not a law in the same sense that the term is used in physics, e.g., the second law of thermodynamics. Instead, it describes the most likely distribution of genotypes within a population. However, for the Hardy-Weinberg law to apply, the population must meet certain criteria:

1. The population is sufficiently large that genetic drift does not occur. To understand genetic drift, consider a small population composed of only 10 mating pairs. If one member of this population of 20 people has a variant allele at some autosomal locus, the frequency of that allele is 1/40 in this population. If, by chance, that allele is not transmitted to any offspring, the allele will disappear from the population within a generation. On the other hand, if the person carrying the variant allele happens to transmit the allele to all of his or her offspring, the frequency of the allele may be greatly increased in the next generation. These dramatic changes in the frequency of an allele in this population are caused by the small size of the population. If the population consisted of 2 million people and 100,000 had the variant allele, the likelihood of such dramatic intergenerational changes in gene frequency in this large population would be much less.

2. There is no migration into or out of the population. Different populations may have different frequencies of alleles at a given locus and so migration and mating between populations will alter the frequencies of alleles within a population. Migration is not simply a geographical flow of people across national borders but includes admixture between ethnic groups that occupy a shared land region. For example, the Duffy blood system has three common alleles, FY*A, FY*B, and FY*O. The FY*O allele does not encode an antigen because of a promoter mutation that abolishes gene transcription. Nearly all sub-Saharan African populations are Fy(a–b–), i.e., homozygous for FY*O, and this phenotype has been shown to confer resistance to infection with *Plasmodium vivax (17)*. In the United States, the frequency of non-Fy(a–b–) alleles among African Americans is approx 0.2, indicating that FY+ alleles have been introduced into this population through mating with Caucasians in the last several hundred years *(18)*.

3. There is random mating of individuals without regard to their genotypes. For example, the expected likelihood of two carriers mating according to Hardy-Weinberg equilibrium is $2pq \times 2pq$. If the actual frequency of such matings were increased, then predictions of the frequency of genotypes in future generations based on the Hardy-Weinberg principle would be wrong. Preferential mating between individuals with similar genetic traits is known as assortative mating and commonly involves traits such as height and intelligence. Assortative mating of carriers of genetic diseases leads to a higher frequency of affected homozygotes among offspring. Inbreeding or consanguinity has the same tendency to increase the proportion of affected homozygotes in offspring of such matings. In general, the rarer a recessive disease in the population, the more frequently are parents of affected children related to each other.

4. No genotype has a significant reproductive advantage or disadvantage. This depends on the fitness associated with an allele. In genetic terminology, fitness (f) is a measure of an individual's capacity to reproduce. A subject with $f = 1$ has a similar number of offspring to other members of the general population. Often, individuals with genetic disorders have reduced fitness. For example, patients with type II osteogenesis imperfecta have very high childhood mortality, and so $f = 0$. This is an autosomal dominant disorder, and therefore most cases represent new mutations. Germline mosaicism in a parent accounts for a recurrence risk of 7% in future pregnancies *(19)*. The coefficient of selection *(s)* is defined as the proportional reduction in the gametic contribution of a particular genotype to the next generation *(16)*.

$$s = 1 - f \qquad (2)$$

In the case of autosomal recessive disorders, the heterozygotes may have a selective advantage that maintains a mutant allele at a high frequency. A good example of this is seen in sickle cell anemia. Homozygotes with the sickle cell mutation have a reduced fitness, but heterozygotes have a relative survival advantage in regions where malaria is found because of resistance to the parasite.

5. Mutation does not lead to a significant change in the frequency of alleles within the population.

A consideration of these criteria shows they are commonly not met in human populations. Despite this limitation, Hardy-Weinberg is important because it provides a means to solve clinically important calculations on gene frequencies in populations. It also allows for a comparison of experimental data of genotypes with what would be expected in a population that was in Hardy-Weinberg equilibrium, and this comparison is useful for understanding and examining deviations from an expected result.

Examples of Calculations Involving Hardy-Weinberg Principles

Hardy-Weinberg principles are frequently used in genetic calculations for clinical purposes. Examples of these calculations include the following.

Example 1. An autosomal recessive disease is observed to affect 1 in 10,000 people. What is the frequency of mutant alleles? What is the carrier frequency?

In autosomal recessive diseases, affected individuals carry two disease alleles. Using the designations p and q for the frequencies of the wild-type and mutant alleles, respectively, the frequency of diseased patients, q^2, is 1/10,000 and therefore q, the frequency of the mutant allele, is 1/100.

Because $p + q = 1$, $p = (1 - q)$, which is 99/100 or $\cong 1$. The carrier frequency is $2pq$, which is $\cong 1/50$.

Knowing the carrier frequency allows us to predict the frequency of affected individuals in a population, as in the following example.

Example 2. If the carrier frequency for an autosomal recessive disorder is 1/20, what is the frequency of affected individuals?

In a population with random mating, we expect that the frequency of mating of carriers will be $2pq \times 2pq$ or, in this case, $1/20 \times 1/20 = 1/400$. One-fourth of the offspring of these matings will be affected, giving us a predicted 1/1600 affected individuals in the population.

Example 2 demonstrates the importance of random mating in a population for Hardy-Weinberg principles to apply. If, for example, carriers were much less likely (or much more likely) to mate with other carriers, then the predicted frequency of affected individuals would deviate from the above estimate.

Knowing the distribution of genotypes in a population allows us to determine whether the population is in Hardy-Weinberg equilibrium for the locus in question. For example, in a survey of the frequency of the β-globin sickle (S) allele and its wild-type counterpart (A) in 12,387 people in west Africa, the following numbers of genotypes were observed:

A/A 9365
A/S 2993
S/S 29

From these data, the frequency of the A and S alleles can be determined as follows:

In this population of 12,387 people, there are 24,774 alleles. Each A/A homozygote has two A alleles, and each A/S heterozygote has one A allele. The total number of A alleles is therefore 21,723. The total number of S alleles is 3051. The frequency of the A allele in this population is 21,723/24,774 or 0.877. The frequency of the S allele is 0.123.

Knowing the frequency of each allele in the population, we can determine the *expected* frequency of each genotype by using the Hardy-Weinberg equation. If $p = 0.877$ and $q = 0.123$, then we *expect* the following frequencies of genotypes:

$$A/A\ (p^2) = 0.877^2 = 0.769$$

$$A/S\ (2pq) = 2 \times 0.877 \times 0.123 = 0.215$$

$$S/S\ (q^2) = 0.123^2 = 0.015$$

Multiplying each genotype frequency by the number of people in the population gives the *expected* numbers of people with each genotype:

$$A/A = 0.769 \times 12{,}387 = 9526$$

$$A/S = 0.215 \times 12{,}387 = 2663$$

$$S/S = 0.015 \times 12{,}387 = 186$$

Comparison of the *observed* genotype data with the *expected* numbers of each genotype shows that there is a marked decrease in the number of observed S/S homozygotes and an increase in the number of observed heterozygotes relative to what one would expect for a population in Hardy-Weinberg equilibrium. The statistical significance of these differences can be determined by a chi square test, which, in this case, indicates that the observed data differ very significantly from the expected results, confirming that the observed population is not in Hardy-Weinberg equilibrium with respect to alleles at the β-globin locus. In this case, the high mortality associated with the S/S genotype and the relative survival advantage of A/S heterozygotes in a malarial region explain these findings.

Bayesian Calculations of Risk

In genetics, the risk of having a disease can be assessed in various ways. For diseases that are characterized by a simple mendelian type of inheritance, the risk depends on the pattern of inheritance of the disease, as outlined previously. However, laboratory data are increasingly available that modify the risk of an individual's having a disease. Combining the risk based on the inheritance pattern with the modified risk based on laboratory data is achieved by performing a bayesian analysis.

Example 3. Consider the couple shown in Fig. 8. They want to know their risk of having a child affected with cystic fibrosis (CF), an autosomal recessive disease that is caused by mutations in the cystic fibrosis transmembrane conductance *(CFTR)* gene on chromosome 7. Both members of the couple are Caucasian, and this population has a CF carrier frequency of 1/29. Neither has a family history of cystic fibrosis. What is the probability of their fetus's having CF?

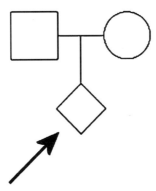

Fig. 8. The parents seek counseling regarding genetic risk of an autosomal recessive disorder to the fetus. See text for discussion.

The probability of either parent being a carrier is 1/29. The probability that both are carriers is $1/29 \times 1/29 = 1/841$. For an autosomal recessive disease such as CF, the probability of any offspring of a mating of two carriers being affected is 1/4. The combined probability of both parents being carriers and their child being affected is therefore $1/841 \times 1/4 = 1/3364$, which is the incidence of CF among Caucasian newborns.

Following recommendations from the American College of Obstetrics and Gynecology, the mother decides to undergo genetic testing for a panel of 25 mutations that includes 80% of all known *CFTR* mutations in Caucasians. Her test indicates that she does not have any of the 25 mutations. What is the revised probability that their child will have CF?

This is a typical problem that can be solved by a simple bayesian calculation. In this case we have two independent pieces of information to consider:

1. the *a priori* probability of being a carrier and
2. the probability of being a carrier without having a mutation identified in this testing procedure.

The term *a priori* means information that was available before any testing was performed. In this case it is the known frequency of carriers in the population, and the information that the patient has no family history of CF. We also know that the mechanism of inheritance is autosomal recessive and that CF carriers are asymptomatic.

The probability of being a carrier, yet not having a mutation identified by the panel of 25 mutations, is based on experimental observation. From studies of *CFTR* mutations in affected patients, we know what percentage of mutations will be detected by the panel of 25 mutations.

This percentage varies among ethnic populations because of variations in the frequencies of mutant alleles.

A bayesian calculation is performed as shown below. In step 1, we list the two mutually exclusive possibilities for the mother's genetic status, i.e., carrier and noncarrier. In step 2, we list the *a priori* probability of her being a carrier (1/29). The probability of her not being a carrier is 1 – (1/29). In step 3, we list the conditional probabilities of her being a carrier and having a negative test result. Because we know that the test detects 80% of carriers, we know that it fails to identify 20% of carriers. We assume that the probability of a noncarrier having a negative result for *CFTR* mutations is 1. In step 4, we multiply the *a priori* and conditional probabilities for each genetic possibility (i.e., carrier or noncarrier). This value is known as the joint probability. Finally, in step 5, we determine the probability that the mother is a carrier. This probability is expressed as the ratio of the joint probability of being a carrier to the sum of the joint probabilities of being a carrier and of not being a carrier. This value is known as the posterior probability. In the illustration below, the posterior probability of the mother's being a carrier is 1/141. The probability of her not being a carrier could be determined by either calculating the posterior probability of this, or by subtracting the probability of her being a carrier from 1, i.e., 1 – (1/141).

	Carrier	Not a carrier
Step 1. List mutually exclusive possibilities.	Carrier	Not a carrier
Step 2. List a priori probability of each	1/29	28/29
Step 3. Conditional probability (i.e., of having a negative mutation test)	20/100	1
Step 4. Multiply line 2 and line 3 Joint probability	(1/29)(20/100) = 20/2900	(28/29)(1) = 2800/2900
Step 5. Calculate posterior probability	(20/2900)/[(20/2900) + (2800/2900)] =20/2820 =1/141	

Because the mutation detection test did not show any mutations, the likelihood of the mother's being a carrier is reduced from 1/29 to 1/141. The probability that both parents are carriers is therefore $1/29 \times 1/141 =$ 1 in 4089, and the chance of their child's having CF is approx 1 in 16,300, compared with 1 in 3364 before testing. If the father were tested and also found not to carry one of the panel of mutations, the risk of this couple having a child with CF would be $1/141 \times 1/141 \times 1/4 = 1/79{,}524$.

Example 4. Consider another couple who are Ashkenazi Jewish and who do not have a family history of CF. The frequency of CF carriers in this population is also approx 1/29, but because of a different distribution of mutations in this population, genetic testing can detect 97% of all mutations. What is the likelihood that an Ashkenazi Jewish mother who has no family history of CF and who is negative on *CFTR* mutation testing would have a child with CF?

	Carrier	Not a carrier
A priori probability	1/29	28/29
Probability of having a negative mutation test	3/100	1
Joint probability	(1/29)(3/100) = 3/2900	(28/29)(1) = 28/29
Final probability	(3/2900)/[(3/2900) + (2800/2900)] =3/2803 =1/934	

In this case, the probability that the mother is a carrier is 1/934. The probability of the couple having a child with CF is $1/29 \times 1/934 \times 1/4 =$ 1 in 108,344. Because mutation testing offers a higher detection rate in this population than in the northern European Caucasian population, this couple can be assured that their chance of having a child with CF is extremely small.

Example 5. What if the Caucasian mother described above is found to have a CF mutation, such as the common ΔF508? In this case, the national recommendations call for testing of the father. If his test result is negative, what is the probability of the couple having a child with CF?

The probability that a Caucasian with a negative mutation test on the recommended panel is a CF carrier is 1/141 (see above). Knowing his wife is a carrier means that the risk of having a CF-affected child is $1/141 \times 1 \times 1/4 = 1/564$.

Now let's consider scenarios that involve a positive family history. In the family shown in Fig. 9, the father of a fetus has two siblings with cystic fibrosis. What is this man's risk of being a carrier? For autosomal recessive diseases, the risk to a child of carrier parents is $1/4$ of being affected, $1/4$ of being a carrier from the mother, $1/4$ of being a carrier from the father, and $1/4$ of being genetically normal at the locus in question (Fig. 3). Therefore the chance of being a carrier is 2/4 or $1/2$. However, in this case we know that the man does not have CF. He can have one of only three possible genotypes: he might be a carrier by having inherited a mutation from his mother, or be a

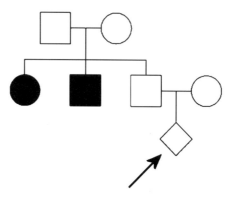

Fig. 9. A father, who has two siblings with cystic fibrosis, seeks genetic counseling regarding the risk of the fetus's having this disease.

carrier by having inherited a mutation from his father, or he might be genetically normal. Of these three genotypes, two involve his being a carrier; therefore his risk of being a carrier is 2/3. His chance of being genetically normal at the locus in question is 1/3.

The risk of the fetus's having CF is therefore 2/3 × 1/29 (the mother's risk of being a carrier) × $^1/_4$ = 1/174. If the mutations in the affected siblings of the man were known, he could be tested for these mutations, and his genetic status for CF could be determined.

Empirical Risks

A common task in genetic counseling is advising parents of a child with a genetic disorder of the recurrence risk for future children. When genetic diseases have a known inheritance pattern, it is usually possible to calculate the risk of recurrence, and if the results of genetic testing are available, the calculation can be refined by bayesian analysis. For some disorders that do not follow simple mendelian genetic patterns of inheritance, it may be possible to give an estimate of the risk of recurrence from empirical observation of other families with the disorder. For example, cleft lip with or without cleft palate (CL/P) is a common developmental anomaly that may be seen in both syndromic forms (i.e., with other developmental anomalies) and in isolated cases. Isolated CL/P has a poorly understood etiology, but familial clustering of cases indicates that heritable factors are contributory. Observation of recurrence rates in large numbers of families with isolated CL/P indicates that the recurrence rate in families with an affected child or parent is approx 4%, whereas if both a parent and a child have CL/P, the recurrence risk is 17% *(20)*. Such estimates depend on the accuracy of the diagnosis of nonsyndromic CL/P in affected family members.

New Mutations, Germline Mosaicism, and Recurrence Risks

In families in which a child with a genetic disease has a new mutation, the risk of recurrence in subsequent children is usually extremely low. Occasionally, however, more than one child in a family has a mutation that cannot be demonstrated in either parent. This is highly suggestive of germline mosaicism in a parent. In this situation, the germinal cells of a parent include a population of cells that harbor the mutation and that give rise to gametes with the mutation. This phenomenon might arise from a mutation that occurred during embryogenesis in the parent leading to the parent's being a mosaic with both somatic and germline mosaicism. Depending on the relative abundance of the mutation in tissues, particularly in white blood cells, which are the most common source of DNA for genetic analysis, the mutation may not be detectable by routine methods. Alternatively, a population of cells containing the mutation may be confined to the gonad (pure germline mosaicism) and may give rise to gametes with the mutation. When discussing recurrence risks for future pregnancies, the possibility of parental germline mosaicism should be considered, especially in the case of diseases such as osteogenesis imperfecta type II, tuberous sclerosis, Duchenne muscular dystrophy, and hemophilia A and B, in which germline mosaicism has been frequently documented *(21,22)*. The presence of germline mosaicism for a disease-causing mutation greatly increases the likelihood of recurrence of the disease in future children. For diseases with reduced penetrance or variable expression, both parents should be thoroughly examined for subtle features of the disease in question. Identification of a mildly affected parent greatly increases the risk of recurrence.

REFERENCES

1. Wexler NS, Young AB, Tanzi RE, et al. Homozygotes for Huntington's disease. Nature 1987;326:194–7.
2. Hagberg B, Aicardi J, Dias K, Ramos O. A progressive syndrome of autism, dementia, ataxia, and loss of purposeful hand use in girls: Rett's syndrome: report of 35 cases. Ann Neurol 1983;14:471–9.

3. Amir RE, Van den Veyver IB, Wan M, Tran CQ, Francke U, Zoghbi HY. Rett syndrome is caused by mutations in X-linked MECP2, encoding methyl-CpG-binding protein 2. Nat Genet 1999;23:185–8.

4. Trappe R, Laccone F, Cobilanschi J, et al. MECP2 mutations in sporadic cases of Rett syndrome are almost exclusively of paternal origin. Am J Hum Genet 2001;68:1093–1.

5. Schanen C. Rethinking the fate of males with mutations in the gene that causes Rett syndrome. Brain Dev 2001;23 Suppl 1:S144–6.

6. Wallace DC. Mitochondrial DNA sequence variation in human evolution and disease. Proc Natl Acad Sci USA 1994;91:8739–46.

7. Wilkie AO. The molecular basis of genetic dominance. J Med Genet 1994;31:89–98.

8. Merscher S, Funke B, Epstein JA, et al. TBX1 is responsible for cardiovascular defects in velo-cardio-facial/DiGeorge syndrome. Cell 2001;104:619–29.

9. Lindsay EA, Vitelli F, Su H, et al. Tbx1 haploinsufficieny in the DiGeorge syndrome region causes aortic arch defects in mice. Nature 2001;410:97–101.

10. de Vries A, Flores ER, Miranda B, et al. Targeted point mutations of p53 lead to dominant-negative inhibition of wild-type p53 function. Proc Natl Acad Sci USA 2002;99:2948–53.

11. Davies S, Ramsden DB. Huntington's disease. Mol Pathol 2001;54:409–13.

12. Fang P, Lev-Lehman E, Tsai TF, et al. The spectrum of mutations in UBE3A causing Angelman syndrome. Hum Mol Genet 1999;8:129–35.

13. Shaffer LG, Agan N, Goldberg JD, Ledbetter DH, Longshore JW, Cassidy SB. American College of Medical Genetics statement of diagnostic testing for uniparental disomy. Genet Med 2001;3:206–11.

14. Spence JE, Perciaccante RG, Greig GM, et al. Uniparental disomy as a mechanism for human genetic disease. Am J Hum Genet 1988;42:217–26.

15. Hermann R, Laine AP, Johansson C, et al. Transient but not permanent neonatal diabetes mellitus is associated with paternal uniparental isodisomy of chromosome 6. Pediatrics 2000;105:49–52.

16. Emery AEH. Methodology in Medical Genetics. An Introduction to Statistical Methods, Churchill Livingstone, Ediburgh, 1986.

17. Miller LH, Mason SJ, Clyde DF, McGinniss MH. The resistance factor to *Plasmodium vivax* in blacks. The Duffy-blood- group genotype, FyFy. N Engl J Med 1976;295:302–4.

18. Lautenberger JA, Stephens JC, O'Brien SJ, Smith MW. Significant admixture linkage disequilibrium across 30 cM around the FY locus in African Americans. Am J Hum Genet 2000;66:969–78.

19. Cole WG, Dalgleish R. Perinatal lethal osteogenesis imperfecta. J Med Genet 1995;32:284–9.

20. Curtis EJ, Fraser FC, Warburton D. Congenital cleft lip and palate. Am J Dis Child 1961;102:853–7.

21. Zlotogora J. Germ line mosaicism. Hum Genet 1998;102:381–6.

22. Leuer M, Oldenburg J, Lavergne JM, et al. Somatic mosaicism in hemophilia A: a fairly common event. Am J Hum Genet 2001;69:75–87.

23. Ozturk IC, Killeen AA. An overview of genetic factors influencing plasma lipid levels and coronary artery disease risk. Arch Pathol Lab Med 1999;123:1219–22.

3   Mutation

The term *mutation* has various meanings *(1)*. In genetics, it means a change in a DNA sequence without regard to the effect of that change on the health of the organism. In clinical usage, however, the term generally implies a deleterious sequence alteration that causes disease. Genes undergo mutation, giving rise to new alleles, and these mutations are the basis of evolutionary change. The term polymorphism is generally used to indicate an allele that is present in at least 1% of the population and is neutral with respect to survival of the organism.

A mutation arising in a nongermline cell is known as a somatic mutation. It may be silent or it may lead to an abnormal phenotype for the cell and its daughter cells. The clinical effect of a somatic mutation depends partly on the gene and cell involved, but perhaps the most dangerous effect is loss of normal regulation of cell growth, leading to tumor formation. Somatic mutations are the critical events underlying the development of most neoplasms.

A mutation that arises in a germ cell may be transmitted to future offspring, in whom it will be present in all cells. Depending on the mutation and the gene involved, it may confer a selective advantage to the offspring, cause disease, or have no physiological consequence. Its presence may be recognized if it gives rise to a new phenotype that was not previously present in the family. This might happen if the new phenotype is manifested as a dominant trait or as an X-linked recessive trait in males. If the new mutation gives rise to a phenotype that manifests as an autosomal recessive trait, it may not be evident for many generations, until mating with another carrier gives rise to an individual who harbors mutations of both alleles of the involved locus.

EFFECT OF GENDER ON RATES AND TYPES OF MUTATION

The rate of *de novo* germline mutations, other than chromosomal aneusomies, is generally higher in males than in females, but it

From: *Principles of Molecular Pathology*
Edited by: A. A. Killeen © Humana Press Inc., Totowa, NJ

varies between genes and depends on the type of mutation. However, some general observations can be made. The rate of single nucleotide substitutions is much higher in males than in females. For example, *de novo* point mutations in the *RET* proto-oncogene that give rise to multiple endocrine neoplasia types 2A and 2B are almost exclusively of paternal origin, as are mutations in the fibroblast growth factor receptor 3 gene that give rise to achondroplasia *(2–4)*. Mutations that give rise to hemophilia A, an X-linked disorder, arise more frequently in males than in females; however, there are gender differences. The frequent inversion mutation and point mutations in the factor VIII gene arise more commonly in males, whereas deletions arise more commonly in females *(5)*.

Chromosomal nondisjunction leading to the common trisomies, i.e., trisomies 21, 13, and 18, occurs predominantly during maternal meiosis. In the case of trisomy 21 and trisomy 13, nondisjunction usually occurs during meiosis I, whereas nondisjunction leading to trisomy 18 usually occurs during meiosis II *(6,7)*. Conversely, Klinefelter's syndrome (47, XXY) is caused by nondisjunction that occurs with similar frequency during paternal and maternal meiosis, with most cases arising because of nondisjunction during paternal meiosis I *(8)*. Although the factors that contribute to nondisjunction are poorly understood, advanced maternal age and chromosome-specific increases or decreases in the rate of recombination between homologous chromosomes during meiosis are associated with nondisjunction.

The reason commonly offered to explain the differences between the types of mutations that arise predominantly in males versus females is related to the number of mitotic cell divisions between conception and the production of gametes. In females, it is estimated that there are 23 cell divisions between conception and production of a haploid ovum. Meiosis I is arrested for several decades between the fetal stage of development and adulthood and is not completed until ovulation. In contrast, spermatogenesis occurs throughout life in males after puberty and involves continual cell divisions. A sperm produced by a 20-year-old man is estimated to be derived from over 150 cell divisions, whereas a sperm produced by a 40-year-old man is derived from over 600 cell divisions *(9)*. This continual cell division leads to accumulation of mutations with time, and an expected higher rate of mutation in offspring of older men than of younger men. Such an age effect has been demonstrated in several diseases including achondroplasia, Apert's syndrome, Marfan's syndrome, polyposis coli, and basal cell nevi *(10,11)*.

In the case of some unstable trinucleotide repeat disorders, the gender of the parent transmitting the mutation can have a significant impact on the risk of expansion of the repeat. For example, expansion of the CGG repeat in the *FMR1* gene, which causes fragile X syndrome, is more common during meiosis in females, whereas expansion of the CAG repeat in the *IT15* gene, which causes Huntington's disease, is more common in males *(12,12a)*.

ALLELIC HETEROGENEITY

Allelic heterogeneity means that multiple mutant alleles at a single locus are associated with a common clinical phenotype. For example, more than 1000 mutations that cause cystic fibrosis have been described in the *CFTR* gene. An important feature of allelic heterogeneity is that different mutations may have different effects on the function of the gene product and on the phenotype. For example, some *CFTR* mutations are associated with pancreatic sufficiency, whereas others are associated with pancreatic insufficiency. Some mutations in the β-globin gene are associated with absence of production of any protein product (β^0-thalassemia), whereas others cause hemoglobinopathies such as sickle cell anemia.

Allelic heterogeneity is very common in genetic diseases and can pose technical challenges in molecular diagnostics. It is relatively easy to test for a few mutations that cause a disease. It is more difficult and expensive to screen genes for multiple possible mutations. Techniques that can be used for these purposes are discussed in Chapter 4.

LOCUS HETEROGENEITY

Locus heterogeneity means that a clinical phenotype can be the result of mutations at different genetic loci. This may be seen in situations in which several gene products function cooperatively, so that abnormalities in any of the genes produce a similar clinical

Table 1
Codon Patterns and Frequencies of *APOE* Alleles in Caucasians

Allele	Codon 112	Codon 158	Frequency (%)
ε2	Cys	Cys	0.05
ε3	Cys	Arg	0.75
ε4	Arg	Arg	0.20

effect. For example, phenylketonuria is caused by lack of activity of hepatic phenylalanine hydroxylase activity. This deficiency can arise from mutations in the phenylalanine hydroxylase gene itself, or from mutations in the gene for dihydropteridine reductase, which is involved in producing tetrahydrobiopterin, an essential cofactor for phenylalanine hydroxylase.

Another example of locus heterogeneity is found among families with early-onset (i.e., <60 years of age) familial Alzheimer disease (EOFAD). In this disorder, mutations in the genes for presenilin-1 *(PS1)*, presenilin-2 *(PS2)*, and amyloid precursor protein *(APP)* have been described *(13)*. These genes are located on chromosomes 14, 1, and 21, respectively.

In contrast to families with EOFAD, most patients with Alzheimer disease are over 60 years of age and do not have a strong family history of the disease. In the general population, the most significant known genetic risk factor for Alzheimer disease is the presence of the ε4 allele of the apolipoprotein E gene, *APOE. APOE* has three common polymorphisms within the population, ε2, ε3, and ε4, that differ at two codons, 112 and 158 (Table 1). Compared with the most frequent genotype (ε3/ε3), the odds ratios of developing Alzheimer disease among Caucasian subjects with genotypes that include ε4 are ε2/ε4, 2.6; ε3/ε4, 3.2; and ε4/ε4, 14.9. For genotypes ε2/ε2 and ε2/ε3, the odds ratio is reduced to 0.6 *(14)*. The effect of the ε4 allele on the risk of developing Alzheimer disease varies among different populations, being stronger among Japanese but weaker among Hispanics and possibly among African Americans *(14)*. The ε4 allele has been shown to exert a dose-dependent effect on the age of onset of the disease: patients who develop Alzheimer disease who have two copies of the ε4 allele develop the first symptoms an average of 6 yr earlier than patients without this allele *(15,16)*.

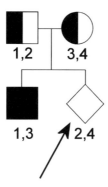

Fig. 1. Principle of linkage analysis. The inheritance of a disease-causing mutation can be inferred from the pattern of inheritance of markers at a nearby polymorphic locus. In the illustration, the parents are heterozygous for an autosomal
recessive disease. They have an affected son and seek genetic information regarding a fetus (symbolized here by a diamond). At a polymorphic locus close to the
disease locus, the father has the genetic markers identified as 1 and 2, and the
mother has markers 3 and 4. The affected son has inherited marker 1 from his
father and 3 from his mother. The inference of this observation is that markers 1
and 3 are on chromosomes that carry disease-causing mutations. Testing of the
fetal sample reveals that the fetus has markers 2 and 4, inherited from the father
and mother, respectively. Because neither of these markers is found in the affected
son, the prediction is that the fetus has not inherited a disease-causing mutation.
Factors that could lead to an erroneous prediction include genetic recombination
between the disease locus and the polymorphic locus being tested, nonpaternity,
and misdiagnosis in the affected son, for example, incorrect diagnosis of steroid
21-hydroxylase deficiency when the correct diagnosis should be 11β-hydroxylase
deficiency. The genes responsible for these enzymes are encoded on different
chromosomes; therefore polymorphic markers near the gene locus of one enzyme
cannot be used to track the familial inheritance of the gene for the other enzyme.

Locus heterogeneity is of importance in molecular diagnostics
because it requires that several genes be examined when one is searching for possible disease-causing mutations. Locus heterogeneity may
lead to erroneous diagnostic results when test strategies are used that
are based on genetic linkage within families if the correct locus
responsible for a disease is not recognized in the proband (Fig. 1). For
example, markers in the HLA region on 6p can be used for linkage
studies in families with congenital adrenal hyperplasia caused by
steroid 21-hydroxylase deficiency. However, if a proband in a family
has the steroid 11β-hydroxylase deficiency form of congenital adrenal
hyperplasia, which has many clinical features in common with the 21-
hydroxylase deficiency form, then the use of chromosome 6 markers

for family linkage studies would give unreliable results. The reason for this is that the 11β-hydroxylase gene is encoded on chromosome 8.

MUTATIONS IN A GENE RESULTING IN DIFFERENT DISEASES

Occasionally, different mutations in a single gene can give rise to different phenotypes. An example of this is provided by different mutations in the cystic fibrosis gene, *CFTR*. Mutations in *CFTR* have been found in otherwise healthy males with infertility caused by congenital bilateral absence of the vas deferens (CBAVD). These patients do not have other features of cystic fibrosis such as pulmonary or pancreatic disease. However, the vast majority of males with typical cystic fibrosis have CBAVD, so isolated CBAVD arising from *CFTR* mutations represents a very restricted expression of the cystic fibrosis phenotype.

A more striking example is seen in Hirschsprung's disease, which is characterized by failure of development of autonomic ganglia in the large bowel, leading to intestinal obstruction or impaired bowel motility in infants. Some patients with Hirschsprung's disease have mutations in the *RET* proto-oncogene *(17)*. Mutations in *RET* are also seen in families with the familial cancer syndromes multiple endocrine neoplasia (MEN), types 2A and 2B (*see* Chap. 6). Therefore, mutations in a single gene, *RET,* are associated with diseases as seemingly unrelated as Hirschsprung's disease and MEN 2.

A final example of mutations in a single gene causing different diseases is seen with mutations in the lamin A/C gene, *LMNA,* on chromosome 1q. This gene encodes lamin A and C proteins that are produced by alternative splicing of a common transcript. These proteins associate with chromatin and other proteins in the inner nuclear membrane. Different mutations in *LMNA* give rise to Emery-Dreifus muscular dystrophy, type I (EMD1), which is an X-linked form of muscular dystrophy associated with cardiac conduction abnormalities; EMD2, which is an autosomal recessive form of the disease; a familial cardiomyopathy syndrome known as CMD1A; a form of lipodystrophy known as familial partial lipodystrophy, which is characterized by loss of fat in the extremities and accumulation of fat around the face and neck, and which shows an autosomal dominant inheritance pattern; and, finally, a recessive

form of Charcot-Marie-Tooth disease, CMT2A *(18,19)*. This extra-
ordinary range of phenotypes from mutations in the one gene is
probably an effect of mutations in different functional domains of
the lamin A/C protein.

PENETRANCE

Penetrance is a measure of the number of individuals with a specific genotype who express the corresponding phenotype. If every-
one with the genotype expresses the phenotype, then the penetrance
is 100% and is said to be complete. For some genetic diseases, the
penetrance is incomplete. For example, in the case of retinoblastoma, an autosomal dominant disease, families with high- and low-
penetrance forms of the disease are recognized, and these
differences in familial penetrance are related to specific mutations
in the retinoblastoma gene *(20)*.

Penetrance can vary with age and gender. For example, Huntington's disease, an autosomal dominant trait, shows age-dependent
penetrance. Symptoms usually do not appear until adulthood, and
there is an increasing likelihood of developing symptoms with
increasing age in subjects who have the mutation that causes Huntington's disease. As an example of the effect of sex on gene penetrance, hereditary mutations in the breast cancer genes, *BRCA1* and
BRCA2, confer a lifetime risk of developing breast cancer of up to
50–80% in females, whereas the risk of breast cancer in males with
a *BRCA2* mutation is about 6% *(21)* and is lower for males with a
BRCA1 mutation *(22)*.

EXPRESSIVITY

Expressivity refers to the degree of expression of the phenotype
arising from a specific genotype. Whereas penetrance is a measure of
whether any symptoms appear in association with a genotype, expressivity is an assessment of the extent to which symptoms appear.
Expression of a phenotype may be influenced by other genetic factors
or by environmental effects. For example, the classic form of congenital adrenal hyperplasia resulting from mutations in the steroid 21-
hydroxylase gene, *CYP21,* is an autosomal recessive disorder that
impairs production of adrenal steroids. Approximately two-thirds of

patients have a tendency to lose sodium in the distal renal tubule as a result of aldosterone insufficiency. This phenotype is known as salt wasting. The remaining one-third of patients are able to produce sufficient aldosterone to avoid salt wasting. Although certain genotypes are invariably associated with salt wasting, families have been described in which siblings with identical *CYP21* genotypes show variable expression of the salt-wasting phenotype *(23)*.

Modifier Genes

Why do subjects with identical genotypes at a major disease locus have differences in penetrance and expression of a genetic trait? The influence of environmental factors that affect disease manifestation can vary from one person to another and thereby modify the manifestation of a major genetic locus. For example, cigarette smoking exacerbates the pulmonary phenotype in patients with α_1-antitrypsin deficiency. Increasingly, the existence of other genes that influence a major genetic trait is being recognized. These genes are known as modifier genes. By themselves, they do not cause disease, but they can modify the clinical expression of a major disease locus. For example, siblings with cystic fibrosis who share the same mutations at the *CFTR* locus may be discordant for certain clinical features such as meconium ileus, the severity of pulmonary disease, and the presence of liver disease. Genetic factors have been implicated in such discordance: an unidentified locus on chromosome 19 has been implicated in the development of meconium ileus, and polymorphisms in a number of specific genes have been shown to affect the pulmonary phenotype. The latter include tumor necrosis factor-α, transforming growth factor-β, glutathione transferase M1, α_1-antitrypsin, several genes encoding antibacterial proteins, and mannose binding protein *(24)*.

In addition to differences between subjects that arise from environmental exposures and modifier genes, there are also examples of major disease genes that have more than one mutation on a single allele. For example, at least six phenylalanine hydroxylase alleles are known that have two mutations, and other polymorphisms within the *PAH* gene are known *(25)*. Alleles with more than one mutation are known as complex alleles. It should be noted that a second mutation may occasionally have a beneficial effect on the phenotype caused by a deleterious mutation. For example, a *CFTR* allele containing both the ΔF508 and R553Q mutations was observed to be associated with lower sweat chloride values than are typically associated with alleles that have just the ΔF508 mutation *(26)*.

MUTATION RATES ACROSS THE GENOME

Hot Spots

Certain regions of the genome are more likely to undergo mutation than are others. CpG dinucleotides are very common sites for mutations and represent one of the best characterized mutation hot spots in DNA. Methylation of cytosine at carbon 5 produces 5-methylcytosine, and this epigenetic modification in regulatory regions of genes is associated with downregulation of gene transcription, as described in Chapter 1. Spontaneous deamination of 5-methylcytosine forms thymine (Fig. 10 in Chapter 1). Many human diseases are caused by C→T transitions occurring at CpG dinucleotides *(27)*. For example, achondroplasia is caused by mutations in the fibroblast growth factor receptor 3 gene, *FGFR3*. More than 95% of these mutations are a G→A transition that causes a Gly→Arg substitution in the receptor *(4)*. The G→A transition is the result of a C→T transition on the complementary strand occurring at a CpG dinucleotide.

Genetic sequences that are duplicated are a common site for gene deletion and gene duplication arising from misalignment and unequal crossing over during meiosis (Fig. 2). Important examples of this include deletions of the α-globin genes in α-thalassemia, deletion of the steroid 21-hydroxylase gene in congenital adrenal hyperplasia, and deletion/duplication of the *PMP22* gene in hereditary neuropathy with liability to pressure palsy/Charcot-Marie-Tooth disease, type 1A.

Meiotic misalignment and unequal crossing over involving repetitive DNA sequences have also been implicated as the mechanism of mutation in several diseases. For example, among French Canadians with Tay-Sachs disease, misalignment of Alu sequences and unequal crossing over has been shown to cause deletions of 7.6 kb of the hexosaminidase A gene, *HEXA,* and is the most common mutation in this gene in this ethnic group *(28)*. A frequent 9.5-kb deletion involving exons 16–18 of the low-density lipoprotien (LDL) receptor gene that is common in the Finnish population is

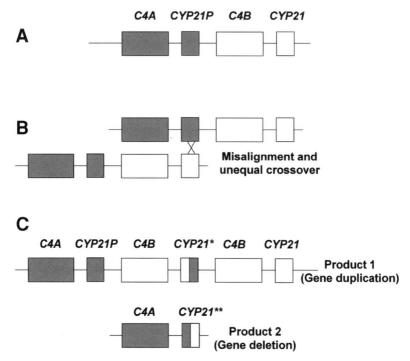

Fig. 2. Origin of gene deletions at the steroid 21-hydroxylase locus. (**A**) The functional steroid 21-hydroxylase gene *(CYP21)* and a pseudogene *(CYP21P)* shown in a tandem arrangement with the genes encoding complement 4 proteins, C4A and C4B. This represents the usual configuration of these genes. (**B**) During meiosis, misalignment of these duplicated sequences followed by unequal crossing over may occur. (**C**) The products formed from this process. These are a chromosome containing duplications of *C4B* and *CYP21* (product 1) and a chromosome in which the *C4B* and *CYP21* genes are deleted (product 2). Note that because of the location of the crossover, the *CYP21* gene in product 2 (indicated by a double asterisk) is a hybrid that contains 5′ sequences derived from the pseudogene and 3′ sequences from the functional gene. In the common deletion that gives rise to congenital adrenal hyperplasia, the hybrid includes pseudogene mutations that render the gene nonfunctional. Product 1, which contains a *CYP21* duplication, is not associated with a clinical phenotype.

believed to have originated from recombination events involving Alu elements in that gene *(29)*.

Another mechanism of mutation is known as gene conversion. In a gene conversion, a sequence of DNA from one gene replaces the sequence from another, homologous gene without a reciprocal exchange of genetic information (Fig. 3). An example of gene conver-

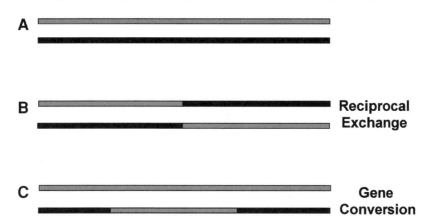

Fig. 3. Different effects of a reciprocal exchange and a gene conversion event. **(A)** Segments from two DNA molecules. **(B)** A reciprocal exchange of genetic sequence between the two DNA segments, as might occur during crossing over at meiosis. **(C)** A gene conversion product. There is a conversion of genetic sequence of one DNA molecule to that of the other without a reciprocal exchange.

sion as a frequent mutation mechanism occurs at the steroid 21-hydroxylase *(CYP21)* locus. Mutations in this gene are responsible for most cases for congenital adrenal hyperplasia, an autosomal recessive disorder *(30)*. The region contains a steroid 21-hydroxylase pseudo-gene *(CYP21P)* that contains several mutations. *CYP21* is commonly mutated by gene conversion events that transfer deleterious sequences from the highly homologous pseudogene into the functional gene.

In addition to mutations involving CpG dinucleotides and regions involving gene duplications, many individual genes show mutation hot spots at specific sites. For example, an acquired G→T transversion in codon 249 of the *TP53* gene is found in the majority of patients with hepatocellular carcinoma associated with aflatoxin B1 ingestion in parts of China and Africa *(31)*. Aflatoxin is produced by some species of *Aspergillus* and is ingested as a contaminant of certain foods. Hepatocellular cancers arising in populations that are not exposed to aflatoxin do not show this particular mutation.

Founder Mutations

In certain geographically isolated or ethnic populations, particular mutations are found with increased frequency relative to other populations. A common explanation for this is that the population is

Table 2
Examples of Founder Mutations

Population	Gene	Mutation(s)	Disease
Ashkenazim	BRCA1	185delAG, 5382insC	Hereditary breast/ovarian cancer
Ashkenazim	HEXA	4-bp insertion, exon 11	Tay-Sachs disease
Celtic	HFE	C282Y	Hereditary hemochromatosis
Finns	LDLR	Partial gene deletion	Familial hypercholesterolemia
French Canadians	HEXA	Partial gene deletion	Tay-Sachs disease
Icelanders	BRCA2	999del5	Hereditary breast/ovarian cancer
Yupik Eskimos	CYP21	Intron 2 splice mutation	Congenital adrenal hyperplasia

descended from a relatively small group of individuals, at least one of whom harbored the mutation in question. Thus, the prevalence of the mutation was increased in the gene pool of this group and has been maintained because of breeding within the group. Such a mutation is called a *founder mutation* and the phenomenon is known as a *founder effect*. Examples of founder mutations are shown in Table 2.

MUTATIONS AND THEIR EFFECTS

Point Mutations

Point mutations are single nucleotide substitutions. A substitution in which a purine is replaced by another purine (e.g., G→A) or in which a pyrimidine is replaced by another pyrimidine (e.g., C→T) are known as *transitions*. Substitution of a purine by a pyrimidine (or vice versa) is known as a *transversion*. The effect of a single nucleotide substitution on a gene depends on where the substitution occurs. If a mutation alters one of the three nucleotides in a codon, there are several possible consequences:

1. No change in the amino acid encoded because of redundancy of the genetic code. This kind of mutation is known as a silent mutation.
2. An alteration in the amino acid encoded. This kind of change is termed a missense mutation. Missense mutations may be conservative or noncon-servative depending on the amino acid substitution. A conservative sub-

stitution involves the replacement of an amino acid by another of similar physicochemical properties, for example, replacement of valine by isoleucine. On the other hand, replacement of an amino acid by proline often causes significant change in the structure and function of proteins because of the disruption that proline induces in protein tertiary structure.

3. Replacement of a codon for an amino acid by that of a stop codon. In nuclear DNA there are three stop codons. This kind of mutation is known as a nonsense mutation. The resulting protein is truncated and may be nonfunctional. A protein truncation assay can sometimes reveal this type of mutation (*see* Chap. 4).

Splice Mutations

Mutations at intron splice junctions can prevent splicing of an intron. The dinucleotides GT and AG are almost invariably present at the 5′ and 3′ ends of introns. Additional nucleotides adjacent to these constitute the 5′ (or left) and 3′ (or right) splice recognition sites. Mutations of these critical nucleotides may disrupt normal splicing of the intron. If the intron is not removed, then the resulting mRNA contains additional sequences from the intron. Translation of this abnormal mRNA typically results in a nonfunctional protein that contains extra amino acids. In addition, the abnormal mRNA may have a shorter half-life than its normal counterpart. If a splicing mutation leads to removal of an exon, then the resulting protein will lack the amino acids encoded by that exon. For example, a common mutation giving rise to phenylketonuria is a mutation (GT→AT) in intron 12 of the phenylalanine hydroxylase gene (*see* Chap. 5). This mutation causes skipping of exon 12 during splicing of the mRNA transcript *(32)*. The protein produced by the mRNA does not have phenylalanine hydroxylase activity.

Mutations in exons, in addition to causing missense or nonsense mutations, can mimic a splice donor or acceptor site. When this happens, a portion of the exon is incorrectly spliced out during mRNA processing, and the resulting protein is generally nonfunctional. The mutation that causes hemoglobin E is representative of this type of mutation (Fig. 4). This mutation is present in exon 1 of the β-globin gene. Incorrect splicing at this position leads to loss of a portion of exon 1 from the final mRNA, resulting in a nonfunctional protein. This splicing error does not occur in all transcripts because the splicing apparatus correctly splices some transcripts.

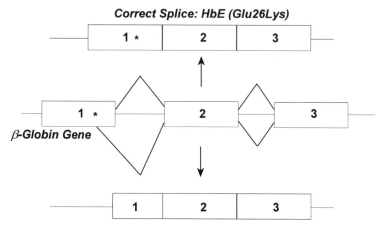

Fig. 4. Effect of the hemoglobin E mutation. The HbE mutation in exon 1 (middle, indicated by an asterisk) has two effects. The mutation generates an alternative splice signal in exon 1 that is used in the majority of transcripts. This splice error leads to a protein that cannot function as a globin (bottom). In the remaining transcripts, the splicing is normal, but the transcript encodes a missense mutation (top).

When correct splicing occurs, the mRNA encodes a globin with a missense mutation, Glu26Lys. The single mutation therefore has two effects. First, because of the splice error, it causes a thalassemia because of the abnormal ratio of production of α-globin chains to β-globin chains. Second, it causes a hemoglobinopathy because of the novel properties of the hemoglobin arising from the missense mutation.

Mutations in Promoter and Other Noncoding Sequences

Mutations in promoter elements generally downregulate gene transcription. For example, a mutation in the factor IX gene promoter, −20 T→A (the Leyden mutation), gives rise to deficiency of factor IX, leading to hemophilia, and is inherited as an X-linked recessive trait.

Mutations in the 3′ untranslated (3′ UT) region of genes may alter the stability of the mRNA. A frequent mutation in the 3′ UT region of the prothrombin gene, G20210A, is associated with an increased level of prothrombin that appears to be responsible for an increased risk of venous thrombosis (*see* Chap. 5).

Diseases Caused by Unstable Trinucleotide Repeats

Trinucleotide repeats are a type of repetitive DNA in which a three-base sequence is repeated in a head-to-tail fashion e.g., [...CGGCGGCGG...]. Over a dozen hereditary disorders are known to be caused by an unusual form of mutation in which the number of copies of a trinucleotide repeat varies between generations (Table 3). These are known as unstable trinucleotide repeat or dynamic mutations. The trinucleotide repeats may be located in coding or noncoding regions of a gene, and the normal number of copies of a repeat is characteristic of each locus. When the normal range of repeat number is exceeded, disease may be manifest. An increase in the number of copies of the trinucleotide repeats, which is termed expansion, takes place during meiosis, and, depending on the disease, there is often a tendency for expansion to occur more frequently during meiosis in one or other sex.

In the case of some of the trinucleotide repeat diseases, for example, fragile X syndrome, alleles that are larger than normal are in a range that is not associated with disease but are prone to undergo further expansion to a range that is associated with disease. This intermediate range is termed *premutation.* Because the number of copies of a trinucleotide repeat can increase from one generation to the next, later generations in a pedigree with an unstable trinucleotide repeat disorder are more likely to contain affected individuals than are earlier generations. This phenomenon is known as *anticipation.*

All the trinucleotide repeat disorders behave as dominant traits in the presence of a full expansion, with the exception of Friedreich's ataxia, which is a recessive disease. SCA8 is unique in that the gene does not encode a protein but appears to encode an antisense RNA molecule that may interact with a transcript from the complementary strand *(33).*

Unstable trinucleotide repeat diseases can be grouped on the basis of where the unstable repeat is situated in a gene. Diseases caused by expansion of repeats in noncoding regions include fragile X syndromes (*FRAXA* and *FRAXE*), Friedreich's ataxia, myotonic dystrophy, and spinocerebellar ataxia, types 8 and 12. Diseases caused by expansion of repeats in coding regions include Huntington's disease, spinobulbar muscular atrophy (Kennedy's disease), dentatorubal-pallidoluysian atrophy (DRPLA), and spinocerebellar ataxia, types 1–3, 6 and 7.

Table 3
Unstable Trinucleotide Repeat Diseases

Disease	Gene/chromosome	Protein	Trinucleotide	No. of Repeats Normal	Disease
Fragile-X	*FRAXA*/Xq27.3	FMRP	CGG	6–54	>230
Fragile-XE	*FRAXE*/Xq28	FMRP-2	GCC	6–35	>200
Friedreich's ataxia	*X25*/9q13	Frataxin	GAA	7–34	>100
Myotonic dystrophy	*DMPK*/19q13	DMPK	CTG	5–37	>50
SCA-8	*SCA8*/13q21	(Anti-sense RNA)	CTG	16–37	>110
SCA-12	*SCA12*/5q31-q33	PP2A-PR55b	CAG	7–28	66–78
Polyglutamine disorders					
Kennedy's disease	*AR*/Xq13-21	Androgen receptor	CAG	9–36	38–62
Huntington's disease	*HD*/4p16.3	Huntingtin	CAG	6–35	36–121
DRPLA	*DRPLA*/12p13.31	Atrophin-1	CAG	6–35	49–88
SCA-1	*SCA1*/6p23	Ataxin-1	CAG	6–44	39–82
SCA-2	*SCA2*/12q24.1	Ataxin-2	CAG	15–31	36–63
SCA-3	*SCA3*/14q32.1	Ataxin-3	CAG	12–40	55–84
SCA-6	*SCA6*/19p13	Ca channel α_{1A}	CAG	4–18	21–33
SCA-7	*SCA7*/13p12-13	Ataxin-7	CAG	4–35	37–306

Abbreviations: SCA, spinocerebellar ataxia; DRPLA, dentatorubral-pallidoluysian atrophy

The *CAG repeat disorders* are a subset of unstable trinucleotide repeat diseases in which the trinucleotide repeat is in the coding region of a gene. Because CAG encodes glutamine, expansion of this trinucleotide results in the presence of an extended polyglutamine tract in a protein. These abnormal proteins tend to form aggregates in the nucleus and are considered to be *gain of function* mutations because the protein formed has a toxic effect on cells. The mechanism of toxicity, and why only certain cells (generally neurons) are affected by this toxicity, are not fully understood *(34)*.

In addition to the trinucleotide repeat instability, intergenerational instability has also been found in tetranucleotide and pentanucleotide repeats. Known examples are associated with myotonic dystrophy, type 2, resulting from a tetranucleotide repeat expansion *(35)*, and with SCA10, resulting from a pentanucleotide repeat expansion *(36)*.

Assessing the Significance of a Point Mutation

When analyzing the relationship between a disease phenotype and a mutation in a specific gene, particularly a point mutation, there are several principles for assessing the significance of a mutation *(1)*.

1. Mutations that introduce frameshifts or nonsense mutations may result in a phenotype because of the magnitude of the effect on the protein. However, nonsense mutations near the carboxyl end of a protein are less likely to be deleterious than those that occur earlier in the protein.
2. Segregation of the mutation with the phenotype within a family is supporting evidence that the mutation is disease-causing.
3. If an assessment of the prevalence of the mutation within a normal population shows it to be rare (e.g., <1%), whereas it is frequent in the disease population, then this information would tend to indicate that it is disease-causing or in close linakge with a disease-causing mutation.
4. Missense mutations that alter amino acids that are conserved in a protein across different species are likely to be of greater functional importance than are mutations in nonconserved amino acids.
5. Missense mutations that change the type of amino acid (e.g., hydrophobic, acidic, basic) are more likely to be functionally significant than those that are conservative.
6. Finally, experimental analysis of expression of the mutant gene in vitro can provide important information on the significance of the mutation.

Insertions

Insertions of DNA can range in size from a single base pair to millions of base pairs. Larger insertions may be visible as cytogenetic abnormalities. Insertions in the coding regions disrupt gene function and may cause a frame shift mutation. For example, a common mutation in the *BRCA1* gene, 5382insC, involves insertion of a single cytosine at nucleotide 5382, located in exon 20. This introduces a frame shift mutation. The new reading frame includes a premature stop codon in exon 24 *(37)*. This mutation is commonly associated with familial breast and ovarian cancer in Poland and Russia and in Ashkenazi Jewish populations *(38–41)*. Another example of a small insertion is seen in the hexosaminidase A gene, which is mutated in patients with Tay-Sachs disease. A 4-bp insertion is the most common mutation seen in the Ashkenazi population, among whom this disease is more common than in other ethnic groups *(42)*.

Occasionally, an Alu or Line-1 (L1) repeat sequence can become inserted into a gene, causing loss of function of the gene. A few patients with an L1 insertion in the factor VIII gene causing hemophilia have been reported *(43)*. Insertion of an Alu repeat into a gene giving rise to disease was first reported in a patient with neurofibromatosis, type I *(44)*, and since that report additional patients with a variety of genetic diseases have been described in whom the basis of mutation involves an Alu insertion in a gene *(45)*. An Alu insertion in an intron of the angiotensin-converting enzyme (ACE) gene is the basis of a frequent insertion/deletion (I/D) polymorphism at this locus in the general population. The I allele is associated in a dose-dependent manner with lower ACE activity in serum *(46)*.

Another common insertion mutation is found in the promoter of the uridine diphosphate glucuronosyltransferase 1A1 gene *(UGT1A1)*. This gene encodes the hepatic enzyme that is responsible for glucuronidation of bilirubin. Mutations in this gene give rise to Gilbert's syndrome, which is a benign form of hyperbilirubinemia, and to Crigler-Najjar syndrome, types 1 and 2 (*see* Chap. 9). Gilbert's syndrome is relatively common, being present in up to 7% of Caucasians *(47)*. The promoter region of this gene contains six copies of a TA dinucleotide repeat in the motif $(TA)_6TAA$. Most subjects with Gilbert's syndrome have seven copies of the TA dinucleotide i.e., $(TA)_7TAA$. The additional TA dinucleotide decreases the efficiency of transcription of the gene. Gilbert's syndrome and both forms of Crigler-Najjar syndrome are inherited as autosomal recessive traits.

Deletions

Like insertions, deletions of DNA sequences can be as small as a single base pair or sufficiently large to be visible by conventional cytogenetic analysis. Numerous diseases are caused by gene deletions of various sizes. Deletion of 3 base pairs is responsible for the most common mutation in cystic fibrosis, the ΔF508 mutation. Deletions that remove a number of nucleotides that is not a multiple of 3 from an exon result in a frameshift mutation. Deletion of one or more exons is the usual mutation found in patients with Duchenne's muscular dystrophy. Deletions of whole genes are found in most patients with α-thalassemia and in approx 25% of patients with congenital adrenal hyperplasia owing to steroid-21 hydroxylase deficiency. It is interesting to note that in both α-thalassemia and 21-hydroxylase deficiency, the genetic locus has undergone duplication. These duplicated genes appear to be susceptible to misalignment and unequal crossing over during meiosis, giving rise to gene deletions.

Chromosome Microdeletions

Chromosome microdeletions refer to deletions of millions of base pairs of DNA. When deletions are this large, they can eliminate several genes. Most of the known microdeletions range from 1.5 to 3.5 Mb and are associated with specific clinical syndromes. The syndrome may be caused by loss of a single gene among those that are deleted. For example, Angelman's syndrome is associated with a deletion of approx 3.5 Mb, and the phenotype is believed to result from loss of the *UBE3A* gene, which lies within the deleted region. Alternatively, the phenotype may result from the loss of more than one gene within the deleted region. These kinds of syndromes are also called *contiguous gene syndromes.* An example of a contiguous gene syndrome is Williams syndrome (WS), which is caused by a deletion of approx 1.5 Mb in 7q11.23. This disorder is characterized by infantile hypercalcemia, dysmorphic features, mental retardation or learning disability, a characteristic impairment of visual-spatial ability, distinctive personality, and an arteriopathy that includes supravalvular aortic stenosis (SVAS). The last of these can be found as a heritable disorder without other manifestations of WS and is associated with mutations in the elastin gene, *ELN,* which is contained in the region of the microdeletion in WS *(48).* It is believed that the other manifestations of WS arise from loss of other genes in the deleted region.

Other examples of microdeletion syndromes are shown in Table 4. Although some microdeletions can be detected with conventional G-banding, the preferred method for detection of most microdeletions is fluorescence *in situ* hybridization (FISH).

Increases in Gene Copy Number

A number of disorders arise from increases in gene copy number. Examples of these include the usual mutation in Charcot-Marie-Tooth type 1a disease (CMT1A), which is a duplication of the peripheral myelin protein-22 gene *(PMP22)* gene on chromosome 17. CMT1A is characterized by motor and sensory neuropathy and is inherited as an autosomal dominant trait.

An increase in copy number of the *CYP2D6* gene, which encodes the cytochrome P450 responsible for metabolism of many drugs, leads to the ultraextensive metabolizer (UEM) phenotype. Subjects with this phenotype have a greatly increased rate of metabolism of certain drugs and may require much higher than normal dosages to achieve a therapeutic effect (*see* Chap. 9).

Increases in the number of copies of specific oncogenes are commonly found in certain tumors. For example, increases in *MYCN* (the N-*myc* oncogene) copy number are seen in up to 25% of pediatric neuroblastomas, in which setting the increased gene dosage confers an adverse prognosis *(49)*. *MYCN* amplifications are seen in extrachromosomal structures called double minutes or in homogeneously staining regions (hsrs) of chromosomes in cytogenetic studies. Increased levels of Myc, the protein that is encoded by *MYCN,* appear to promote tumor development through interaction with a transcriptional factor, Max, and aberrant activation of transcription of genes involved in cell growth *(50)*.

Increases in expression of the *HER2/neu* gene are found in approx 20–30% of breast cancers and confer an adverse prognosis relative to tumors that do not show such increased expression. In nearly all cases, increased expression is a result of gene amplification. *HER2/neu* is a member of the epidermal growth factor receptor family of genes that play important roles in cell growth, migration, and differentiation. Detection of amplification of this marker is a potential indication for therapy with trastuzumab (Herceptin), a commercially available antibody directed against the overexpressed HER2/neu protein *(51)*. The development of this therapy marks the

Table 4
Some Disorders Associated with Chromosomal Microdeletions

Disorder	Chromosome	Gene	Major features
Alagille's syndrome	20p11.23–p12.1	*Jag1*	Deficiency of intrahepatic bile ducts; cardiac, vertebral, ocular anomalies; characteristic facies
Angelman's syndrome	15q11–q13	*UBE3A*	Mental retardation, seizures, ataxia, microcephaly
DiGeorge's syndrome	22q11.2	*Tbx1* (?)	Hypocalcemia, immunodeficiency, cardiac anomalies
Langer-Gideon syndrome	8q24.11	*EXT1, TRPS*	Mental retardation, microcephaly, multiple exostoses, cone-shaped epiphyses, sparse hair, facial anomalies, excess skin
Male infertility	Yq11	*AZF a-c*	Azoospermia, severe oligozoospermia
Miller-Dieker syndrome	17p13.3	*LIS1*	Lissencephaly, agyria, mental retardation, facial anomalies, multiple abnormalities of brain, heart, kidneys, GI tract
Prader-Willi syndrome	15q11–q13	*SNRPN* (?)	Hypotonia, hypogonadism, behavioral abnormalities, obesity
Smith-Magennis syndrome	17p11.2	Unknown	Aggressive, self-injurious behavior, midface hypoplasia, delayed development, short stature, brachydactyly

first availability of a specific agent directed against an oncogene that is involved in development of a solid tumor. Amplification can be detected by FISH or by immunohistochemistry, but these two approaches do not always yield a consistent result, partly because of inherent differences between these methods and partly because of intraobserver differences in interpretation of immunohistochemistry studies *(52)*.

In addition to increases in gene copy number arising from expansion of individual genes, increases in gene copy number are also seen in chromosomal aneusomies in which extra copies of entire chromosomes are present.

Translocations

Translocations involve breakage followed by exchange and rejoining of portions of two or more chromosomes. Specific, recurring translocations are found in many hematological malignancies, and their presence provides important diagnostic and prognostic information. The recent World Health Organization (WHO) classification of hematological malignancies categorizes certain forms of malignancy on the basis of detection of highly characteristic translocations *(53)*. Such acquired translocations confer a selective advantage on the cell because of alteration in the regulation of cell growth, for example, because of activation of an oncogene that is present at the fusion point in the translocation. This is discussed further in Chapter 6, and specific examples of translocations involved in hematological malignancies are described in Chapter 8.

Robertsonian Translocations

Robertsonian translocations involve breakage and fusion of two acrocentric chromosomes (i.e., chromosomes 13, 14, 15, 21, and 22) near their centromeres, with resulting loss of their short arms. The short arms of the acrocentric chromosomes contain genes that encode ribosomal RNAs, and because these genes are duplicated on several different chromosomes, the loss of these genes in a Robertsonian translocation is not deleterious. Among the more common Robertsonian translocations are 13q14q and 14q21q. Subjects with a Robertsonian translocation that involves chromosome 21 are at increased risk of having an offspring with Down syndrome, and this effect is independent of maternal age.

Approximately 4% of Down syndrome patients have a Robertson-ian translocation. Identification of a Robertsonian translocation in a patient with Down syndrome should prompt a cytogenetic evaluation of the parents and genetic counseling to discuss the recurrence risks.

Inversions

An inversion involves breakage of a chromosome in at least two places followed by rotation and rejoining of the involved segment. Inversions may be submicroscopic or visible by cytogenetic study. At a chromosomal level, inversions are characterized as either paracentric, in which case the inverted segment is contained within a chromosomal arm, or pericentric, in which case the inverted segment spans the centromere because a break occurred on each arm. The clinical effect of an inversion may arise from changes in gene structure at the boundaries of the inversion, or from production of gametes with unbalanced karyotypes following meiosis.

If one member of a chromosome pair has an inversion, then alignment of the homologous chromosomes during meiosis requires the formation of an inversion loop for pairing to occur. The effects of crossing over depend on whether the inversion is pericentric or paracentric. If crossing over occurs within the inversion loop of a paracentric inversion, the possible results are the production of gametes with one of the following chromosome complements: a normal chromosome, a chromosome carrying the inversion, a dicentric chromosome, and an acentric chromosome. The latter two are unstable and incompatible with life; thus fetuses that come to term have either a normal karyotype or have a chromosome containing the inversion, which is associated with a balanced karyotype.

However, if the inversion is pericentric, the possible gametes formed include a normal chromosome, a chromosome with the inversion, and two chromosomes, each of which is missing a portion of one arm and containing a duplication of a portion of the other arm. These latter chromosomal anomalies may be compatible with life but are commonly associated with severe phenotypic abnormalities. The risk of having a child with an unbalanced karyotype is

Chromosome 16

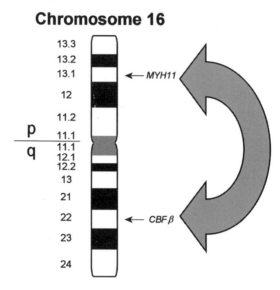

Fig. 5. Generation of the inversion on chromosome 16 commonly seen in acute myeloid leukemia (FAB-M4Eo subtype). The locations of the *MYH11* and *CBFB* genes are shown. Breakage at both genes and inversion of the intervening segment leads to formation of fusion genes.

therefore greater for a parent with a pericentric inversion than for one with a paracentric inversion.

An acquired inversion, inv(16), is present in most patients with the M4Eo type of acute myeloid leukemia *(54)*. This inversion fuses the core binding factor β gene *(CBFB)* on 16q with the smooth muscle myosin heavy chain gene (*SMMHC,* also called *MYH11*) on 16p (Fig. 5). The fusion protein produced by this translocation has a dominant inhibitory effect on a transcriptional factor, Runt-related transcription factor 1 (RUNX1, also known as AML1), and is involved in development of certain forms of leukemia *(55)*. This is discussed further in Chapter 8.

Approximately 40–50% of patients with severe hemophilia A have an inversion of 400–500 kb of DNA in Xq extending from intron 22 of the *FVIII* gene to regions close to the Xq telomere *(56,57)*. This inversion arises from an intrachromosomal recombination between a sequence in intron 22 of *FVIII,* (int22h-1) and homologous sequences (int22h-2 nd int22h-3) that are situated toward the telomere (Fig. 6). This inversion moves the first 22 exons

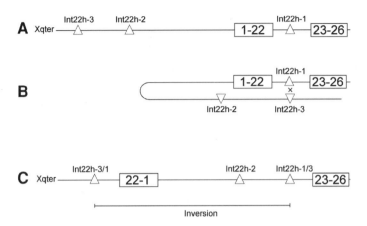

Fig. 6. The inversion mutation in the factor VIII gene. (**A**) The region of the gene up to the end of exon 22 and the region from exon 23 to 26 are shown as rectangles. Intron 22 contains a region (int22h-1) that has homology to two regions located further upstream, toward the telomere of Xq. (**B**) Recombination between one of the more upstream regions of homology and int22h-1 can lead to an inversion of most of the FVIII gene. (**C**) The resulting mutation does not encode functional factor VIII protein.

on *FVIII* toward the telomere and disrupts the gene so that no factor VIII protein can be produced.

NUMERICAL CHROMOSOMAL ABNORMALITIES

Nondisjunction

During meiosis and mitosis, chromosomes separate during cell division so that daughter cells have the correct complement of chromosomes (Fig. 7). Failure of normal segregation of chromosomes is known as nondisjunction and leads to aneuploidy, with cells containing either too few or too many chromosomes. During meiosis, if nondisjunction occurs during the first meiotic division (meiosis I), the resulting gamete will either have both copies of a chromosome or will be lacking a chromosome (Fig. 8). At fertilization, a gamete with two copies of a chromosome will lead to a zygote with trisomy for that chromosome, whereas a gamete that is missing a chromosome will lead to a zygote with monosomy for that chromosome. If nondisjunction occurs during meiosis II (Fig. 9), the gametes with two chromosomes have two copies of one of the parental chromosomes, although

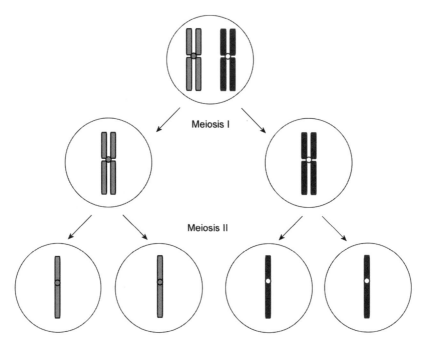

Fig. 7. Meiosis reduces the number of chromosomes from 46 to 23. In this illustration, a pair of homologous chromosomes is shown. In meiosis I and II, there are two rounds of cell division, leading to formation of gametes that are haploid. Note that the cell at the top of the figure has undergone a round of chromosome replication. In females, only one gamete is formed because at each round of meiosis, one daughter cell is destined to become a polar body.

these may not be exact copies because of recombination occurring during crossing over. Most nondisjunction occurs during meiosis I.

Nondisjunction is the usual mechanism underlying common chromosomal aneuploidy syndromes at birth: trisomy 21, trisomy 13, and trisomy 18. Other aneuploid karyotypes are found in spontaneous abortions, but the pattern of involved chromosomes in aneuploidy in spontaneous abortions is very different from that observed in live-born babies. For example, the most common trisomy seen in spontaneous abortions is trisomy 16, but this is lethal *in utero* and therefore is not seen in full-term newborns.

Isochromosomes

An isochromosome refers to a chromosome that has two copies of either the short or long arm fused at or near the centromere.

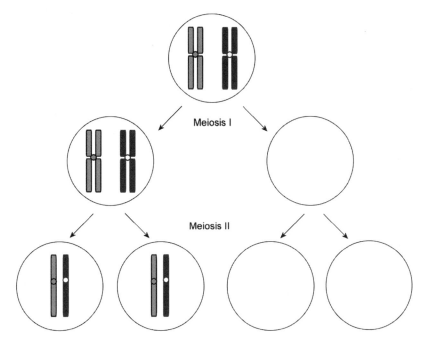

Fig. 8. Nondisjunction occurring during meiosis I. The resulting gametes have either two copies of a chromosome or are missing a chromosome. Nondisjunction at meiosis I leads to a gamete with copies of both parental chromosomes.

The uninvolved arm of the chromosome is missing. Certain isochromosomes are found as recurring abnormalities associated with specific tumors. For example, i(12p) is frequently found in testicular germ cell tumors in young males where its presence appears to confer increased invasive potential *(58,59)*. In childhood medulloblastomas, i(17q) is a common finding, and the association with tumorigenesis may be caused by loss of 17p (which contains the *TP53* tumor suppressor gene) *(60)*. Isochromosome 17q is also commonly present in blast crisis of chronic myelogenous leukemia *(61)*.

Ring Chromosomes

A ring chromosome can be formed by two breaks within a chromosome, followed by joining of the free ends of the central portion of the chromosome. Ring chromosomes are therefore associated with loss of genetic information from the termini of the involved

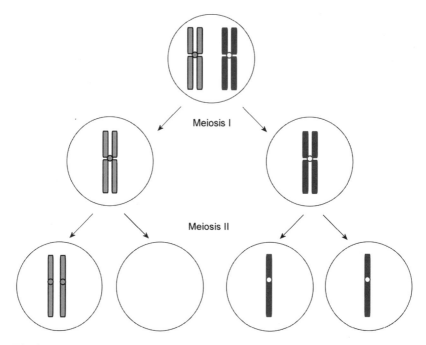

Fig. 9. Nondisjunction occurring during meiosis II. Following nondisjunction, the resulting gametes may contain two copies of a chromosome or may be missing a chromosome. If a gamete contains two copies of a chromosome, these are both copies of a single parental chromosome.

chromosome. If a normal copy of the chromosome is present, then the cell is monosomic for the regions that are lost in the ring. If the ring chromosome is supernumerary to two normal chromosomes, then the cell is trisomic for the genetic material in the ring. The clinical features of constitutional ring chromosomes therefore depend on the chromosome involved and on the number of normal copies of that chromosome that are also present.

Ring chromosomes are seen as a frequent abnormality in some types of cancer. Dermatofibrosarcoma protuberans is associated with translocations or supernumerary ring chromosomes containing portions of chromosome 17 or 22 in 80% of cases *(62)*. These result in fusion of the collagen type I α 1 gene *(COLIA1)* on chromosome 17 with the platelet-derived growth factor B-chain gene *(PDGFB)* on chromosome 22 *(63)*. The result appears to be overexpression of PDGF, a mitogenic signaling molecule.

Chromosomal Abnormalities in Molar Pregnancy

Partial and complete hydatidiform moles occur with a frequency of approximately 1 in 1500 pregnancies in the United States; they are more common (1 in 250 pregnancies) in Asia. These moles have a risk of becoming invasive tumors.

A complete hydatidiform mole (CHM) consists of hyperplastic trophoblastic tissue without evidence of fetal development. The chromosomes in a CHM are of paternal origin. This entity can arise by fertilization of an enucleate (empty) ovum in one of two scenarios. The ovum may be fertilized with a single sperm, the chromosomes then undergoing duplication to form a diploid cell that forms trophoblastic tissue. In this scenario, the sperm must carry the X chromosome in order for the resulting cell to be viable. Alternatively, an enucleate ovum is fertilized by two sperm (X/X or X/Y), giving rise to a diploid cell that forms trophoblastic tissues.

A partial hydatidiform mole (PHM) is produced when two sperm fertilize a normal ovum. PHMs can also arise from fertilization of an ovum by a single sperm that subsequently undergoes chromosomal duplication. In either case, the resulting cell is triploid (i.e., the karyotype is 69, XXX or 69, XYY). In this situation, both trophoblastic and fetal tissues can develop, and very rarely a fetus with triploidy can survive to term, although the postnatal life expectancy is extremely short. Approximately 16% of spontaneous abortions show triploidy.

REFERENCES

1. Cotton RG, Scriver CR. Proof of "disease causing" mutation. Hum Mutat 1998;12:1–3.
2. Schuffenecker I, Ginet N, Goldgar D, et al. Prevalence and parental origin of de novo RET mutations in multiple endocrine neoplasia type 2A and familial medullary thyroid carcinoma. Le Groupe d'Etude des Tumeurs a Calcitonine. Am J Hum Genet 1997;60:233–7.
3. Carlson KM, Bracamontes J, Jackson CE, et al. Parent-of-origin effects in multiple endocrine neoplasia type 2B. Am J Hum Genet 1994;55:1076–82.
4. Bellus GA, Hefferon TW, Ortiz de Luna RI, et al. Achondroplasia is defined by recurrent G380R mutations of FGFR3. Am J Hum Genet 1995;56:368–73.
5. Becker J, Schwaab R, Moller-Taube A, et al. Characterization of the factor VIII defect in 147 patients with sporadic hemophilia A: family studies indicate a mutation type-dependent sex ratio of mutation frequencies. Am J Hum Genet 1996;58:657–70.
6. Eggermann T, Nothen MM, Eiben B, et al. Trisomy of human chromosome 18: molecular studies on parental origin and cell stage of nondisjunction. Hum Genet 1996;97:218–23.

7. Bugge M, Collins A, Petersen MB, et al. Non-disjunction of chromosome 18. Hum Mol Genet 1998;7:661–9.

8. Jacobs PA, Hassold TJ, Whittington E, et al. Klinefelter's syndrome: an analysis of the origin of the additional sex chromosome using molecular probes. Ann Hum Genet 1988;52:93–109.

9. Crow JF. The origins, patterns and implications of human spontaneous mutation. Nat Rev Genet 2000;1:40–7.

10. Risch N, Reich EW, Wishnick MM, McCarthy JG. Spontaneous mutation and parental age in humans. Am J Hum Genet 1987;41:218–48.

11. Rolf C, Nieschlag E. Reproductive functions, fertility and genetic risks of ageing men. Exp Clin Endocrinol Diabetes 2001;109:68–74.

12. Nolin SL, Lewis FA 3rd, Ye LL, et al. Familial transmission of the FMR1 CGG repeat. Am J Hum Genet 1996;59:1252–61.

12a. Zuhlke C, Riess O, Bockel B, Lange H, Thies U: Mitotic stability and meiotic variability of the (CAG)n repeat in the Huntington disease gene. Hum Mol Genet 1993;2:2063–7.

13. Martin JB. Molecular basis of the neurodegenerative disorders. N Engl J Med 1999;340:1970–80.

14. Farrer LA, Cupples LA, Haines JL, et al. Effects of age, sex, and ethnicity on the association between apolipoprotein E genotype and Alzheimer disease. A meta-analysis. APOE and Alzheimer Disease Meta Analysis Consortium. JAMA 1997;278:1349–56.

15. Holmes C. Genotype and phenotype in Alzheimer's disease. Br J Psychiatry 2002;180:131–4.

16. Meyer MR, Tschanz JT, Norton MC, et al. APOE genotype predicts when—not whether—one is predisposed to develop Alzheimer disease. Nat Genet 1998;19:321–2.

17. Edery P, Lyonnet S, Mulligan LM, et al. Mutations of the RET proto-oncogene in Hirschsprung's disease. Nature 1994;367:378–80.

18. Shalev A. Discovery of a lipodystrophy gene: one answer, one hundred questions. Eur J Endocrinol 2000;143:565–7.

19. De Sandre-Giovannoli A, Chaouch M, Kozlov S, et al. Homozygous defects in LMNA, encoding lamin A/C nuclear-envelope proteins, cause autosomal recessive axonal neuropathy in human (Charcot-Marie-Tooth disorder type 2) and mouse. Am J Hum Genet 2002;70:726–36.

20. Harbour JW. Molecular basis of low-penetrance retinoblastoma. Arch Ophthalmol 2001;119:1699–704.

21. Easton DF, Steele L, Fields P, et al. Cancer risks in two large breast cancer families linked to BRCA2 on chromosome 13q12–13. Am J Hum Genet 1997;61:120–8.

22. Ford D, Easton DF, Stratton M, et al. Genetic heterogeneity and penetrance analysis of the BRCA1 and BRCA2 genes in breast cancer families. The Breast Cancer Linkage Consortium. Am J Hum Genet 1998;62:676–89.

23. Witchel SF, Bhamidipati DK, Hoffman EP, Cohen JB. Phenotypic heterogeneity associated with the splicing mutation in congenital adrenal hyperplasia due to 21-hydroxylase deficiency. J Clin Endocrinol Metab 1996;81:4081–8.

24. Salvatore F, Scudiero O, Castaldo G. Genotype-phenotype correlation in cystic fibrosis: the role of modifier genes. Am J Med Genet 2002;111:88–95.

25. Scriver CR, Waters PJ. Monogenic traits are not simple: lessons from phenylketonuria. Trends Genet 1999;15:267–72.

26. Dork T, Wulbrand U, Richter T, et al. Cystic fibrosis with three mutations in the cystic fibrosis transmembrane conductance regulator gene. Hum Genet 1991;87:441–6.
27. Cooper DN, Youssoufian H. The CpG dinucleotide and human genetic disease. Hum Genet 1988;78:151–5.
28. Myerowitz R, Hogikyan ND. A deletion involving Alu sequences in the beta-hexosaminidase alpha-chain gene of French Canadians with Tay-Sachs disease. J Biol Chem 1987;262:15396–9.
29. Aalto-Setala K, Helve E, Kovanen PT, Kontula K. Finnish type of low density lipoprotein receptor gene mutation (FH- Helsinki) deletes exons encoding the carboxy-terminal part of the receptor and creates an internalization-defective phenotype. J Clin Invest 1989;84:499–505.
30. White PC, Speiser PW. Congenital adrenal hyperplasia due to 21-hydroxylase deficiency. Endocr Rev 2000;21:245–91.
31. Reeves ME, DeMatteo RP. Genes and viruses in hepatobiliary neoplasia. Semin Surg Oncol 2000;19:84–93.
32. Marvit J, DiLella AG, Brayton K, Ledley FD, Robson KJ, Woo SL. GT to AT transition at a splice donor site causes skipping of the preceding exon in phenylketonuria. Nucleic Acids Res 1987;15:5613–28.
33. Nemes JP, Benzow KA, Moseley ML, Ranum LP, Koob MD. The SCA8 transcript is an antisense RNA to a brain-specific transcript encoding a novel actin-binding protein (KLHL1). Hum Mol Genet 2000;9:1543–51.
34. Cummings CJ, Zoghbi HY. Fourteen and counting: unraveling trinucleotide repeat diseases. Hum Mol Genet 2000;9:909–16.
35. Liquori CL, Ricker K, Moseley ML, et al. Myotonic dystrophy type 2 caused by a CCTG expansion in intron 1 of ZNF9. Science 2001;293:864–7.
36. Matsuura T, Yamagata T, Burgess DL, et al. Large expansion of the ATTCT pentanucleotide repeat in spinocerebellar ataxia type 10. Nat Genet 2000;26:191–4.
37. Miki Y, Swensen J, Shattuck-Eidens D, et al. A strong candidate for the breast and ovarian cancer susceptibility gene BRCA1. Science 1994;266:66–71.
38. Gayther SA, Harrington P, Russell P, Kharkevich G, Garkavtseva RF, Ponder BA. Frequently occurring germ-line mutations of the BRCA1 gene in ovarian cancer families from Russia. Am J Hum Genet 1997;60:1239–42.
39. Gorski B, Byrski T, Huzarski T, et al. Founder mutations in the BRCA1 gene in Polish families with breast-ovarian cancer. Am J Hum Genet 2000;66:1963–8.
40. Fodor FH, Weston A, Bleiweiss IJ, et al. Frequency and carrier risk associated with common BRCA1 and BRCA2 mutations in Ashkenazi Jewish breast cancer patients. Am J Hum Genet 1998;63:45–51.
41. Struewing JP, Hartge P, Wacholder S, et al. The risk of cancer associated with specific mutations of BRCA1 and BRCA2 among Ashkenazi Jews. N Engl J Med 1997;336:1401–8.
42. Myerowitz R, Costigan FC. The major defect in Ashkenazi Jews with Tay-Sachs disease is an insertion in the gene for the alpha-chain of beta-hexosaminidase. J Biol Chem 1988;263:18587–9.
43. Kazazian HH Jr, Wong C, Youssoufian H, Scott AF, Phillips DG, Antonarakis SE. Haemophilia A resulting from de novo insertion of L1 sequences represents a novel mechanism for mutation in man. Nature 1988;332:164–6.
44. Wallace MR, Andersen LB, Saulino AM, Gregory PE, Glover TW, Collins FS. A de novo Alu insertion results in neurofibromatosis type 1. Nature 1991;353:864–6.
45. Deininger PL, Batzer MA. Alu repeats and human disease. Mol Genet Metab 1999;67:183–93.

46. Rigat B, Hubert C, Alhenc-Gelas F, Cambien F, Corvol P, Soubrier F. An insertion/deletion polymorphism in the angiotensin I-converting enzyme gene accounting for half the variance of serum enzyme levels. J Clin Invest 1990;86:1343–6.
47. Tukey RH, Strassburg CP. Human UDP-glucuronosyltransferases: metabolism, expression, and disease. Annu Rev Pharmacol Toxicol 2000;40:581–616.
48. Morris CA, Mervis CB. Williams syndrome and related disorders. Annu Rev Genomics Hum Genet 2000;1:461–84.
49. Bown N. Neuroblastoma tumour genetics: clinical and biological aspects. J Clin Pathol 2001;54:897–910.
50. Maris JM, Matthay KK. Molecular biology of neuroblastoma. J Clin Oncol 1999;17:2264–79.
51. Leyland-Jones B. Trastuzumab: hopes and realities. Lancet Oncol 2002;3:137–44.
52. Anonymous. Clinical laboratory assays for HER-2/neu amplification and overexpression: quality assurance, standardization, and proficiency testing. Arch Pathol Lab Med 2002;126:803–8.
53. Harris NL, Jaffe ES, Diebold J, et al. The World Health Organization classification of neoplastic diseases of the hematopoietic and lymphoid tissues. Report of the Clinical Advisory Committee meeting, Airlie House, Virginia, November, 1997. Ann Oncol 1999;10:1419–32.
54. Liu PP, Hajra A, Wijmenga C, Collins FS. Molecular pathogenesis of the chromosome 16 inversion in the M4Eo subtype of acute myeloid leukemia. Blood 1995;85:2289–302.
55. Speck NA, Gilliland DG. Core-binding factors in haematopoiesis and leukaemia. Nat Rev Cancer 2002;2:502–13.
56. Lakich D, Kazazian HH Jr, Antonarakis SE, Gitschier J. Inversions disrupting the factor VIII gene are a common cause of severe haemophilia A. Nat Genet 1993;5:236–41.
57. Bowen DJ. Haemophilia A and haemophilia B: molecular insights. Mol Pathol 2002;55:1–18.
58. Murty VV, Chaganti RS. A genetic perspective of male germ cell tumors. Semin Oncol 1998;25:133–44.
59. Rosenberg C, Van Gurp RJ, Geelen E, Oosterhuis JW, Looijenga LH. Overrepresentation of the short arm of chromosome 12 is related to invasive growth of human testicular seminomas and nonseminomas. Oncogene 2000;19:5858–62.
60. Gilbertson R, Wickramasinghe C, Hernan R, et al. Clinical and molecular stratification of disease risk in medulloblastoma. Br J Cancer 2001;85:705–12.
61. Hernandez-Boluda JC, Cervantes F, Costa D, Carrio A, Montserrat E. Blast crisis of Ph-positive chronic myeloid leukemia with isochromosome 17q: report of 12 cases and review of the literature. Leuk Lymphoma 2000;38:83–90.
62. Naeem R, Lux ML, Huang SF, Naber SP, Corson JM, Fletcher JA. Ring chromosomes in dermatofibrosarcoma protuberans are composed of interspersed sequences from chromosomes 17 and 22. Am J Pathol 1995;147:1553–8.
63. Simon MP, Pedeutour F, Sirvent N, et al. Deregulation of the platelet-derived growth factor B-chain gene via fusion with collagen gene COL1A1 in dermatofibrosarcoma protuberans and giant-cell fibroblastoma. Nat Genet 1997;15:95–8.

4   Methods in Molecular Pathology

SOURCES OF NUCLEIC ACIDS

All nucleated cells contain DNA and RNA. Common sources of DNA obtained for clinical use include blood, bone marrow, and tissue samples such as biopsies and tissues removed during surgical resections. Buccal scrapings and hair roots may also be used. In forensic applications, semen and vaginal fluids are common sources of DNA.

Clinical specimens for DNA extraction from blood and bone marrow are normally collected in tubes containing anticoagulants such as ethylenediaminetetra-acetic acid (EDTA) or citrate. Tissue samples should generally be transported in saline to the laboratory and extracted without delay or stored frozen until processed. Tissues for nucleic acid extraction should not be placed in formalin or other fixatives because these will make subsequent extraction more difficult. If RNA is to be purified, extraction should be performed immediately, or the tissue should be frozen in liquid nitrogen to preserve RNA, which is highly labile.

It is possible to extract DNA from formalin-fixed, paraffin-embedded tissues. This is quite useful for analysis of stored samples in archival material. Before nucleic acids can be extracted, the paraffin must be removed and the tissues treated with proteinase to break down the protein cross links formed during formalin fixation. The quality of these preparations is variable and depends on the age of the tissue and the length of time it was exposed to formalin. Although DNA obtained from fixed tissues is usually unsuitable for Southern analysis because of degradation, it is often possible to amplify this DNA by techniques such as polymerase chain reaction. RNA isolations from tissues fixed in formalin, although they have been reported, are usually much less successful. RNase activity in tissues is often substantial, and the delay as formalin penetrates tissues often allows for significant degradation of RNA before RNases

From: *Principles of Molecular Pathology*
Edited by: A. A. Killeen © Humana Press Inc., Totowa, NJ

are inactivated. If DNA is stored under appropriate conditions, it is stable for many years.

EXTRACTION TECHNIQUES

Extraction of DNA and RNA involves several steps including lysis of cells, removal of proteins and other cellular components, and purification of the nucleic acids. Because of the ubiquitous presence of nucleases, particularly RNases, some precautions are necessary to minimize degradation of DNA and RNA during extraction. These include the use of EDTA, which chelates Mg^{2+}, an essential cofactor for many DNases, and guanidine isothiocyanate, which inactivates RNase. Solutions used for RNA extraction are usually made with water that has been treated with diethyl pyrocarbonate (DEPC), which also destroys RNases.

Protein removal can be accomplished either by extraction with organic solvents, such as phenol and chloroform, or by selective precipitation of proteins with high concentrations of salt. The latter method is often preferred because of the toxicity and waste disposal costs associated with the use of organic solvents.

Having removed contaminating proteins, nucleic acids can be precipitated from solution using high concentrations of alcohols such as ethanol or isopropanol. The precipitate is usually washed with 70% ethanol, and the nucleic acid is then resuspended in a buffer. Specific protocols for extraction of nucleic acid from a variety of sources are described in ref. *1*.

MEASUREMENT OF NUCLEIC ACID CONCENTRATION

The bases in nucleic acids absorb light in the ultraviolet portion of the spectrum with an absorption maximum at approx 260 nm. This property is used to quantify nucleic acids in solution by spectrophotometry. Contaminating proteins can be detected by measuring the absorption at 280 nm, the wavelength at which the aromatic amino acid residues phenylalanine, tyrosine, and tryptophan absorb strongly. The ratio of absorption at 260 nm/280 nm is commonly used to determine the purity of DNA and RNA preparations. Ratios of at least 1.8 indicate minimal contamination by proteins.

Other general methods for nucleic acid quantification exist *(2)*. Several fluorescent dyes are available that bind DNA with a result-

ing increase in their fluorescence efficiency. These include SYBR®
Green I and ethidium bromide. The latter is commonly used to stain
nucleic acids that have been separated by electrophoresis in agarose
or polyacrylamide gels. Some colorimetric methods utilize dyes that
undergo changes in absorption in the visible wavelengths on binding of nucleic acids *(3)*.

INTEGRITY OF NUCLEIC ACID PREPARATIONS

Nucleic acids can undergo degradation during their isolation or
storage, resulting in the formation of smaller fragments. This can be
caused by nuclease action or by mechanical shearing and affects the
quality of the subsequent analysis to an extent that depends on the
type of technique to be used. For example, extremely high molecular weight DNA is critical for pulsed-field gel electrophoresis,
whereas conventional Southern analysis requires reasonably high
molecular weight DNA for optimal results. Although methods that
amplify nucleic acids, such as polymerase chain reaction, are less
susceptible to template degradation, even these can be adversely
affected by fragmentation of the template.

The presence of degraded DNA or RNA can be identified by
electrophoretic separation followed by ethidium bromide staining of
an aliquot of the purified sample. Degraded DNA appears as a
smear of fragments of differing molecular weights, whereas intact
DNA appears as a single high molecular weight band. Intact RNA
isolated from eukaryotic cells shows the presence of the 28S and
18S ribosomal subunits.

SOUTHERN BLOTTING

Southern blotting takes its name from Dr. E.M. Southern, who
described it in 1975 *(4)*. This technique involves a series of steps
including restriction (cutting) of genomic DNA with restriction
enzymes, separation of the restricted fragments by electrophoresis,
transfer of the fragments to a solid membrane, and detection of fragments of interest. These steps are outlined in Figs. 1 and 2.

Restriction of DNA

Restriction refers to cutting of DNA by restriction enzymes.
These enzymes are isolated from bacteria and are usually named

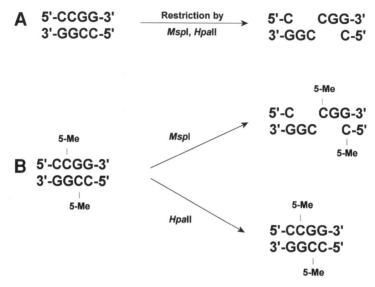

Fig. 1. Restriction enzyme cutting. (**A**) Restriction by the enzymes *Msp*I and *Hpa*II. These cut DNA within the sequence CCGG. (**B**) The different effects of these enzymes on a methylated restriction site. *Msp*I cuts, but *Hpa*II does not, because of methylation of the site.

according to the bacterial species from which they are obtained. For example, the first restriction enzyme isolated from *Escherichia coli* is *Eco*RI. These enzymes cut DNA at specific sequences known as restriction sites. These sites are short—typically 4–8 bp in length— and are frequently palindromes, which means that the sequence on one strand is identical to that on the complementary strand when read in the same orientation (e.g., 5′→3′). Numerous restriction enzymes are available from commercial suppliers. In the case of most restriction enzymes, DNA cutting takes place within the recognition sequence, but some enzymes cut at a nearby position. Examples of restriction enzymes and their recognition sequences are shown in Table 1. A comprehensive database of restriction enzymes, REBASE, is maintained at http://rebase.neb.com *(5)*

Note that both *Hpa*II and *Msp*I recognize the same sequence and cut at the same position (Fig. 1). Different enzymes that cut at the same sequence are known as isoschizomers. There are many examples of enzymes isolated from different species of bacteria that share the same recognition and cutting sites. Although they both recognize the same sequence, *Hpa*II and *Msp*I differ with respect to the effect

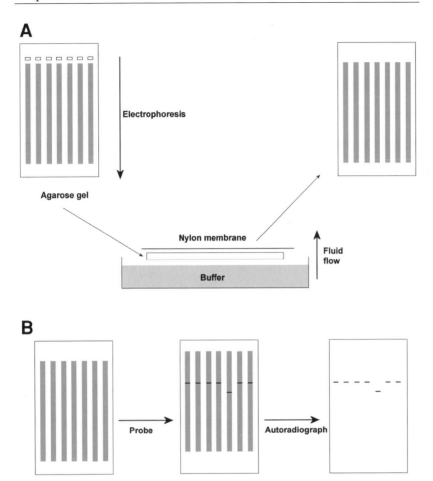

Fig. 2. Illustration of Southern blot principle. **(A)** Restricted DNA is loaded into wells of a suitable gel matrix (e.g., agarose or polyacrylamide) and electrophoresed. This separates DNA molecules on the basis of size. Following electrophoresis, a nylon membrane is placed over the gel in a apparatus that allows fluid to flow through the gel, moving DNA fragments onto the membrane, where they lodge. The membrane now has the DNA fragments arranged in the same respective locations as in the gel. **(B)** A labeled probe is applied that hybridizes to its complementary sequences on the membrane. After washing to remove nonspecifically bound probe, the membrane is exposed to X-ray film to produce an autoradiograph.

Table 1
Examples of Restriction Enzymes

Enzyme	Recognition sequence (5′-3′)[a]	Bacterium
DdeI	C^TNAG	Desulfovibrio desulfuricans
EcoRI	G^AATTC	Escherichia coli
HpaII	C^CGG	Haemophilus parainfluenzae
MspI	C^CGG	Moraxella species
TaqI	T^CGA	Thermus aquaticus

[a] The cutting position for each enzyme is indicated by a caret. In the recognition sequence for DdeI, the letter N means any of the four bases.

of methylation of DNA. *HpaII* is a methylation-sensitive enzyme and will not cut if the cytosine immediately 5′ to the guanine in the recognition sequence is methylated. *MspI* will cut regardless of whether or not the cytosine is methylated. It is possible to determine whether a given piece of DNA is methylated by comparing the fragments produced by restricting the DNA with a methylation-insensitive enzyme and a methylation-sensitive isoschizomer. To use this approach, the region of DNA of interest must contain the recognition site for the restriction enzymes.

When DNA from a human cell is restricted, a very large number of fragments is produced. The number and sizes of these fragments are determined by the distance between restriction sites in genomic DNA. Some restriction sites are more closely spaced, and restriction at these sites results in relatively short fragments of DNA. In other parts of the genome, the distance between restriction sites is greater. The fragments produced by cutting at these sites are longer.

The number of restriction sites in human genomic DNA for a restriction enzyme depends on several factors. Among these are the length of the restriction recognition sequence—8 bp sequences are found less commonly than 4 bp sequences, for example. Recognition sites that include the dinucleotide CG (such as those of *TaqI*, *MspI*, and *HpaII*) are found less commonly because of the low frequency of this particular dinucleotide relative to that of other dinucleotides. This effect is a result of the tendency of CG dinucleotides to undergo mutation to TG (*see* Chap. 3). Conversely, the dinucleotide TG is found more frequently than would be expected by chance. In addition, restriction enzymes that include CG dinu-cleotides in their recognition sequences are more likely to give rise to polymorphic patterns when samples from different individuals are restricted than when restriction enzymes that do not include CG in their recognition sequences are used *(6)*.

Gel Electrophoresis of Restricted DNA

DNA molecules can be size separated by electrophoresis in a suitable gel matrix, such as agarose or polyacrylamide. At mildly alkaline pH, DNA molecules are negatively charged because of the presence of ionized phosphate groups along the backbone of both strands of DNA. When they are electrophoresed, DNA molecules migrate toward the positive electrode (anode). Smaller molecules can move more rapidly under these conditions than can larger mole-cules, and so a separation based on size is achieved by electrophore-sis in a gel.

DNA molecules in gels may be visualized by staining with dyes such as ethidium bromide. This dye fluoresces when exposed to ultraviolet light. On binding to DNA, it intercalates between the stacked bases and shows an increase in its relative fluorescence quantum efficiency. Because the length of a DNA molecule deter-mines the number of intercalation sites for ethidium bromide, larger molecules generally fluoresce more intensely.

Transfer to a Solid Support

When electrophoresis is complete, the DNA fragments have been size-separated in the gel. Gels are delicate and difficult to manipu-late without causing breakage. Transferring DNA from a gel to a solid material such as a membrane enables subsequent steps to be performed on a much more robust support. Before transfer, the gel is treated with a dilute solution of hydrochloric acid to hydrolyze the larger DNA fragments so that they can be easily transferred by capillary action of fluid out of the gel and onto the membrane. After treatment with acid, the gel is treated with alkali, which causes denaturation of DNA and formation of single strands. Finally, the transfer step is performed in which capillary flow of buffer washes the DNA fragments from the gel onto the membrane. Most mem-branes in contemporary use are composed of sheets of positively charged nylon. DNA can bind this by electrostatic interactions. The position of DNA fragments on the membrane is a replica of their relative positions in the gel.

Probes and Probing

Essentially all techniques that are involved in recognition of specific DNA sequences exploit the ability of a single-stranded DNA molecule to hybridize to its complementary sequence. In Southern blotting applications, the single-stranded DNA molecules are generally known as probes. A DNA probe is a fragment of DNA that is cloned by polymerase chain reaction or by insertion into a plasmid (a self-replicating DNA structure) and propagated in bacteria. Probes for known DNA sequences (e.g., a gene of interest) are used to identify the location of that sequence in a Southern blot. When a DNA probe is applied to a membrane containing restricted DNA, it will hybridize to its complementary sequence. It is essential that both the membrane-bound DNA and the probe be single stranded for hybridization to occur. As mentioned, the DNA on the membrane is made single stranded by treatment with alkali. The probe may be briefly boiled to denature it before it is applied to the membrane.

Hybridization of the probe to its complementary target is affected by several factors. The factor that is most easily controlled experimentally is the temperature of the hybridization solution—the hotter the temperature, the more specific is the hybridization; however, if the solution is too hot, the probe will not be able to bind to even a perfectly complementary sequence. If the hybridization solution is too cool, the probe can bind nonspecifically to other DNA fragments. The optimum temperature can be predicted from knowledge of the length and base content of the probe, but in practice it is often determined empirically. Other factors that influence the specificity of hybridization include the salt concentration (higher salt concentrations facilitate annealing of complementary DNA molecules by neutralizing the repulsive negative charges on phosphate groups). Denaturing agents such as formamide can be used to increase the specificity of hybridization. Hybridization can be accelerated by including very high molecular weight compounds such as polyethylene glycol (PEG) in the solution. PEG occupies a large fraction of the available solution volume, limiting the effective volume in which the probe is dissolved. The result is to increase the effective probe concentration and therefore the rate of the hybridization reaction.

Detection of Hybridization

To detect hybridization, it is customary to label the probe with a suitable reporter. ^{32}P, a radioactive isotope of phosphorous that is a commonly used reporter, can be incorporated into a probe giving rise to a radioactively labeled probe. Following hybridization with the probe, the membrane is washed to remove nonspecifically bound probe. The location of the restriction fragments to which the probe has hybridized can be determined by exposing X-ray film to the membrane. Various nonisotopic reporter systems, such as chemiluminescent reporters, are also available commercially.

Restriction Fragment Length Polymorphisms

If the restriction sites for the enzyme used to cut genomic DNA are polymorphic, the length of the fragment(s) carrying the gene of interest will vary between members of the population. Such variations are known as restriction fragment length polymorphisms (RFLPs). These polymorphisms are inherited as genetic traits and may provide useful markers for analyzing the inheritance of genetic traits within families (Fig. 3). RFLPs are also used in some applications for sample identification, e.g., in forensic analysis (*see* Chap. 10).

Applications of Southern Blotting

Southern blotting is used for several kinds of analysis. Changes in gene dosage (i.e., deletions or amplifications) can often be demonstrated by Southern blotting and appear as alterations in the intensity of bands on a Southern blot. Disease-causing mutations that alter restriction enzyme recognition sites may be detected by Southern blotting as variations in the length of restriction fragments generated from normal and mutated genes. RFLP markers used for linkage studies may be detected by Southern blotting. If a variable-number tandem repeat marker is flanked by restriction sites, cutting with the restriction enzyme generates fragments that vary in length from different chromosomes. This is used for sample identification, e.g., in forensic analysis (*see* Chap. 10). Finally, cutting of DNA with a methylation-sensitive enzyme can reveal regions of the genome that are methylated. This approach is used in, for example, identification of abnormal methylation of the *FRAXA* gene in patients with fragile X syndrome (*see* Chap. 5).

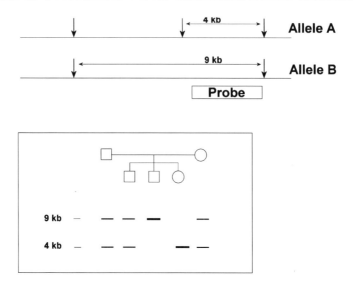

Fig. 3. Example of inheritance of restriction fragment length polymorphisms (RFLPs). Two alleles are shown that differ with respect to a restriction enzyme site (arrows). The probe used in the Southern blotting hybridizes to the region shown. Inheritance of these alleles in a family is shown in the box. Both parents are heterozygous for the A and B alleles. The children have inherited one allele from each parent. The second and third children are homozygous for the B and A alleles, respectively.

Northern Blotting

Northern blotting is similar in technique to Southern blotting, the major difference being that RNA rather than DNA is analyzed. In addition, RNA is not treated with restriction enzymes prior to electrophoresis. Northern analysis is commonly used to demonstrate the presence of particular gene transcripts in tissue extracts. Probe hybridization demonstrates the presence of a transcript in a semi-quantitative fashion. In addition, Northern analysis can be used to determine the size of an RNA transcript.

Pulsed-Field Gel Electrophoresis

DNA molecules that are larger than approx 30–50 kb cannot be efficiently separated using conventional gel electrophoresis because such large molecules move very slowly through a gel matrix under the influence of a constant, uniform electrical field, and separations tend to be poor. Pulsed-field gel electrophoresis (PFGE) is a modification in which the orientation of the electrical field is regularly alternated or pulsed. DNA molecules in such a field are forced to change direction regularly, which dramatically improves the separation of very large molecules. Various geometric arrangements of the electrodes have been used in PFGE *(7)*.

PFGE is used in Southern blot applications such as determining the gene dosage of the peripheral myelin protein 22 gene, *PMP22*. Duplications of a 1.5-MB segment of DNA including this gene are responsible for most cases of Charcot-Marie-Tooth disease (OMIM 118220), a neuromuscular disease associated with reduced nerve conduction velocities *(8)*. Deletions of the same gene cause hereditary neuropathy with liability to pressure palsies (OMIM 162500) *(9)*. PFGE is also used in clinical diagnostics to compare the genomes of micro-organisms for identification purposes, for example, in establishing the origin of outbreaks of infection *(10)*. The Centers for Disease Control and Prevention runs a program to make rapid PFGE available for investigation of outbreaks of infections by food-borne micro-organisms. This program is known as PulseNet (www.cdc.gov/pulsenet).

AMPLIFICATION TECHNIQUES

Amplification techniques are in wide use in clinical laboratories. By comparison with Southern blotting techniques, amplification methods are much faster, require less DNA, can be automated, and may be less expensive. Amplification techniques are broadly grouped into two categories: target amplification and signal amplification. Target amplification involves increasing the number of copies of a target DNA or RNA by in vitro synthesis of nucleic acids. The alternative approach to is to amplify a signal generated when the target DNA or RNA is present, without increasing the abundance of nucleic acid. Both target and signal amplification are commonly used in molecular diagnostics to detect and quantify specific nucleic acids. Both approaches can also be used to detect mutations in nucleic acids.

Target Amplification Techniques
POLYMERASE CHAIN REACTION

Polymerase chain reaction (PCR) was the first target amplification technique to be developed and was described by Kary Mullis, who won a Nobel prize for this work in 1993 *(11)*. It is one of the

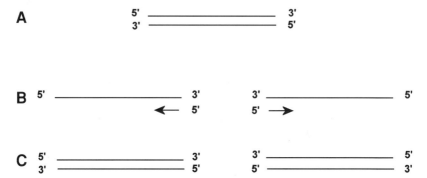

Fig. 4. Principle of PCR. (**A**) A DNA template molecule to be amplified. (**B**) The two strands of the template have been separated, and one member of a pair of primers is annealing to each strand. These flank the region to be amplified. The primers are extended by a DNA polymerase in the direction indicated by the arrows. (**C**) The first cycle of PCR has been completed. There are now two copies of the template present. Each of these can be copied during the next round of PCR, thereby doubling the number of copies of the template sequence. This process is repeated many times.

most widely used methods in clinical and research testing in molecular pathology.

The principle of PCR is shown in Fig. 4. The reaction mixture consists of the DNA to be amplified (known as the template), a pair of oligonucleotides that function as primers, the four deoxyribonucleotide triphosphates (dNTPs) that are the building blocks for DNA synthesis, a DNA polymerase, suitable concentrations of magnesium, and buffer. Other reagents such as betaine, dimethyl sulfoxide (DMSO), and 7-deaza-dGTP may be added to improve the amplification efficiency. Their use is largely empirical and they are not essential for all PCR amplifications. Several thermostable DNA polymerases are commonly used that are obtained from thermophilic micro-organisms. These enzymes are not inactivated by exposure to near-boiling temperatures. The oligonucleotide primers are typically 18–30 nucleotides in length, single-stranded DNA molecules that are custom synthesized. The sequence of each primer is complementary to one of the strands of the target DNA, and the pair of primers flank the region of template DNA to be amplified. The primers become incorporated into the final PCR product.

PCR begins by heating the reaction solution to 94°C. At this temperature the complementary strands in genomic DNA separate completely. The solution is then cooled to a suitable temperature, typically around 55°C, at which the primers anneal to their complementary sequences. The choice of annealing temperature is critical to the specificity of the reaction. If the temperature is too low, nonspecific hybridization of the primers results in undesired priming of genomic sequences other than the primary target of interest. If the temperature is too high, the primers cannot hybridize to the target. This effect of temperature parallels that described for probe hybridization in Southern blotting.

Following primer annealing, the DNA polymerase extends the primers by adding nucleotides in a 5′-3′ orientation. This synthesis of DNA is accelerated by increasing the temperature of the reaction to the optimum for DNA polymerase activity, which is 72°C for the commonly used DNA polymerase from *Thermus aquaticus* (*Taq* polymerase).

After sufficient time for extension has occurred, the solution is reheated to 94°C and the process is repeated. One cycle of amplification consists of heat denaturation of DNA, primer annealing, and primer extension by DNA polymerase. During each cycle, the number of copies of the target DNA sequence is, in theory, doubled. Thus, PCR amplification results in a geometric increase in the number of copies of the target DNA. The theoretical yield of PCR product is:

$$P = T(1 + E)^n$$

where P is the number of PCR molecules synthesized, T is the number of template molecules present at the beginning of the amplification, E is the amplification efficiency, and n is the number of cycles performed. The value of E can vary between 0 and 1. In the exponential phase of DNA synthesis, the value of E approaches the theoretical maximum, 1, in which case doubling of the number of copies of the target DNA occurs. In later cycles of PCR, the value of E decreases toward 0, resulting in a plateau of DNA synthesis (Fig. 5). After 30 cycles, the number of copies of the target DNA has been increased by about 1 billion-fold (10^9) and is now sufficiently abundant that the amplified DNA fragments, termed amplicons, are easily demonstrated in gels with simple staining techniques.

Amplicons have the same sequence as the target sequence in genomic DNA. If a mutation is present in the template DNA, it will also be present in the amplicons. Occasionally, the DNA poly-

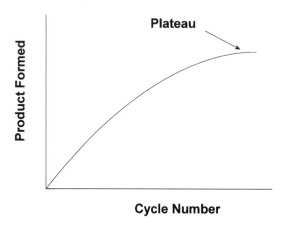

Fig. 5. Plateau effect in PCR. With increasing numbers of cycles, there is no longer a doubling of the amount of DNA synthesized during each cycle, and so a "plateau" is reached. Note that the amount of product formed is shown on a logarithmic scale.

merase incorporates an incorrect base as it copies the template. Such misincorporations are generally not of significance in diagnostic applications of PCR.

MULTIPLEX PCR

A PCR reaction can simultaneously amplify multiple targets if the appropriate primers are added to the reaction. A multiplex PCR reaction can be used to detect the presence of more than one target DNA. For example, simultaneous amplification of several exons in the Duchenne's muscular dystrophy gene on the X chromosome is used to detect the presence of exon deletions in affected males (Fig. 6).

QUANTIFICATION OF SPECIFIC NUCLEIC ACIDS BY PCR

PCR is commonly used to measure the concentration of specific nucleic acids such as HIV-1 and hepatitis C virus (HCV) for monitoring response to treatment. Although direct amplification by PCR with end-point detection is a reliable qualitative technique for detecting the presence of a nucleic acid in a sample, it is of little value for quantitative purposes *(2)*. The amount of PCR product generated depends not only on the initial concentration of target DNA, but also on the efficiency of each cycle of the reaction. Reliable measurement of the efficiency of the reaction is not a simple task. Moreover, in the case of RNA targets, an initial reverse tran-

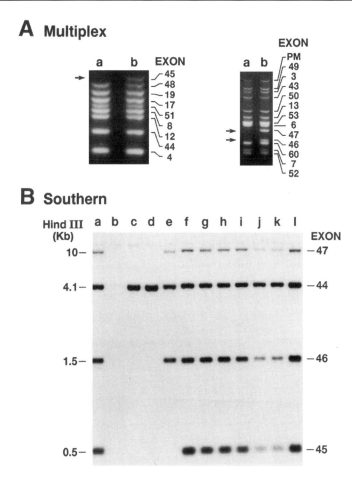

Fig. 6. Dystrophin DNA analysis for deletion and duplication mutations. (**A**) Multiplex PCR analysis. For the two multiplex PCR panels shown, lanes represent: (a) a patient deleted in exons 46 through 48, and (b) a normal male control. Arrows point to deleted exons. (**B**) Southern analysis of *Hind*III fragments using cDNA probe 47-4B. Patient samples are in lanes b–k; male control (a), male patients (b–f); female patients (g–k); female control (l). Patient b is deleted for exons 44–47; patients c and d are deleted for exons 45–47; patient e is deleted for exon 45 only; patient f, no deletion detected. Carrier analysis of female relatives (lanes j and k) of affected male in lane c identifies the familial deletion. (Reproduced with permission from ref. *32*.)

scription must be performed to generate a cDNA that can function as a template for the PCR reaction. Determining the efficiency of the reverse transcription step is also technically challenging.

These difficulties in quantification by PCR can be overcome by including in the reaction an internal control, the concentration of which is known. The internal control should participate in the reaction in the same manner as the target nucleic acid of interest, including both reverse transcription (if the target is a RNA molecule) and amplification during PCR cycles. By measuring the ratio of product formed from the target to that from the internal control, it is possible to determine the initial amount of target nucleic acid present in the sample. This forms the basis for widely used clinical laboratory methods for quantification of targets such as HIV-1 and HCV.

NUCLEIC ACID SEQUENCE-BASED AMPLIFICATION

Nucleic acid sequence-based amplification (NASBA) is an isothermal target amplification system *(12)*. The principles of NASBA are illustrated in Fig. 7. NASBA is particularly suitable for amplifying RNA targets, although the basic procedure can be adapted to amplification of DNA.

If RNA is the template, the NASBA reaction begins with annealing of a single-strand DNA oligonucleotide primer to the 3′ end of the RNA to be amplified. This primer has two separate regions: the 3′ end has a sequence that is complementary to the template RNA to which it hybridizes, and the 5′ end contains the binding sequence of T7 bacteriophage RNA polymerase. This primer is extended by the action of avian myeloblastosis virus reverse transcriptase (AMV-RT). This is a standard reverse transcription reaction that results in the formation of a double-stranded molecule consisting of the original RNA template hybridized to the newly synthesized complementary DNA (cDNA). The latter is complementary to the RNA except at its 5′ end, where it has the T7 RNA polymerase binding site.

Following reverse transcription, the original RNA template is selectively hydrolyzed by the action of RNase H, leaving just the cDNA molecule. A second oligonucleotide primer binds to the 3′ end of the cDNA and is extended by the action of AMV-RT. This reaction is possible because, in addition to being an RNA-dependent DNA polymerase (i.e., a reverse transcriptase), AMV-RT can also function as a DNA-dependent DNA polymerase. After extension of the second primer is complete, a double-stranded DNA molecule exists that has the T7 RNA polymerase binding sequence at one end. T7 RNA polymerase then binds at this recognition site and this begins the process of synthesis of a large number of RNA molecules by T7 RNA polymerase.

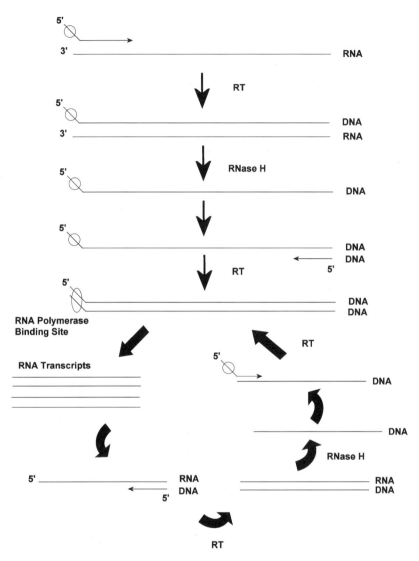

Fig. 7. Nucleic acid sequence-based amplification (NASBA) procedure. The principle of this reaction is described in the text. RT, reverse transcription.

Each of these newly synthesized RNA molecules can serve as the template for a reverse transcription reaction using the second primer. Once again, the RNA member of the resulting RNA/DNA duplex is hydrolyzed by RNase H. This allows the first primer to anneal, and this is extended by the action of AMV-RT, resulting in additional double-stranded DNA molecules containing the T7 RNA polymerase binding site. These molecules are used by T7 RNA polymerase to synthesize additional RNA molecules. This cyclical action results in geometric amplification of the number of copies of the RNA. The entire NASBA process is isothermal and takes place at 41°C.

Detection of the amplified RNA molecules can be achieved by a variety of methods. A common method involves the use of electrochemiluminescence (ECL). This method uses a paramagnetic particle to which a capture oligonucleotide is bound. This captures the amplified RNA molecule, which is then attached through the capture probe and the magnet to an electrode. An electrochemiluminescent probe containing ruthenium (Ru) is bound by hybridization at the free end of the amplified RNA molecule. When a voltage is applied to the electrode, oxidative reactions occur that result in light emission by the ruthenium reporter. This light is measured by a photomultiplier tube and is proportional to the amount of RNA present. In this way, NASBA is suitable for quantitative measurements of specific RNA molecules. Internal controls at different concentration levels can be coamplified in the reaction, allowing for generation of a standard curve. Detection of NASBA-amplified RNA molecules can also be performed by using molecular beacons on real-time PCR instruments.

NASBA is a proprietary technology belonging to bioMérieux (Marcy-Étoile, France). Several commercial assays for infectious agents that use the NASBA technology are available under the NucliSens brand. These include quantitative assays for HIV-1 and a qualitative assay to detect cytomegalovirus (CMV) replication.

TRANSCRIPTION-MEDIATED AMPLIFICATION

Transcription-mediated amplification (TMA) functions by a similar principle to NASBA *(13)*. The major difference is that in TMA the enzyme that is used for reverse transcription also has intrinsic RNase H activity. Therefore TMA uses two enzymes, whereas NASBA uses three enzymes. TMA is a proprietary process belonging to Gen-Probe (San Diego, CA). Commercial assays for several infectious agents and for *BCR-ABL* are available.

LIGASE CHAIN REACTION (LCR)

Ligase chain reaction (LCR) uses a thermostable DNA ligase to join two pairs of oligonucleotides that are brought together in a head-to-tail arrangement when they bind to their respective targets

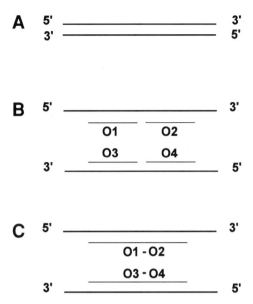

Fig. 8. Ligase chain reaction (LCR) principle. **(A)** The template DNA. **(B)** The two strands of the template have been separated by heating, and, following cooling to the appropriate annealing temperature, a pair of oligonucleotides binds to each template strand. **(C)** The bound oligonucleotides are ligated by a thermostable ligase. In the next round of LCR, the original template and these newly ligated oligonucleotides are separated and each can bind new oligonucleotides, which in turn are ligated. Repeating this process leads to an exponential increase in the number of ligated oligonucleotides.

(Fig. 8) *(14)*. An LCR amplification involves initial melting of DNA at 94°C, cooling to a suitable annealing temperature to allow the pairs of oligonucleotide probes to hybridize to their targets, and ligation of the adjacent oligonucleotides by the activity of the DNA ligase. Each of these newly ligated pairs of oligonucleotides is capable of hybridizing with their complementary oligonucleotides, leading to ligation of the latter in the next cycle of LCR.

LCR produces ligated oligonucleotides. As such, the technique is easily adapted to the qualitative detection of nucleic acids in clinical samples, e.g., micro-organisms. Detection of these can be accomplished by demonstrating the presence of ligated oligonucleotides following LCR. In a widely used commercial system for detecting Neisseria *gonorrhea* and Chlamydia *trachomatis,* the Abbott LCx, a pair of oligonucleotides is each labeled at their 5′ ends with different antigens. Detection of LCR products involves the use of a bound antibody to capture one of the oligonucleotides to a solid support. A second labeled antibody, directed against the antigen on the second oligonucleotide, is added to the reaction. The presence of the ligated oligonucleotides in the sample results in linking the labeled antibody to the solid phase. Detection of the labeled antibody linked to the solid phase indicates that the LCR reaction was successful, which indicates that the target DNA was present in the sample.

LCR is a proprietary technology of Abbott Laboratories (Chicago, IL) and is marketed as LCx. Several assays for infectious agents such as *N. gonorrhea* and *C. trachomatis* are commercially available.

STRAND DISPLACEMENT AMPLIFICATION

Strand displacement amplification (SDA) is an isothermal procedure for amplifying specific nucleic acids *(15)*. An SDA assay can be considered to occur in two phases. In the first phase, an amplifiable target is synthesized from template DNA contained in the sample. In the second phase, the synthesized target is exponentially amplified. The process begins with denaturation of the template DNA by heating to 94°C, and then cooling to allow two primers to anneal (Fig. 9) to either strand of the target. These primers are designated B1 (for bumper) and S1, which contains one strand of the recognition site for the restriction enzyme *Bso*BI. Only the 3' region of S1 is complementary to the target; the 5' region contains the recognition site. B1 anneals 5' to S1, which, in turn, anneals 5' to the region of the target to be amplified.

The reaction solution contains exo⁻ *Bst* DNA polymerase and the four nucleotides dATP, dGTP, dUTP (which can be incorporated in place of dTTP), and thio-dCTP. Extension of both primers occurs; however, the nascent strand that is primed by S1 is displaced as the B1 primer is extended. This displaced strand is shown as S1-ext in Fig. 9 (reactions labeled A). A parallel set of reactions occurs with the other template stand using primers B2 and S2, shown on the right side of Fig. 9. The displaced S1-primed strand then acts as a template that binds primers B2 and S2. Extension and displacement occurs, producing a strand that has *Bso*BI sites at each end (Fig. 9, reactions labeled B). Again, parallel reactions occur, as shown on the right side of Fig. 9. The strands that have a *Bso*BI recognition site at each end can bind the complementary primer (S1 on the left

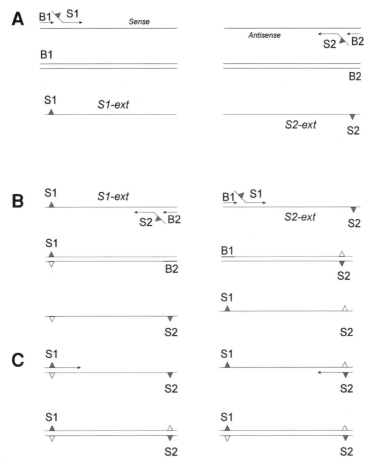

Fig. 9. (A–C) Strand displacement amplification (SDA). The initial reactions are shown. See text for details.

and S2 on the right in Fig. 9). Extension of these completes the first phase of SDA by forming an amplifiable target. It is important to note that strands that are extended incorporate thio-dCTP. The *Bso*BI recognition sites are described as hemiphosphorothioate, meaning that one strand has a thioate linkage between adjacent nucleosides, whereas the strand that was initiated with the comple-mentary primer (S1 or S2) contains a normal phosphate linkage at this position.

The second phase of SDA begins with restriction by *Bso*BI (Fig. 10). This enzyme recognizes the hemiphosphorothioate recognition

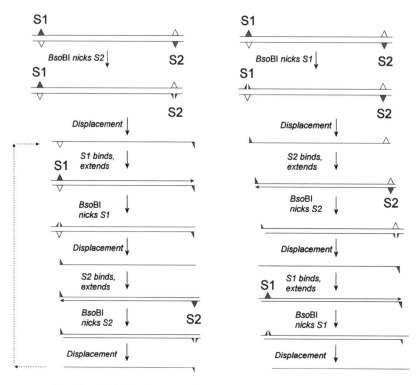

Fig. 10. SDA. The later reactions are shown. See text for details.

site but only cuts the strand containing the phosphate linkage, thereby generating a single-stranded nick. Again, exo⁻ *Bst* polymerase extends from the nicked site and displaces the existing strand. The displaced strand can bind the complementary primer (either S1 or S2), which is then extended by the polymerase. In addition, the recessed 3′ ends that are formed by primer binding are filled in by the action of the polymerase, thereby creating the hemiphosphorothioate recognition site. Nicking of the newly synthesized strand again results in extension from the nicked site and strand displacement. This process continues in an exponential reaction, leading to amplification of the target produced at the end of the first phase of SDA.

In a commercial implementation of the SDA assay (the BDProbeTecET, Becton Dickinson), detection of the amplified DNA is achieved using fluorescence resonance energy transfer (FRET) technology. A single-stranded DNA detection probe containing a stem-loop structure approximates bound fluorescein and rhodamine molecules so that the energy of excited fluorescein is transferred to rhodamine, thereby minimizing fluorescent light emission. The 3' end of the probe is complementary to a displaced strand from the exponential amplification phase from the SDA reaction. Extension and displacement of the probe occur, as shown in Fig. 10. Binding and extension of the downstream primer, S2, have two effects. First, the fluorescein and rhodamine are physically separated as the stem-loop structure is converted to being a piece of a duplex DNA molecule. Second, the *Bso*B1 site is formed and cut by the enzyme. This liberates a small DNA molecule containing the fluorescein, which can fluoresce because it is no longer adjacent to rhodamine. Monitoring of the fluorescence readings during the reaction allows for detection and quantification of the amount of target DNA present in the sample.

TARGET AMPLIFICATION AND CONTAMINATION

In general, a disadvantage of target amplification methods is that they are prone to contamination of subsequent samples by the products of an earlier reaction. For example, opening a reaction tube in which PCR has been performed can lead to formation of an aerosol that contains large numbers of amplicons. Each amplicon is capable of being reamplified and giving a positive signal in a subsequent PCR analysis. Extreme care must therefore be taken in the laboratory to minimize the risk of contamination of samples by the products of prior target amplification reactions.

Signal Amplification Techniques

BRANCH DNA

Branch DNA (bDNA) analysis is a quantitative technique that is used primarily to quantify levels of certain viruses, such as HIV-1 and HCV, in biological samples. The principle of a bDNA assay is shown in Fig. 11. In this example, the target is an RNA virus molecule. The target RNA is liberated from the virus, and capture extender and label extender molecules are allowed to hybridize to the target. Capture extenders and label extenders are single-strand DNA oligonucleotides that have sequence complementarity to regions of the target RNA. The capture extenders also have a region that can hybridize to immobilized DNA oligonucleotides (capture probes) on the wall of a microtiter plate well. If the target RNA is present in

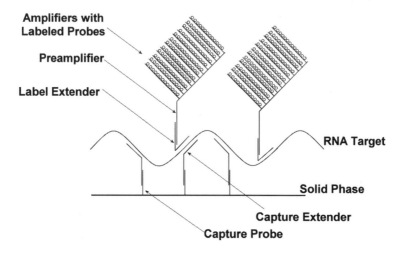

Fig. 11. Branch DNA (bDNA). See text for details.

the sample being tested, it will bind to the microtiter plate via the capture probes and the capture extenders. The label extenders can also hybridize to another set of oligonucleotides called preamplifier molecules. These, in turn, hybridize to amplifier molecules. The result of these steps is that multiple amplifier molecules are bound to the wall of the microtiter plate if the target RNA is present in the sample being analyzed.

Detection of the amplifier molecules is by the addition of oligonucleotide-linked alkaline phosphatase molecules, which bind to the amplifier molecules. Addition of a chemiluminescent substrate for alkaline phosphatase generates a chemiluminescent signal that is measured with a photodetector. The intensity of the emitted light is proportional to the number of target RNA molecules in the sample.

bDNA is a proprietary technology of Bayer. Commercially available assays include quantitative tests for HIV-1, HCV, and HBV.

HYBRID CAPTURE

The Hybrid Capture system utilizes a monoclonal antibody that selectively recognizes RNA/DNA duplexes. It has been developed to recognize targets such as human papillomavirus (HPV) DNA. The principle of the Hybrid Capture system is shown in Fig. 12. DNA isolated from the specimen (e.g., a cervical swab) is extracted, dena-

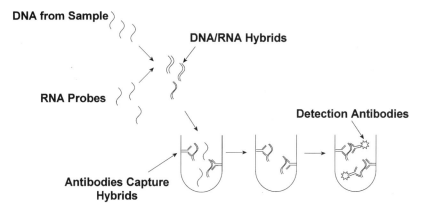

Fig. 12. Hybrid capture assay. See text for details.

tured, and then allowed to hybridize to a synthetic RNA probe that is complementary to the target DNA. Hybridization of the probe to the target leads to the formation of a RNA/DNA duplex that is captured by immobilized antibody to the wall of a microtiter plate. This antibody recognizes RNA/DNA duplexes, but not RNA or DNA single-stranded molecules or homoduplexes. A detection antibody, which also recognizes RNA/DNA duplexes and is conjugated to alkaline phosphatase, then binds to the immobilized duplex. Addition of a chemiluminescent substrate results in emission of light in proportion to the number of copies of the target present in the sample. Hybrid Capture is a proprietary technology of Digene (Gaithersburg, MD).

REVERSE TRANSCRIPTION

During gene transcription, the usual direction of flow of genetic information is from DNA to RNA. Several enzymes are known that can synthesize DNA using RNA as a template. Such enzymes are called reverse transcriptases, and the process they catalyze is called reverse transcription (RT) because the direction of information flow is the reverse of normal. Because many laboratory techniques, notably PCR and other cloning schemes, are designed to work with DNA as a template, it is a common prerequisite for such techniques to convert a RNA sequence to its cDNA sequence using RT. Examples of applications in which RT is performed include detection or quantification of gene expression, or of RNA viruses such as HIV-1 or HCV.

For gene expression studies, total cellular RNA can be used for RT, or the RNA can be enriched for messenger RNA (mRNA). The latter represents only a small fraction—about 2–5%—of the total cellular RNA but is composed of molecules that are often of the greatest biological interest. mRNA can be purified by passing total cellular RNA over a column containing bound oligo-dT (i.e., a DNA molecule composed of approx 18 dT residues). The poly-A tail present in most mRNAs binds specifically to the oligo-dT, while the other RNA molecules pass through the column. The enriched mRNA can then be eluted from the column.

In order to perform an RT reaction, a reverse transcriptase is needed. Enzymes in clinical laboratory use include Moloney murine leukemia virus (MMLV) and AMV. Other reagents required for a RT reaction are dNTPs, which serve as the building blocks for the complementary DNA molecule, a suitable buffer, the RNA template, and primers to serve as an anchor for new DNA synthesis.

RT PRIMERS

Three types of reverse transcription primer are commonly used:

1. Oligo-dT is used to prime synthesis of cDNA from mRNA selectively. Most mRNA molecules have a 3′ tail consisting of poly-A; oligo-dT can hybridize to this. This approach is used to prime synthesis of expressed genes.
2. Random hexamers. These are random sequences composed of six nucleotides that can be used to prime DNA synthesis at many positions in RNA. This results in synthesis of a large number of cDNA molecules. Each mRNA may be represented by multiple different cDNA molecules.
3. Target-specific primers. These are designed to hybridize selectively to an RNA molecule of interest. Under conditions of suitable stringency, only a particular RNA molecule will be reverse transcribed.

MUTATION DETECTION

Different mutation detection strategies are used to detect specific mutations or to find unknown mutations. The mutation that causes sickle cell anemia is the same in every patient with this disease; therefore a method to test for this specific mutation would be used to identify patients carrying the mutation. On the other hand, hundreds of different mutations in *BRCA1* and *BRCA2* have been associated with hereditary breast cancer. Detection of these in patient samples requires a different laboratory approach. Some approaches are suitable for both kinds of mutation detection. Methods in common use are described here, but it should be noted that there are many reported variations *(16)*.

Methods to Identify Known Mutations

METHODS BASED ON PCR

PCR is widely used in mutation detection because of its rapidity and simplicity. The region of the target gene containing the suspected mutation is amplified. Mutation detection can be accomplished in several ways including RFLP analysis, allele-specific amplification, and detection of mutations by allele-specific oligonucleotides.

PCR RESTRICTION FRAGMENT LENGTH POLYMORPHISM ANALYSIS

If a mutation alters a restriction enzyme site, then that mutation can be demonstrated by incubating the PCR product with the restriction enzyme and analyzing the sizes of the resulting fragments. This size determination can be accomplished by several methods. The most commonly used method in clinical laboratories is electrophoresis in a suitable gel, typically agarose or polyacrylamide, followed by staining of the gel with ethidium bromide and visualizing the fragments. DNA fragments of known size are run in parallel for size comparison. An example of this approach is shown in Fig. 13. Separations and sizing of fragments by capillary electrophoresis is also in reasonably common use. Other techniques in use include determination of fragment size by mass spectrometry.

PCR WITH MUTAGENIC PRIMERS

The PCR-restriction enzyme digestion approach is quite useful if a mutation creates or destroys a naturally occurring restriction enzyme site. It can also be used if a mutation does not alter such a site. By using mutagenic primers, it is often possible to create a restriction enzyme site in the PCR product depending on whether the template DNA contains the mutation of interest. The principle of this approach is shown in Fig. 14. One of the primers used for PCR contains one or more nucleotide substitutions toward its 3′ end, the end of the primer that is extended by the DNA polymerase during PCR. These substitutions are designed in such a way that the sequence of the PCR product contains (or doesn't contain) a restriction site depending on whether or not the patient sample contains

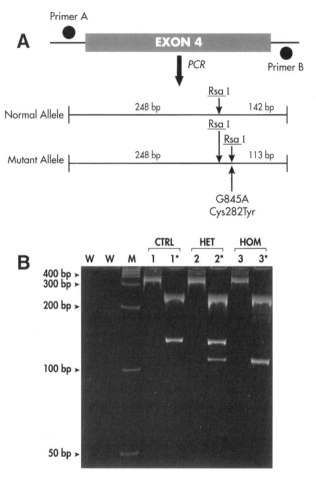

Fig. 13. PCR RFLP detection of Cys282Tyr in *HFE*. (**A**) Schematic of the 390-bp amplicon of *HFE* encompassing exon 4 and nucleotide 845 (cDNA sequence). Primers A and B are located in flanking intron sequences. The G845A mutation generates a new *Rsa*I recognition site, as shown in the mutant allele. (**B**) Photograph of ethidium bromide-stained 12.5% polyacrylamide gel demonstrating PCR RFLP analysis for Cys282Tyr in *HFE*. W denotes water (reagent) controls. M denotes molecular weight markers. Lanes 1, 2, and 3 show undigested 390-bp amplicons from wild-type (CTRL), heterozygous mutant (HET), and homozygous mutant (HOM) individuals. Lanes 1*, 2*, and 3* show *Rsa*I digestion products from the 390-bp amplicons shown in lanes 1, 2, and 3, respectively. *Rsa*I digestion of a wild-type allele yields fragments of 248 and 142 bp. *Rsa*I digestion of a mutant allele yields fragments of 248, 113, and 29 bp. (The 29-bp fragment is not seen.) (Reproduced with permission from ref. *1*).

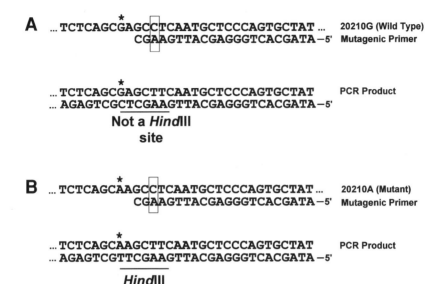

Fig. 14. Mutagenic primer usage to create a restriction site. (**A, B** The sequence of the prothrombin (factor II) gene is shown around the site of the G→A transition that is associated with increased thrombotic risk (indicated by an asterisk). This mutation does not alter a naturally occurring restriction enzyme recognition sequence. The sequence of a mutagenic primer for PCR is shown below the prothrombin gene sequence. This primer contains a mispaired base, indicated by a box. This nucleotide alteration becomes incorporated into PCR products with each cycle of PCR. At completion of PCR, the products amplified by the mutagenic primer contain a *Hind*III site (AAGCTT) if the 20210A mutation was present, but not if the original template did not contain this mutation. The second member of the pair of PCR primers is not shown in this illustration.

the mutation of interest. The mutagenic primer provides part of the restriction site; the patient's DNA template provides the remaining essential sequence to form the complete restriction site.

This approach has some limitations. Altering the sequence of a primer may alter its specificity for binding to the template DNA and therefore its ability to prime the target of interest efficiently or selectively. Following restriction, the size of the PCR product is reduced by approximately the length of the mutagenic primer, which is usually only about 18 or so nucleotides in length. Such a length change may be difficult to detect if it represents a minor alteration in the overall length of the PCR product. Finally, for cer-

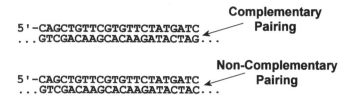

Fig. 15. Allele-specific amplification. In the upper part of the diagram the 3′ end of a primer forms a complementary base pair with a target DNA sequence. This primer can be extended during PCR. In the lower part of the diagram the 3′ end of a primer has a base pair mismatch with the target DNA sequence. This primer cannot be extended. Successful PCR amplification with the primer can therefore be used to detect the presence of one or other sequence in a DNA sample, in this case, the sequence in the upper part of the illustration. The second member of the pair of PCR primers is not shown in this illustration.

tain mutations, it may not be possible to design a mutagenic primer to create a restriction site.

ALLELE-SPECIFIC PCR AMPLIFICATION

Allele-specific amplification [also called the amplification refractory mutation system (ARMS)] is based on the inability of many DNA polymerases to extend a primer if the base at the 3′ end of the primer does not form a perfect match with the corresponding base in the DNA template (Fig. 15). Extension can take place only if a perfect match exists. If one primer is specific for a given mutation at its 3′ end, geometric amplification during PCR can occur only if the target DNA contains this mutation. In a typical allele-specific analysis, two PCR reactions are performed in parallel. One uses a primer that is specific for the mutation, and the other uses a primer specific for the corresponding wild-type allele. Both reactions also use a common second primer. Successful amplification of genomic DNA in only one sample indicates that the DNA is homozygous for that allele. Amplification in both reactions indicates heterozygosity for both wild-type and mutant alleles. Because absence of amplification of the target is a possible outcome, it is usual to coamplify a second, unrelated target using a second pair of primers in the same reaction. Amplification of this second target provides assurance that both amplifiable DNA and the PCR reagents were indeed present in the reaction and therefore that absence of amplification of the primary target is not caused by technical artifact.

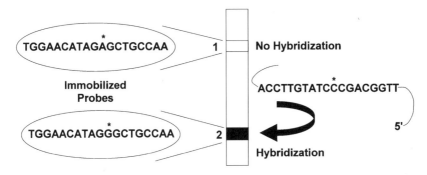

Fig. 16. Reverse allele-specific oligonucleotide (ASO) principle. Two oligonu-cleotides are immobilized on a solid phase. Under the right stringency conditions, the PCR product, shown on the right, can hybridize to the probe with which it has perfect sequence complementarity. Detection of hybridization can be achieved using various techniques such as labeling the PCR product with a radioactive iso-tope and performing autoradiography.

ALLELE-SPECIFIC OLIGONUCLEOTIDE PROBES

An allele-specific oligonucleotide (ASO) probe is used to detect the presence of mutations by specific hybridization of the probe to amplified DNA. In this technique, the gene of interest is amplified by PCR, denatured, and then applied to a membrane. Genomic DNA can also be used, but the large amounts of genomic DNA required make this somewhat impractical. The ASO probe, which is single-stranded DNA, generally 18–30 nucleotides in length, is allowed to hybridize to the immobilized DNA under stringency con-ditions such that the probe can hybridize only if there is perfect sequence complementarity with the target DNA. Under the correct stringency conditions, a mismatch of even a single nucleotide within an oligonucleotide probe of approx 20 nucleotides can inhibit hybridization by altering the optimum annealing temperature of the oligonucleotide. To detect hybridization, the probe can be labeled and detected with a variety of systems, e.g., a radioactive label and autoradiography. For each allele to be detected (i.e., wild-type and mutant), a specific probe is used.

A more commonly used variation of the ASO technique is to immobilize the probe on a membrane or other solid support and allow the amplified, denatured DNA to hybridize to the probe (Fig. 16). This approach is known as *reverse ASO*. It has the advantage that multiple probes, designed to detect different mutations in the same amplified DNA fragment, can be applied to the solid support. This allows for multiple mutations to be detected simultaneously. In this technique, the amplified DNA fragments are labeled so that hybridization can be detected. This approach can be used in microarrays containing hundreds or thousands of immobilized oligonucleotides to detect many mutations.

OLIGONUCLEOTIDE LIGATION ASSAY

An oligonucleotide ligation assay (OLA) utilizes two oligonucleotides that anneal to the target DNA in a head-to-tail fashion, as in ligase chain reaction (Fig. 8). The target DNA of interest is first amplified by PCR. If the 3′ end of the first oligonucleotide is perfectly hybridized to the target DNA, then it can be ligated by a DNA ligase to the 5′ end of the adjacent oligonucleotide. If the target DNA contains a mutation that prevents the 3′ end of the first primer from hybridizing at this position, then ligation does not occur. Detection of ligation can be made by several methods, such as observing the change in molecular weight of the ligated oligonucleotides by polyacrylamide gel or capillary gel electrophoresis.

REAL-TIME PCR

Some thermal cyclers allow for continuous monitoring of the production of PCR products as the reaction proceeds during each cycle. This is known as real-time PCR monitoring, and it can be used to perform quantitative PCR or for qualitative identification of genetic variants. The thermal cycler contains the necessary light source, optics, filters, and detectors to perform fluorescence measurements. The chambers in which each PCR is performed have an optically clear segment to enable fluorescence readings to be made.

For quantitative measurements in real-time PCR, two general approaches are available. Nonspecific quantitative monitoring of a PCR product is performed by observing the fluorescence of a double-stranded DNA-binding dye such as SYBR® Green I. This dye fluoresces in proportion to the amount of DNA in a reaction vessel. As DNA is synthesized in each cycle, more DNA is available to bind the dye, and so the fluorescence increases until the PCR reaction reaches the plateau phase. A limitation of the use of SYBR Green I is that any PCR product that is amplified is capable of binding the dye, resulting in increased fluorescence. The PCR primers

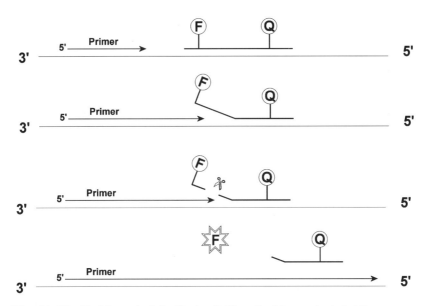

Fig. 17. The TaqMan principle. During PCR, a TaqMan probe hybridizes to one of the strands that is being amplified. The probe contains a fluorescent reporter (F) and a quencher (Q). The quencher prevents fluorescence by the reporter when the two molecules are physically in close proximity. *Taq* polymerase extends a primer during PCR, and the enzyme's 5′-3′ exonuclease activity degrades the TaqMan probe. This separates the fluorescent reporter from the quencher, allowing the former to fluoresce. Increases in fluorescence therefore indicate that the sequence to which the TaqMan probe hybridizes are present in the sample and are being amplified by PCR. Measurements of increases in fluorescence during PCR can be used for quantitative PCR assays.

and reaction conditions must be chosen so as to ensure specificity of the reaction if reliable quantification is to be achieved. The second real-time PCR monitoring approach involves the use of target-specific probes, namely, TaqMan probes and molecular beacons.

TaqMan. Real-time PCR can be used to quantify a specific DNA PCR product by use of FRET probes *(17)*. This form of real-time PCR increases the specificity of the reaction considerably over that achieved by use of SYBR Green I. The principle of FRET technology is shown in Fig. 17. A FRET probe is an oligonucleotide that has a fluorophore at its 5′ end and a fluorescence quencher at its 3′ end. The distance between these is such that when the fluorophore is excited, its energy is absorbed by the quencher, and so the overall fluorescence of the reaction is low. The middle region of the

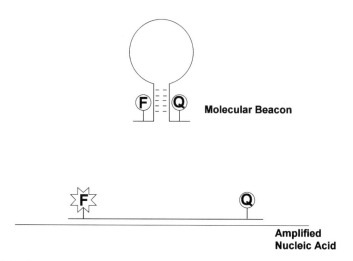

Fig. 18. The molecular beacon principle. A molecular beacon is an oligonu-cleotide that contains a fluorescent reporter (F) and a quencher (Q) at its ends. **(A)** Because of sequence complementarity near the ends, the structure forms a hairpin. The central part is complementary to a target DNA that is amplified by PCR. **(B)** If the target DNA is present, the molecular beacon hybridizes to it, thus separating the reporter and quencher. The former is now able to fluoresce.

oligonucleotide is designed to hybridize specifically to the region of DNA being amplified. As the target is replicated, the TaqMan probe hybridizes to its complementary sequence. As the PCR primer is extended by *Taq* polymerase to the hybridized probe, the poly-merase removes the FRET probe by 5′-3′ nuclease cleavage. This releases the free fluorophore into solution, where its fluorescence is unimpeded by the quencher. The fluorescence of the reaction there-fore increases, and this increase is in proportion to the amount of amplified product present. This allows for real-time monitoring of the amplification of a specific DNA target. Because the rate of amplification is dependent on the amount of template at the begin-ning of PCR, the reaction can be used to quantify a nucleic acid tar-get. Coamplification of an internal control can be monitored by use of a specific TaqMan probe.

Molecular Beacons. A molecular beacon, like a TaqMan probe, is an oligonucleotide that contains a fluorophore and a quencher (Fig. 18). These are at the ends of a stem-loop structure. The loop is com-plementary to a sequence in a target nucleic acid, and the stem con-tains a short stretch of complementary sequences such as the structure

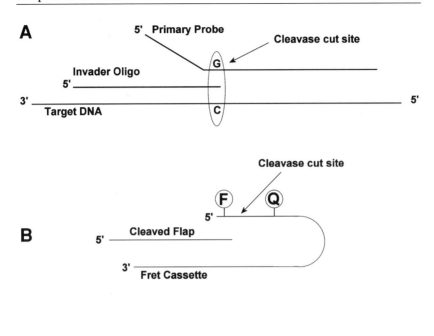

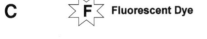

Fig. 19. Invader principle. **(A)** A primary probe is hybridizing to its target sequence in DNA. The Invader probe overlaps by 1 bp. This arrangement is recognized by Cleavase, which cuts the primary probe, liberating the "5'-flap." **(B)** The liberated flap functions as an Invader oligonucleotide in a second reaction with a FRET cassette. Cleavase cuts the FRET cassette, leading to separation of the fluorescent reporter (F) from the quencher (Q). **(C)** The former can now fluoresce.

folds as shown. The fluorophore and the quencher are physically adjacent when the structure is folded, and this inhibits fluorescence. When the target nucleic acid is present, the loop can hybridize to its complementary sequences. This results in disruption of the stem-loop structure and physical separation of the quencher from the fluorophore, which results in an increase in fluorescence of the solution.

Invader®. Invader is a homogenous, isothermal mutation detection system produced by Third Wave Technologies (Madison, WI) *(18)*. It is used to identify single-nucleotide polymorphisms and point mutations in genomic DNA. The principle of Invader is shown in Figure 19. An Invader reaction uses two probes, a primary probe and an Invader probe. The primary probe contains a 3' region that can anneal to the target region in genomic DNA and a 5′ region that is not complementary to the target and therefore does not hybridize to the target. The latter region of the primary probe is termed the *flap*. At the junction between these two regions is the base that is complementary to the base in the target DNA that is to be identified as being present or absent. In Fig. 19, this is a C in the target DNA, and the primary probe contains the complementary G. The Invader probe is complementary to the target DNA 5′ of the base to be tested and extends in a 3′ direction to overlap that base. If this base is present in the target DNA, the primary probe is cut by an enzyme known as Cleavase. This liberates the flap region from the primary probe. The temperature at which the Invader reaction takes place is close to the T_m of the primary probe, and the residual portion of this probe dissociates from the template and is replaced by another intact primary probe. The T_m of the Invader probe is designed to be at least 10°C higher than that of the primary probe, and therefore the Invader probe remains bound to the target as a series of primary probes binds and are cleaved.

The liberated flap then participates in a second Invader reaction that involves binding to an oligonucleotide containing a fluorophore and a quencher. This structure is known as a FRET cassette. When the fluorophore and the quencher molecules are physically adjacent, as in the FRET cassette, fluorescence is diminished. Binding of the flap allows for Cleavase to cut the FRET cassette, thereby separating the fluorophore from the quencher and increasing fluorescence in the reaction well. If the target DNA does not include the base of interest, the primary probe is not cut by Cleavase, and therefore there is no increase in fluorescence.

For each point mutation or SNP to be tested by Invader, two reaction wells are used: one for the wild-type allele and one for the mutant allele or SNP. Each of these uses a unique, allele-specific primary probe. It is not essential that the Invader oligonucleotide be complementary to the base to be tested, and therefore a common Invader probe can be used for both reactions. The ratio of fluorescence produced in both wells is used to determine the genotype.

Approaches to Detect Unknown Mutations

In certain molecular diagnostic assays, the goal is to screen a gene for any of multiple possible mutations. An efficient approach to achieve this goal is to apply a mutation screening technique that

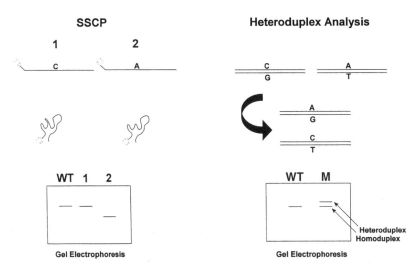

Fig. 20. Single-strand conformation polymorphism (SSCP; left) and heteroduplex principles (right). **(Left)** Two samples of DNA, which differ in their sequence by just one nucleotide, are amplified by PCR. During the amplification, these are labeled, e.g., by incorporation of a radioisotope. Following PCR, the fragments are made single stranded and electrophoresed. Differences in sequence lead to different structures that exhibit differences in electrophoretic mobility in a nondenaturing gel. This enables sequence variants to be identified using this technique. Characterization of the actual sequence variation requires further analysis. **(Right)** A known wild-type control sample and a sample containing a mutation are both amplified by PCR. Following amplification the two products are heated to melt the strands and then allowed to cool. This leads to formation of some heteroduplexes (double-stranded DNA molecules that do not have perfectly complementary sequences). Heteroduplexes migrate more slowly than homoduplexes during electrophoresis. The presence of a heteroduplex band indicates a sequence variant in the sample being tested. Characterization of the actual sequence variation requires further analysis. WT is wild type, M is mutant.

can rapidly identify samples containing a sequence variation, and subsequently to confirm suspected mutations with a definitive method such as sequencing. Two common methods of screening for unknown mutations are single-strand conformation polymorphism (SSCP) analysis and heteroduplex analysis. The principles of these methods are shown in Fig. 20.

SINGLE-STRAND CONFORMATIONAL POLYMORPHISM ANALYSIS

In dilute solutions, single-stranded DNA molecules spontaneously adopt a three-dimensional conformation because of the formation of sequence-specific intramolecular base-pairing. Minor alterations to the sequence of the DNA strand can result in different conformations. These conformational differences alter the electrophoretic mobility of the DNA strand in nondenaturing gels. This principle is used in SSCP analysis. In a typical analysis, a region of DNA to be examined for the presence of mutations is amplified by PCR, and the PCR products are denatured (i.e., made single-stranded) and then electrophoresed in a nondenaturing gel. Control samples containing either the wild-type sequence or known mutations are run in parallel with patient samples. Electrophoretic mobility differences between the wild-type control and a patient sample indicate the presence of a possible mutation. The mutation is then characterized by sequencing.

HETERODUPLEX ANALYSIS

A heteroduplex is a molecule composed of two strands of different sequence. Normally, DNA forms a double-stranded (duplex) molecule with two strands that are complementary to each other. However, a minor degree of noncomplementarity between the paired strands can be tolerated in a molecule that can still exist as a duplex. Such heteroduplexes migrate more slowly during electrophoresis than does a homoduplex (in which there is complete complementarity between strands) of similar size. Heteroduplexes are generated by mixing amplified mutant DNA with amplified wild-type DNA, heating the mixture to separate the strands, and then cooling to allow duplexes to form. Both homoduplexes and heteroduplexes will be produced on cooling. When the products from this procedure are separated by electrophoresis, a heteroduplex band will be visible as a more slowly migrating band than that formed by homoduplex molecules.

DENATURING AND TEMPERATURE GRADIENT GEL ELECTROPHORESIS

The concentration of denaturing agents, or temperature, at which the two strands in a DNA molecule separate ("melt") is determined by the sequence of the DNA. If a DNA molecule is electrophoresed into an environment with an increasing concentration of a denaturing agent, or into a gradient of increasing temperature, small sections of the molecule with the weakest interstrand bonding will begin to separate. This alteration will slow the electrophoretic mobility of the molecule. If molecules with sequence variations are run in parallel lanes in such a gel, these will show different electrophoretic mobilities. The use of progressively denaturing conditions can also be used to increase the separation between homoduplex and heteroduplex molecules in a heteroduplex analysis.

DNA SEQUENCING

DNA sequencing is considered the gold standard for mutation identification. However, the limited sample throughput of many automated DNA sequencers has tended to preclude its routine application in many clinical laboratories. The most common method of DNA sequencing is based on the chain termination method reported by Sanger, who won a Nobel prize in 1980 for this technique *(19)*.

In the chain termination method for DNA sequencing, the piece of DNA to be sequenced is first amplified by PCR or other cloning strategy. The amplified DNA is denatured, and a primer is allowed to anneal to one end of the DNA. This primer functions in essentially the same way as a primer that might be used for PCR, namely, it serves as an anchor and starting point for a DNA polymerase to extend the primer using the sample DNA as a template. Only one primer is used for each sequencing reaction, which means that one of the two strands of DNA is extended. The sequencing reaction includes both dNTPs and one of the four di-deoxynucleotide triphosphates (ddNTPs). The latter do not have the 3'-hydroxyl group that is present in dNTPs. Once a dideoxynucleotide is incorporated in a molecule of DNA, no further extension is possible because there is no available hydroxyl group on the sugar group for the formation of the 3'-5' phosphodiester linkage that is found in nucleic acid polymers. At each position in the template at which the complementary base to the ddNTP is present, the polymerase can incorporate either the ddNTP or the normal dNTP. The relative likelihood of incorporating either nucleotide is dependent on the relative concentrations of ddNTP and dNTP. If the concentration of ddNTP is relatively high, DNA synthesis will tend to terminate early and produce large numbers of shorter molecules. Conversely, if the concentration of ddNTP is relatively low, longer length fragments can be synthesized before synthesis is terminated by a dideoxynucleotide. By controlling the concentrations of dNTP and ddNTP, it is possible to generate a range of fragment sizes.

A sequence analysis can be performed by setting up four separate reactions, each of which contains one of the ddNTPs (i.e., ddATP,

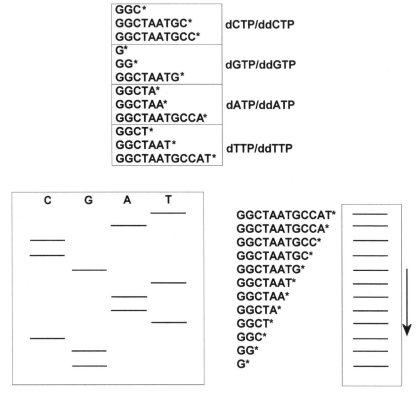

Fig. 21. Chain termination sequencing principle. A series of primer extension reactions is performed using a DNA template to be sequenced (top). The reactions contain mixtures of the deoxynucleotide triphosphates and di-deoxynucleotide triphosphates. Each reaction is terminated when a di-deoxynucleotide is incorporated. Separation of the products of these reactions in polyacrylamide gels enables determination of the sequence of the DNA template by reading the size order of the products (lower left). If each of the four di-deoxynucleotides is labeled with a different fluorescent dye, an automated reading of the products during size separation (e.g., by capillary electrophoresis) can be performed (lower right).

ddCTP, ddGTP, or ddTTP) (Fig. 21). These reactions will generate a range of fragment lengths, each of which terminate in the respective ddNTP. By electrophoretic separation of the products of these reactions in adjacent lanes, it is possible to determine the sequence of one strand of a DNA molecule. An alternative approach, which utilizes only one sequencing reaction, involves the use of chain termination nucleotides that are linked to dyes with different fluorescence

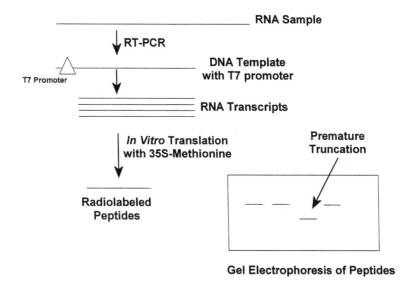

RNA Sample

↓ RT-PCR

DNA Template
with T7 promoter

T7 Promoter

RNA Transcripts

In Vitro Translation
with 35S-Methionine

Premature
Truncation

Radiolabeled
Peptides

Gel Electrophoresis of Peptides

Fig. 22. Protein truncation assay principle. An RNA from the gene of interest is amplified by RT-PCR, incorporating a T7 RNA polymerase promoter. This product is used for in vitro transcription and translation. The peptides produced are labeled by incorporation of ^{35}S-methionine. The size of these peptides is determined by electrophoresis in denaturing gels. A shortened peptide indicates the presence of a truncating mutation in the RNA.

wavelengths. The products of such a reaction are separated by a technique such as capillary electrophoresis. As the separated molecules pass through the detection window, they are excited by UV light, and the identity of the passing fluorophore (and therefore the base) is determined from its emitted light spectrum.

PROTEIN TRUNCATION TEST

The protein truncation test is a method of identifying nonsense mutations in genes *(20)* (Fig. 22). These give rise to premature stop codons that cause early termination of protein synthesis. By performing an in vitro transcription and translation using a cloned gene or cDNA, the length of the translated protein can be determined. The cloned construct contains a T7 RNA polymerase promoter at its 5′ end and a eukaryotic translation initiation codon (AUG). This is used as a template by T7 RNA polymerase to produce RNA. In vitro translation in a suitable system (e.g., a reticulocyte lysate) generates peptides, and the length of the translated peptides can be determined

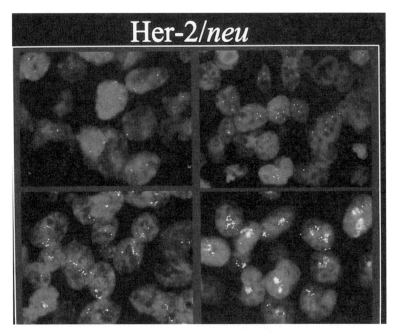

Fig. 23. Four-part photomicrograph of HER2/*neu* gene amplification detection by FISH. (**Upper left**) Unamplified case with a mean signal count of 1.5 signals per nucleus. (**Upper right**) Breast cancer with a borderline result featuring a mean signal count of 4.1 signals per nucleus. (**Lower left**) Significantly amplified breast tumor with a mean signal count of 17.5 signals per nucleus. (**Lower right**) Another example of a significantly amplified breast cancer with a mean HER2/*neu* signal count of 24. 9 signals per nucleus (Reproduced with permission from ref. *1*).

by electrophoresis in a denaturing gel. The presence of a premature truncating mutation is indicated by synthesis of a short peptide. Because of its complexity, the protein truncation test is primarily used as a research tool. It can be used to identify truncating mutations in genes in which this kind of mutation is common, e.g., *BRCA1, BRCA2,* or *DMD (21,22).*

Fluorescence In Situ *Hybridization*

Fluorescence *in situ* hybridization (FISH) is a cytogenetic technique in which a fluorescently labeled probe is hybridized to chromosomes. Probes used in FISH are either fluorescently labeled (direct technique) or contain a hapten such as biotin or digoxigenin that can be detected by a fluorescently labeled conjugate (indirect technique). Hybridization is detected by fluorescence microscopy (Fig. 23).

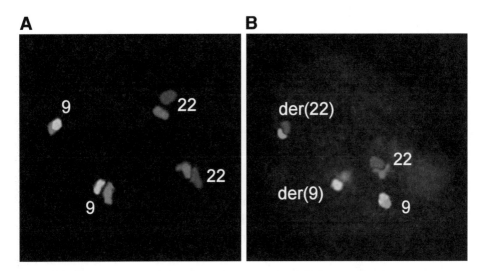

Fig. 24. Four-color FISH detection of the t(9;22) BCR-ABL translocation. (**A**) A normal cell has been hybridized with four FISH probes. The blue and red probes hybridize to sequences in chromosome 22. The yellow and green probes hybridize to sequences in chromosome 9. The der(22) chromosome, which contains the *BCR-ABL* fusion, is shown by the adjacent green and red probes. The der(9) chromosome, which contains the reciprocal ABL-BCR fusion, is shown by the adjacent yellow and blue probes (Courtesy of Cancer Genetics, Inc.).

FISH can be performed on metaphase chromosome preparations (i.e., from cells that can be cultured in vitro) or directly on nondividing cells (interphase FISH) *(23)*. A large number of probes is commercially available that are used for different kinds of applications. For example, probes for α-satellite markers can be used to identify the origin of marker chromosomes. Probes for specific loci or chromosomal regions can be used to demonstrate deletions or amplifications (Fig. 23). FISH is used to demonstrate abnormalities in the subtelomeric regions of chromosomes that are responsible for a number of cases of unexplained mental retardation. By using several probes labeled with different fluorochromes, it is possible to detect chromosomal translocations. In this approach, the probes hybridize to their corresponding sequences on each of the partner chromosomes in the translocation and on the normal chromosomes. The presence of a translocation is indicated by the close proximity of probes that hybridize to the translocation partners (Fig. 24). Among other applications, interphase FISH is used for rapid identification of the common chromosomal aneuploidies in prenatal samples.

Spectral Karyotyping and Multiplex FISH

Spectral karyotyping (SKY) *(24)* and multiplex FISH (M-FISH) *(25)* are related analytical techniques that are developments of FISH. In both techniques, fluorescently labeled probes for each of the 24 chromosomes are applied to metaphase chromosome spreads and visualized using a computerized imaging system. The probes are produced by flow sorting or microdissecting normal chromosomes and then performing PCR on the isolated chromosomes using degenerate primers. For each chromosome, the PCR-generated probes are synthesized so as to contain a unique combination of different fluorophores. In this way, each chromosome is represented by probes that have unique fluorospectroscopic characteristics. In general, N fluorophores can be used to generate $2^N - 1$ unique combinations of labeled probes. Five fluorophores can be used to produce 31 possible combinations of dyes, which are sufficient to label each of the 24 chromosomes with a unique combination of fluorophores.

After hybridization, the labeled probes are bound to the metaphase chromosomes in the sample to be analyzed. The fluorescent probes are excited and the image is captured. By computer analysis of the image, the particular set of probes that is hybridizing to a metaphase chromosome can be identified. The results are displayed in false colors for ease of interpretation, with each chromosome being assigned a unique false color (Fig. 25).

SKY and M-FISH differ primarily in the method by which the image is analyzed. In SKY, an interferometer is used to identify the combination of fluorophores hybridized to each chromosome. In M-FISH, the image is photographed using a set of filters. Computer analysis of the image obtained with each filter is used to determine which probes have hybridized to each chromosome.

USES AND LIMITATIONS OF SKY AND M-FISH

Both techniques are of value for rapid detection of chromosomal aneuploidy and identification of the chromosome involved. Translocations, and the chromosomes involved in translocations, can also be rapidly identified. The origin of marker chromosomes can be established in some cases. However, these techniques are not suit-

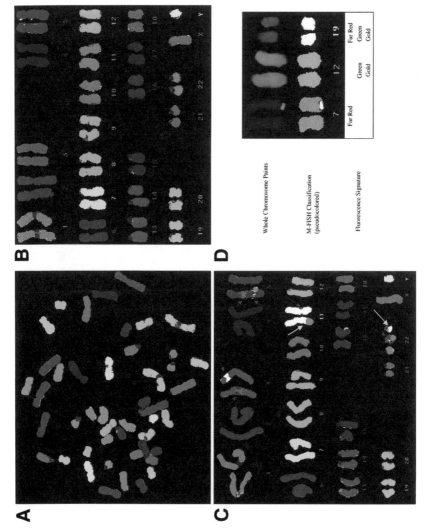

Fig. 25. (**A, B**) M-FISH analysis of a PHA-stimulated whole blood culture, showing a metaphase and a normal male karyotype. (**C**) M-FISH karyotype from a fibroblast culture showing a t(11;22) and an extra chromosome 22. The yellow arrows identify the translocation, and the red arrows indicate areas of chromosome overlaps. (**D**) M-FISH analysis from a whole blood culture involving an unbalanced 7;12 translocation. The translocated chromatin on chromosome 7 appears to be from chromosome 19, owing to the overlapping signals. Individual chromosome 12 painting probe was used to identify correctly the source of the translocated material to chromosome 7 to be chromosome 12 (Reproduced with permission from ref. 23).

133

able for identification of deletions, duplications, or inversions of chromosomal material. For these applications, conventional staining (e.g., G-banding) or FISH are superior. The lower limit of size of DNA from one chromosome that can be visualized by SKY when inserted into another chromosome is approx 1–2 Mb (26).

Determining Methylation of DNA

Methylation of DNA is can be determined by several approaches. Restriction with a methylation-sensitive enzyme generates a pattern of fragments that depends on the methylation status of the DNA. This is the basis of detection of methylation at the fragile X locus, *FMR1*, which is discussed in Chapter 5. Digestion of samples with isoschizomers (restriction enzymes from different species that recognize the same DNA sequence and cut at the same position) can indicate the methylation status of DNA if one of the isoschizomers is methylation-sensitive. As discussed earlier, *Msp*I and *Hpa*II form such a pair of restriction enzymes, *Hpa*II being methylation-sensitive. The use of restriction enzymes to determine methylation status is limited to sequences that are recognized by available restriction enzymes, and detection is normally by Southern blotting.

An alternative approach to determining methylation status that is faster, and requires much less starting material, is PCR following bisulfite treatment of DNA. This technique is known as methylation-specific PCR (27). Treatment with bisulfite converts cytosine residues to uracil residues; during PCR, thymidine is incorporated where uracil was present in the original template DNA. However, 5-methylcytosine is not altered by bisulfite treatment, and, during PCR, cytosine is incorporated where 5-methylcytosine was present in the template. Comparison of the sequence of PCR products amplified from genomic DNA and a parallel sample amplified after treatment with bisulfite demonstrates the location of 5-methylcytosine residues in the template DNA (Fig. 26).

Microarray Technology

Microarray technology is becoming an important tool with several applications of relevance to molecular pathology. The basic principle underlying this technology involves immobilization of probes onto a solid support and detection of hybridization of target nucleic acids in a sample. The probes can be oligonucleotides,

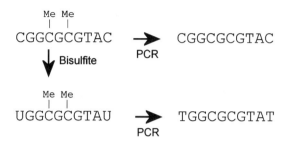

Fig. 26. Determining methylation of DNA by PCR. Bisulfite reacts with cytosine residues in a DNA sample and converts these to uracil residues. During PCR, uracil is replicated as thymidine. Methylated cytosine residues do not react in this way with bisulfite and are replicated as cytosine. Comparison of the sequence of a DNA fragment amplified by PCR following bisulfite treatment allows for identification of cytosines that were methylated in the original DNA template.

cDNAs corresponding to known genes, or cDNAs of unknown expressed RNAs, called expressed sequence tags (ESTs). This principle of microarray technology is similar to that of reverse ASO; however, microarrays utilize thousands of different probes that are immobilized in rows and columns on a small area. The probes may be synthesized directly on a silicon chip using technology derived from the microelectronics field. Affymetrix (Santa Clara, CA) produces a variety of chips (called GeneChips) using this approach. Alternatively, the probes may be spotted onto a solid support using a robotic pipeting device. In either case, the nucleic acids in a sample bind to these probes through sequence complementarity, and this binding is detected, often through the use of florescent labels that have been incorporated into the sample nucleic acid. Detection of hybridization involves the use of microscopy using a suitable imaging system and computer for data analysis.

Microarrays are used in three broad classes of experiment. The first involves examining the expression of genes in tissue extracts through analysis of RNA expression profiles. The second involves determination of sequence variations in DNA, and the third involves comparative genomic hybridization to look for changes in gene dosage because of chromosomal abnormalities.

MICROARRAYS FOR GENE EXPRESSION PROFILING

The pattern of expressed genes, and the relative levels of expression of specific genes, vary between different tissues, for example,

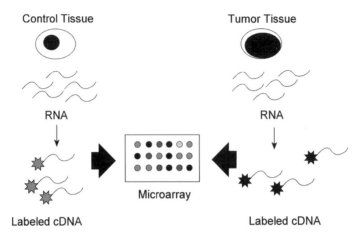

Fig. 27. Gene expression profiling by microarray technology. RNA samples from a tumor specimen and from a control tissue are extracted and reverse transcribed to produce cDNAs. During reverse transcription, these are labeled with different fluorescent dyes, shown as gray and black in this illustration. After mixing, the cDNAs are hybridized to a microarray containing immobilized probes for target genes of interest. If an RNA is equally abundant in both the tumor sample and control tissue, the signal produced will be a composite of both dyes. A relatively strong signal from the dye used to label the tumor sample indicates that expression of a particular gene is increased in the tumor sample.

between normal tissue and its malignant counterpart. Such differences in gene expression can be observed using microarray technology as increases or decreases in the abundance of specific mRNA transcripts (Fig. 27). In this kind of experiment, RNA from a tumor sample and from a control tissue are extracted, and cDNAs are prepared by reverse transcription. These reverse transcription reactions incorporate different fluorescent dyes so that cDNA from the tumor and from the control tissue can be distinguished by their fluorescence emission spectra. These cDNAs are mixed and then hybridized to the microarray. A relative increase in expression of a particular gene in a tumor sample leads to an increase in binding of labeled tumor-derived cDNA to the spot in the array that is complementary to the gene of interest. Conversely, a relative decrease in the expression of a gene in a tumor sample manifests as a relative decrease in intensity of fluorescence by the tumor-derived cDNA.

An examination of the profile of gene expression gives data that can be used to generate a molecular classification of tumors that may provide important diagnostic and prognostic information. Such profiles can also reveal activation of certain cellular pathways and can lead to the discovery of new biological markers of malignancy, tumor invasiveness, and response to drug therapy. A landmark study using gene expression profiling demonstrated the ability of this methodology to distinguish acute myeloid leukemia from acute lymphocytic leukemia *(28)*. Numerous studies have examined molecular profiles of gene expression in a variety of other tumors (reviewed in ref. *29*).

High-density microarrays are proving quite useful for discovery of genes and pathways involved in various types of tumors. However, it is unlikely that high-density arrays will be used in routine clinical diagnostics. The more likely scenario for clinical applications is that alterations in expression of a limited number of genes will provide medically important information for diagnosis, classification, and prognosis of tumors. Changes in expression of such a set of genes may be determined by low-density microarrays, by quantitative RT-PCR methods, or by immunohistochemical approaches, when these are feasible.

MICROARRAYS FOR DETERMINING SEQUENCE

By immobilizing multiple oligonucleotide probes from a gene on an array, it is possible to perform a sequence analysis, also known as a mutation microarray analysis. To do this, the oligonucleotides applied to the array are designed to hybridize specifically to a particular allele under standard stringency conditions. For each allele to be detected, e.g., members of a pair of alleles comprising an SNP, a specific oligonucleotide probe is used. The target DNA is commonly amplified by PCR and labeled with a fluorescent tag for ease of detection of hybridization *(30)*.

MICROARRAYS FOR COMPARATIVE GENOMIC HYBRIDIZATION

Comparative genomic hybridization (CGH) is a cytogenetic method that allows for genome-wide detection of gains or losses of chromosomal material. In a CGH experiment, DNA is extracted from a sample (e.g., a tumor specimen) and from a control tissue, and these are labeled with different fluorochromes. These labeled DNAs are then hybridized to a normal 46 X,Y metaphase chromosome preparation. A gain of chromosomal material such as a gene amplification in

a tumor will manifest as an increase in the fluorescence intensity of
the tumor fluorophore in the region of the chromosome with the gain.
A loss of chromosomal material will have the opposite effect. The
specific chromosome with the gain or loss of material can be identified after counterstaining with a suitable dye such as DAPI. This
methodology is relatively labor-intensive and difficult to automate
and has relatively large minimal detectable alterations. The size limitation for detection of chromosomal gains is not less than 2 Mb, and
that for detection of chromosomal loss is not less than 10 Mb *(31)*.

In a microarray CGH procedure, the sample DNA is hybridized
against arrayed probes, instead of a metaphase chromosome spread.
The procedure involves immobilizing clones of chromosomal
regions or cDNAs onto arrays and then hybridizing normal and
tumor-derived DNAs that have been labeled with different fluorochromes. Increases or decreases in DNA from a chromosomal
region in a tumor sample will give rise to increases or decreases in
the fluorescence intensity at the corresponding spots on the microarray *(31)*. Compared with CGH using metaphase chromosomes, the
microarray approach offers higher throughput and the ability to
resolve gains or losses involving smaller regions of the genome.

REFERENCES

1. Killeen AA, ed. Molecular Pathology Protocols. Totowa, NJ: Humana, 2001.
2. Killeen AA. Quantification of nucleic acids. Clin Lab Med 1997;17:1–19.
3. Passmore LJ, Killeen AA. Toluidine blue dye-binding method for measurement of genomic DNA extracted from peripheral blood leukocytes. Mol Diagn 1996;1:329–34.
4. Southern EM. Detection of specific sequences among DNA fragments separated by gel electrophoresis. J Mol Biol 1975;98:503–17.
5. Roberts RJ, Macelis D. REBASE—restriction enzymes and methylases. Nucleic Acids Res 2001;29:268–9.
6. Cooper DN, Schmidtke J. DNA restriction fragment length polymorphisms and heterozygosity in the human genome. Hum Genet 1984;66:1–16.
7. Lahti CJ. Pulsed field gel electrophoresis in the clinical microbiology laboratory. J Clin Lab Anal 1996;10:326–30.
8. Patel PI, Roa BB, Welcher AA, et al. The gene for the peripheral myelin protein PMP-22 is a candidate for Charcot-Marie-Tooth disease type 1A. Nat Genet 1992;1:159–65.
9. Mariman EC, Gabreels-Festen AA, van Beersum SE, et al. Prevalence of the 1.5-Mb 17p deletion in families with hereditary neuropathy with liability to pressure palsies. Ann Neurol 1994;36:650–5.
10. Pfaller MA. Molecular epidemiology in the care of patients. Arch Pathol Lab Med 1999;123:1007–10.

11. Mullis KB. The unusual origin of the polymerase chain reaction. Sci Am 1990;262:56–61, 64–5.
12. Deiman B, van AP, Sillekens P. Characteristics and applications of nucleic acid sequence-based amplification (NASBA). Mol Biotechnol 2002;20:163–79.
13. Hill CS. Molecular diagnostic testing for infectious diseases using TMA technology. Expert Rev Mol Diagn 2001;1:445–55.
14. Wiedmann M, Wilson WJ, Czajka J, Luo J, Barany F, Batt CA. Ligase chain reaction (LCR)—overview and applications. PCR Methods Appl 1994;3:S51–64.
15. Little MC, Andrews J, Moore R, et al. Strand displacement amplification and homogeneous real-time detection incorporated in a second-generation DNA probe system, BDProbeTecET. Clin Chem 1999;45:777–84.
16. Nollau P, Wagner C. Methods for detection of point mutations: performance and quality assessment. Clin Chem 1997;43:1114–28.
17. Kricka LJ. Stains, labels and detection strategies for nucleic acids assays. Ann Clin Biochem 2002;39:114–29.
18. Kwiatkowski RW, Lyamichev V, de Arruda M, Neri B. Clinical, genetic, and pharmacogenetic applications of the Invader assay. Mol Diagn 1999;4:353–64.
19. Sanger F, Nicklen S, Coulson AR. DNA sequencing with chain-terminating inhibitors. Proc Natl Acad Sci USA 1977;74:5463–7.
20. Roest PA, Roberts RG, Sugino S, van Ommen GJ, den Dunnen JT. Protein truncation test (PTT) for rapid detection of translation-terminating mutations. Hum Mol Genet 1993;2:1719–21.
21. Hilton JL, Geisler JP, Rathe JA, Hattermann-Zogg MA, DeYoung B, Buller RE. Inactivation of *BRCA1* and *BRCA2* in ovarian cancer. J Natl Cancer Inst 2002;94:1396–406.
22. Roest PA, Roberts RG, van der Tuijn AC, Heikoop JC, van Ommen GJ, den Dunnen JT. Protein truncation test (PTT) to rapidly screen the DMD gene for translation terminating mutations. Neuromuscul Disord 1993;3:391–4.
23. Fan Y-S. Molecular cytogenetics in medicine. An overview. In: Fan Y-S., ed. Molecular Cytogenetics: Protocols and Applications. Totowa, NJ: Humana, 2002.
24. Schrock E, du Manoir S, Veldman T, et al. Multicolor spectral karyotyping of human chromosomes. Science 1996;273:494–7.
25. Speicher MR, Gwyn Ballard S, Ward DC. Karyotyping human chromosomes by combinatorial multi-fluor FISH. Nat Genet 1996;12:368–75.
26. Speicher MR, Ward DC. The coloring of cytogenetics. Nat Med 1996;2:1046–8.
27. Herman JG, Graff JR, Myohanen S, Nelkin BD, Baylin SB. Methylation-specific PCR: a novel PCR assay for methylation status of CpG islands. Proc Natl Acad Sci USA 1996;93:9821–6.
28. Golub TR, Slonim DK, Tamayo P, et al. Molecular classification of cancer: class discovery and class prediction by gene expression monitoring. Science 1999;286:531–7.
29. Macgregor PF, Squire JA. Application of microarrays to the analysis of gene expression in cancer. Clin Chem 2002;48:1170–7.
30. Hacia JG, Collins FS. Mutational analysis using oligonucleotide microarrays. J Med Genet 1999;36:730–6.
31. Beheshti B, Park PC, Braude I, Squire JA. Microarray CGH. In: Fan YS., ed. Molecular Cytogenetics: Protocols and Applications. Totowa, N.J.: Humana, 2002:191–207.
32. Principles of molecule medicine. Totowa, NJ: Humana, 1998.

5   Inherited Disorders

The molecular bases of numerous inherited diseases are now known, and diagnostic testing for many of these is now widely available. Molecular testing is performed to establish, confirm, or exclude a diagnosis, for screening, or, in some cases, to predict the severity of disease. Of the many genetic diseases that can be investigated by molecular diagnostic techniques, testing for a few has become relatively commonplace in clinical laboratories. These include cystic fibrosis, hereditary hemochromatosis, certain thrombophilias, Huntington's disease, and fragile X syndrome. In this chapter, the molecular pathology of these diseases is reviewed, as are some of the more common mitochondrial disorders that illustrate the principles of molecular pathology of this group of diseases. In addition, because of the widespread implementation of newborn screening programs in most countries, the molecular bases of diseases that are commonly included in these programs are also described.

CYSTIC FIBROSIS

Clinical Features

Cystic fibrosis (CF) is an autosomal recessive disorder caused by mutations in the CF transmembrane conductance regulator *(CFTR)* gene on chromosome 7q31.2. CF affects approximately 1 in 3200 newborns in the United States, most commonly those of northern European ancestry. Approximately 1 in 29 Caucasians is a carrier of this disease. The disease is much less prevalent among African Americans (1 in 15,000) and Asian Americans (1 in 31,000) *(1)*.

CF is characterized by clinical features that include recurrent respiratory symptoms, failure to thrive or malnutrition, steatorrhea, and meconium ileus. Among adult males, obstructive azoospermia, caused by congenital bilateral absence of the vas deferens (CBAVD), is pre-

From: *Principles of Molecular Pathology*
Edited by: A. A. Killeen © Humana Press Inc., Totowa, NJ

sent in >95% of CF patients. Of these symptoms, the most debilitating are recurring pulmonary infections. The average life expectancy of a patient with CF is currently approximately 30 years *(2)*.

Patients with CF have abnormal transport of electrolytes across epithelial surfaces, resulting in the production of viscid mucous that tends to obstruct the bronchial epithelium, the pancreatic ducts, the biliary ducts, and, in males, the vasa deferentia. In the bronchial tree, these electrolyte abnormalities may also alter the functioning of natural antibacterial peptides produced by the epithelium *(3)*. These factors predispose to infection with bacteria such as *Staphylococccus aureus, Haemophilus influenzae,* and, later, *Pseudomonas aeruginosa.* Infection with *Burkholderia cepacia* (a highly drug-resistant, mucoid bacterium, formerly called *Pseudomonas cepacia*) can lead to the commonly fatal cepacia syndrome, which is characterized by *B. cepacia* sepsis and necrotizing pneumonia *(4,5)*. With deterioration in pulmonary function, chronic bronchitis and bronchiectasis develop, with associated thickening of the bronchial walls and the formation of bronchial abscesses. Death is usually caused by respiratory failure and cor pulmonale.

CFTR Protein Function

The CFTR protein is membrane-bound and is a member of the adenosine triphosphate binding cassette (ABC) family of proteins. Members of this family of proteins include the multidrug resistance (mdr) transporters (also called P-glycoprotein) *(6)* and the sulfonylurea receptors (SUR1 and SUR2), which are present on β-cells of the islets of Langerhans and are responsible for mediating the pharmacological action of the sulfonylurea class of hypoglycemic drugs *(7)*.

The CFTR protein has two transmembrane regions, each composed of six α-helices, two nucleotide-binding domains that bind ATP, and a regulatory domain (Fig. 1). The protein functions as a Cl^- ion channel and also as a negative regulator of the amiloride-sensitive epithelial sodium channel (ENaC) *(8)*. The channel is stimulated by ATP and cAMP-dependent protein kinase or protein kinase A. Mutations associated with CF impair Cl^- ion channel activity and remove the negative regulation of ENaCs. These abnormalities lead to changes in the airway surface liquid (ASL), a thin film of liquid that lines the airways, causing production of viscous airways mucus *(8,9)*.

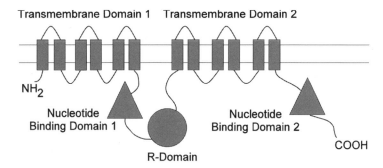

Fig. 1. Schematic showing the structure of the CFTR protein. The R-domain is the regulatory domain.

Table 1
**Cystic Fibrosis Foundation Consensus Panel Criteria
for Diagnosis of Cystic Fibrosis**

1. At least one characteristic phenotypic feature (e.g., chronic sinopulmonary disease, gastrointestinal or nutritional abnormalities) *and either*
2. A history of cystic fibrosis (CF) in a sibling *or*
3. A positive newborn screening test *and* laboratory evidence of a CFTR abnormality, namely, elevated sweat chloride concentrations *or* identification of CF-causing mutations in *CFTR or* characteristic ion transport abnormalities in nasal epithelium

Adapted from ref. *13.*

The channel abnormalities in CF patients can be demonstrated by measuring the potential difference across the nasal epithelium. Patients with CF have baseline nasal transepithelial potential differences of –50 to –70 mV, compared with –30 mV in normal subjects, and show an exaggerated depolarization response to superperfusion with amiloride, a drug that blocks certain sodium channels *(10,11)*. The combination of a maximum basal potential difference ≤30 mV and an amiloride-induced depolarization of ≥50% of baseline is consistent with a diagnosis of CF *(12)*.

Guidelines for Diagnosis

A Cystic Fibrosis Foundation consensus panel has recommended that a formal diagnosis of CF should be based on the presence of a combination of clinical and laboratory findings, as outlined in Table 1 *(13)*.

Table 2
Common *CFTR* Mutations in Northern European Patients

Mutation	Prevalence
ΔF508	0.70
G542X	0.02
G551D	0.02
N1303K	0.01
R553X	<0.01
1717-1G→T	<0.01
W1282X	<0.01

Data from ref. *95.*

IMPORTANCE OF EARLY DIAGNOSIS

Because it is one of the more common genetic diseases in Caucasians, newborn screening for CF has been advocated by some, and it is included in the newborn screening programs of a few states. An important issue to consider in any general screening program is whether early identification of disease leads to a benefit for patients who are identified through the program. In the case of CF, there are limited data available because of the paucity of centers that have offered newborn CF testing for sufficiently long periods to permit comparison of outcomes between patients diagnosed by screening programs and patients diagnosed because of presentation with clinical symptoms. However, a few studies have reported improvements in nutritional status and pulmonary function in children diagnosed by active screening programs *(14)*. These findings provide support for more widespread inclusion of CF testing in newborn screening programs.

Molecular Genetics

Approximately 1000 mutations in *CFTR* that cause CF have been reported *(15)*. The most frequent mutation among Caucasian patients is a deletion of codon 508, which encodes phenylalanine (ΔF508). This mutation is found in 70% of mutated alleles, so 49% (0.7×0.7) of Caucasian patients are homozygous for this mutation. However, the next two most frequent mutations among Caucasians, G542X and G551D, are each found in only approx 2% of CF patients, and other mutations are even less common

Table 3
Common *CFTR* Mutations in Ashkenazi Jewish Patients

Mutation	Prevalence
W1282X	0.48
ΔF508	0.30
G542X	0.12
3849+10kb C→T	0.04
N1303K	0.03

Data from ref. *16*.

(Table 2). This large diversity of mutations poses a challenge to laboratory diagnostic strategies that attempt to provide a comprehensive mutation detection scheme. Among Ashkenazi Jews, a more limited number of mutations is found, allowing a mutation identification rate of 97% by testing a panel of only five mutations (Table 3) *(16)*.

Based on their associated clinical phenotypes, *CFTR* mutations can be divided into those that are milder, defined by sufficiency of pancreatic function (PS), and those that are more severe, defined by pancreatic insufficiency (PI). The latter are much more common. The ΔF508 mutation is considered a severe mutation, and other PI mutations include G542X, G551D, and N1303K. PS mutations include R117H, R334W, and 3489+10kb C→T.

Nonclassic Manifestations of CFTR Mutations

Isolated CBAVD is the cause of infertility in approx 2% of infertile men and is present in 0.8% of all men, being inherited as an autosomal recessive disorder. This disorder is associated with mutations in *CFTR*, particularly the 5T variant of a 5T/7T/9T polythymidine tract polymorphism in intron 8 (IVS8-5T), and an allele containing R117H and IVS8-5T *in cis (17,18)*. The R117H/5T allele is also seen in some patients with classic CF. The length of the poly-T tract is inversely related to the rate of skipping of exon 9 during mRNA processing (i.e., the IVS8-5T variant is associated with the highest degree of skipping). Most CBAVD patients are compound heterozygotes for the IVS8-5T allele and a more severe CF allele, usually ΔF508 *(17)*. Developments in assisted reproductive technologies have enabled some men with CBAVD to have children. These technologies have raised concerns about transmission of mutant CF alleles that might cause classic CF in offspring *(19)*.

In addition to the clear association between CBAVD and *CFTR* mutations, increased prevalences of *CFTR* mutations have been reported in patients with pancreatitis *(20)*, disseminated bronchiectasis *(21)*, and allergic bronchopulmonary aspergillosis *(22)*. Thus, the spectrum of diseases associated with *CFTR* mutations includes not only classic CF, but also several other chronic diseases *(2,23)*.

Testing

SWEAT CHLORIDE TESTING

For decades, measurement of sweat chloride concentrations has been used for laboratory diagnosis of CF. Sweat is collected by iontophoresis, a technique that involves applying a low voltage through an area of skin upon which a drug such as pilocarpine has been applied. Sweat is collected and the chloride concentration is measured. This test can give false-positive results in infants younger than 48 h of age, and therefore testing should be delayed until at least 48 h after birth. Other laboratory analyses of sweat, such as measurements of osmolality or conductivity, are considered to be screening rather than diagnostic and should not replace a quantitative sweat chloride test for diagnostic purposes *(24)*. A sweat chloride concentration value that is >60 mmol/L is consistent with a diagnosis of CF, although a few other diseases are also associated with sweat chloride concentrations of this magnitude *(10)*. A value of >40 mmol/L is considered normal but does not exclude a diagnosis of CF *(10)*. Between 40 and 60 mmol/L is a borderline range that may indicate the presence of CF.

IMMUNOREACTIVE TRYPSINOGEN

Immunoreactive trypsinogen (IRT) was first reported to be elevated in blood from newborns with CF in 1979 *(25)*. It is thought that trypsinogen, which is produced by the exocrine glands of the pancreas, enters the circulation because of obstruction of pancreatic ducts in patients with CF. IRT can be measured in blood spots collected on filter cards for newborn screening tests. Different laboratories use different cutoff levels for determining a positive result, but the value is usually based on the 99th centile of IRT values for each laboratory. As might be expected, with lower cutoff values the test is more sensitive for identifying infants with CF, but also less specific (i.e., more false-positive results are produced). False-positive results are more frequent among African-American infants (who have a lower risk of CF than do Caucasians) and among infants with low Apgar scores at birth *(26)*. As with any laboratory test, the positive predictive value depends on the specificity of the test (i.e., the false-positive rate) and on the prevalence of the disease in the population being tested. Several centers screen with IRT and perform *CFTR* mutation analysis on samples with the highest IRT levels (e.g., ≥99th centile). Newborns with at least one CF-causing mutation are referred for sweat chloride testing. Reported positive predictive values of this approach for detecting the presence of CF from several large CF newborn screening programs range from 15 to 37%, substantially higher than the approx 5–6% positive predictive value of IRT testing alone *(26–28)*.

CFTR MUTATION TESTING

DNA testing is of use in confirming a diagnosis in a suspected CF patient. Knowing the specific mutations present in an affected child is useful for genetic counseling of the parents, who can be offered some guidance on the likely severity of the disease, although the relationship between genotype and phenotype is not always consistent *(29)*. Mutation identification in a proband reveals the mutations present in the family and provides information for determining the CF status in future offspring. As with all autosomal recessive diseases, each child of two carrier parents has a 1-in-4 risk of being affected. Very rarely, patients with CF have uniparental disomy for *CFTR* and adjacent regions of chromosome 7 *(30)*. These patients have inherited two copies of a mutant allele from one parent and no allele from the other parent (*see* Chap. 2). This possibility should be considered in families in which only one parent is found to be a carrier of a *CFTR* mutation and the child is homozygous for that mutation.

Because of the large number of *CFTR* mutations that can cause CF, it is not always feasible to identify both mutations in an affected patient. The success rate depends on the ethnic group involved (although most patients are Caucasian) and on the number of mutations that are tested. Currently, several commercial reference laboratories are offering panels that will identify both mutations in approx 90% of patients in the general population *(10)*. The panel of 25 mutations recommended by the American College of Medical Genetics for carrier screening will detect approx 80% of mutations among Caucasians *(31)*.

SCREENING FOR CF CARRIERS

In 1997, a National Institutes of Health (NIH) Consensus Conference on CF Screening recommended that the following groups be offered CF mutation testing to identify carriers: adults with a positive family history of CF, partners of patients with CF, couples currently planning a pregnancy, and couples seeking prenatal care. Naturally, the latter two groups comprise a very large number of people. In 2001, the American College of Medical Genetics (ACMG) issued recommendations for laboratory standards and population screening for CF carriers, bearing in mind the widely different frequency of CF mutations in different ethnic groups, and the different numbers of mutations that account for the majority of known mutations in these ethnic groups *(31)*. These guidelines distinguish between ethnic groups to which CF carrier testing should be offered and those to which it should be made available. People belonging to non-Jewish Caucasian and Ashkenazi Jewish ethnic groups should be offered CF carrier testing. These are the groups with the highest CF carrier frequencies and the greatest likelihood of mutation identification using a limited panel of mutations. Among other ethnic groups, there are lower carrier rates, and larger panels of mutations must be tested to achieve a satisfactory mutation detection rate (e.g., >80%). For these groups, it is recommended that CF carrier testing be made available and that information about success in detecting mutations in these groups be provided through educational and other means. In 2001, the American College of Obstetrics and Gynecology recommended that CF screening be offered to pregnant Caucasian and Ashkenazi couples and made available to couples in other ethnic groups. This marked the first widespread implementation of screening for carriers of genetic disease.

According to published guidelines, carrier screening should be performed on both members of a couple at the same time (couple-based screening), if possible. Alternatively, a sequential testing strategy can be used in which one partner, usually the woman, is screened; if she is found to be a carrier, then the partner can be tested. The choice of couple-based or sequential testing is decided by the physician and the couple.

Table 4
American College of Medical Genetics Recommended Core Mutation Panel
for General Population CF Carrier Screening

Standard Mutation Panel
ΔF508
ΔI507
G542XG551DW1282X
N1303K
R553X621+1G→T
R117H1717-1G→A
A455ER560T
R1162X
G85E
R334W
R347P 711+1G→T
1898+1G→A
2184delA
1078delT
3849+10kbC→T
2789+5G→A
3659delC
I148T
3120+1G→A
Reflex Tests
I506V,[a]
I507V,[a]
F508C[a]
5T/7T/9Tb[b]

[a] Benign variants. This test distinguishes between a CF mutation and these benign variants. I506V, I507V, and F508C are performed only as reflex tests for unexpected homozygosity for ΔF508 and/or ΔI507.

[b] 5T *in cis* can modify R117H phenotype or alone can contribute to bilateral absence of the vas deferens (CBAVD); 5T analysis is performed only as a reflex test for R117H positives.

Reproduced with permission from ref. *31,* © Lippincott Williams & Wilkins and the American College of Medical Genetics.

Mutations to Test in Carrier Screening Programs The 2001 ACMG guidelines recommended that a panel of 25 mutations, comprising a representation of mutations seen in the general U.S. population with a frequency of $\geq 0.1\%$, be included in the testing panel. These mutations are shown in Table 4. This panel is applicable to the United States. In other countries, local CF carrier frequencies may not justify carrier screening, or an alternative panel of mutations may be more appropriate for carrier screening.

HEREDITARY HEMOCHROMATOSIS

Hereditary hemochromatosis (HH) is an autosomal recessive disease usually caused by mutations in the *HFE* gene on chromosome 6p. Approximately 1 in 200 to 1 in 400 people of northern European ancestry are affected by this disease, and approximately 1 in 10 of the population in the United States and parts of northwestern Europe is a heterozygous carrier. Mutations in *HFE* are very uncommon in other racial groups; however, the existence of other genes that predispose to iron overload disorders has been demonstrated. These disorders include African siderosis, juvenile hemochromatosis, neonatal hemochromatosis, and aceruloplasminemia *(32)*.

Patients with HH accumulate increased amounts of iron because of abnormally high absorption of iron in the duodenum. Whereas normal subjects absorb approx 1–2 mg of iron per day, subjects with HH absorb almost double this amount. In contrast to this active absorption of iron, there exist few physiological mechanisms by which the metal can be excreted from the body. The major routes are losses that occur during shedding of gastrointestinal epithelial cells and, in women, menstrual blood loss. The relative increase in iron absorption in patients with HH over many decades leads to significant iron accumulation and deposition in many tissues, including the liver, spleen, bone marrow, pancreas, pituitary, synovium of joints, and heart. Clinical manifestations include hepatic injury, diabetes resulting from damage to the pancreas, cardiomyopathy, arthritis, and skin discoloration because of iron deposition. Arthritis and fatigue are common presenting symptoms. Because of menstrual blood losses, females are less commonly symptomatic during their reproductive years than are males of similar ages.

Damage to these organs can be recognized by laboratory anomalies such as increased serum transaminase levels, decreased serum albumin, prolongation of prothrombin times, and elevated glucose levels. However, these tests are not specific for hemochromatosis and are not sufficiently sensitive in early disease that a normal result would exclude a diagnosis of hemochromatosis. More specific and sensitive laboratory tests for hemochromatosis include measurement of serum iron, total iron binding capacity (TIBC), and ferritin.

Iron in plasma is bound to transferrin, which is a carrier protein that transports iron in the Fe(III) form and delivers it to tissues. Each transferrin molecule can bind two Fe(III) ions. Cellular uptake of iron involves binding of transferrin to a cell membrane receptor. The transferrin/transferrin receptor complex undergoes endocytosis and the liberated iron is made available for incorporation into heme or non-heme iron-containing proteins, or stored in ferritin. Each ferritin molecule can hold several thousand iron atoms as Fe(III) oxyhydroxide. The ratio of serum iron to TIBC is known as the iron saturation, and this is normally expressed as a percentage, (iron/TIBC) × 100%. Iron saturation values > 60% in males and >50% in females are highly suggestive of hemochromatosis, and increased ferritin levels (>300 µg/L) are common in this disease. Although serum ferritin levels are a measure of the magnitude of iron stores, this protein also rises in acute-phase reactions, and therefore increased serum levels of ferritin are not specific for iron overload disorders.

The degree of liver damage in hemochromatosis is an important prognostic marker. Hepatic injury is characterized by cirrhosis and an increased risk of hepatocellular carcinoma. Iron accumulation can be measured in biopsy samples of liver. The amount of iron/gram of liver tissue (micromoles of iron per gram dry weight) divided by the patient's age is known as the hepatic iron index. Values greater than 1.9 are useful in distinguishing iron overload owing to hereditary hemochromatosis from other causes such as alcoholism and hepatitis C infection.

Genetics

For several decades, it was known that the HH gene locus was near the *HLA* genes on chromosome 6p. A particular HLA class I gene, *A3,* was known to be present in most patients with HH, indicating linkage disequilibrium between this allele and a disease-causing mutation in an unknown gene. In 1996, the *HFE* gene (initially named *HLA-H*) was identified as being responsible for the common form of HH among Caucasians. Surprisingly, the protein encoded by this gene is structurally related to the HLA class I genes *(33).* Like the HLA class I proteins, *HFE* associates with β2-microglobulin in the cell membrane. It is believed that HFE protein regulates iron uptake into cells by interacting with the transferrin receptor in the cell membrane and decreasing the affinity of the receptor for transferrin *(34)*. Once transferrin has bound to its receptor, it is taken into cells by endocytosis, transferrin is degraded, and the iron is liberated. By regulating the binding of transferrin to its receptor, HFE can regulate the amount of iron that is taken into a cell. In this way, HFE acts as a negative regulator of cellular iron stores.

MUTATIONS IN HFE

Homozygosity for an *HFE* missense mutation, Cys282→Tyr (C282Y), is found in approximately 83% of patients with HH. This mutation, which arises from a single point mutation, G→A at nucleotide 845 of *HFE,* replaces a cysteine residue that is critical for formation of an intramolecular disulfide bond in the α3 domain of the protein, and it disrupts binding of HFE to β2-microglobulin. The protein containing this mutation is not expressed on the cell membrane because of a failure of normal processing in the endoplasmic reticulum and Golgi, as well as decreased stability *(35)*. In the absence of HFE protein on the cell membrane, the negative regulation that this protein normally exerts on binding of transferrin to its receptor is removed. This leads to increased cellular uptake and storage of iron, particularly in the tissues described above.

Based on haplotype analysis of other genetic markers around *HFE,* it is believed that the C282Y mutation arose 60–70 generations ago in a Celtic individual *(36)*. Most people of northern European ancestry who carry this mutation (approx 10% of the white population in the United States) are descendents of this single individual.

The second mutation found in *HFE* is His63Asp, which arises from a point mutation, C→G, at nucleotide 187. The replacement of a histidine by aspartate disrupts protein tertiary structure. Although this mutant protein is expressed on the cell surface, it does not interact normally with the transferrin receptor. Approximately 5% of subjects with HH are C282Y/H63D compound heterozygotes. Rarely, subjects with hemochromatosis are homozygous for this mutation. However, given the relatively high frequency of H63D among healthy controls (15% in many populations), it appears to have a lower penetrance than does C282Y. Estimates of the prevalence of C282Y and H63D in different populations are shown in Table 5.

Table 5
Estimated Prevalences (%) of C282Y and H63D in Selected Populations

Population	C282Y	H63D
Northern Europe	3.8	13.6
Irish	10	18.9
Danes	9.2	12.5
British	6.4	12.8
German	3.9	14.8
United States	5.4	13.5
Africa/Middle East	~0	2.6
Indian Subcontinent	0.2	8.4

Data from refs. *96* and *97.*

In addition to C282Y and H63D, several other mutations have been reported in *HFE*. One of these is S65C, which is found in 1–2% of European populations. Its significance remains unclear, and it may be a benign polymorphism. Several other rare mutations have also been described in a few families *(37)*.

Hereditary hemochromatosis is treated by regular (weekly) phlebotomy to remove excess iron, followed by a less intensive maintenance schedule. Each unit (approx 450 mL) of blood removed contains approximately 200–250 mg of iron. A commonly stated goal of therapeutic phlebotomy is a serum ferritin in the low-normal range (approx <50 µg/L). In one study of newly diagnosed patients, this was achieved by an average of 30 phlebotomies *(38)*.

Because of the relatively high frequency of this disease, the serious morbidity and mortality associated with untreated hemochromatosis, and the therapeutic benefits, there is much interest in population screening for this disease. The College of American Pathologists (CAP), the Centers for Disease Control and Prevention (CDC), and the American Hemochromatosis Society (AHS) have issued recommended guidelines for screening for HH *(39–41)*. These recommendations vary with respect to the numbers of people who would be screened. The CDC recommends screening for close family members of affected patients and for those with symptoms. The CAP recommends screening for all people over the age of 20, and the AHS recommends regular universal screening, even in childhood. All these organizations recommend that initial screening be performed by measurement of iron saturation. Importantly, although most recommendations include DNA testing as a follow-up to a positive transferrin saturation screening test, there is no consensus regarding the transferrin saturation that should be interpreted as a positive screening result. Recommendations for transferrin saturation range from 40% (AHS) to 60% (CAP). The choice of the transferrin saturation cutoff point for further evaluation is important. Higher cutoff points will improve the specificity of the test (i.e., reduce false positives) but decrease the sensitivity (i.e., increase false negatives). As a general principle, screening tests should be designed to maximize sensitivity; however, as the cutoff point for a positive transferrin saturation is lowered, the number of subjects with a false-positive screening test and the associated financial costs of confirmatory testing rise. Further study is needed to determine the optimal transferrin saturation that indicates the need for more extensive evaluation of a patient for hemochromatosis.

DNA testing for the common HH mutations is currently not recommended as a screening technique for the general population. Homozygosity for the common mutation, C282Y, is not necessarily indicative of the presence of hemochromatosis because of incomplete penetrance of the gene. Penetrance may be influenced by nongenetic factors such as low dietary iron, blood loss, or possibly other genetic factors. Moreover, as described above, locus heterogeneity is known to exist and so a DNA-based screening approach will fail to detect some affected individuals who have genetic hemochromatosis not caused by *HFE* mutations. DNA testing is useful, however, for investigation of relatives of persons known to carry an *HFE* mutation. Testing of asymptomatic relatives of known patients can be expected to yield a much higher rate of case identification than would be expected from general population screening because of the bias in favor of ascertaining subjects who have an increased likelihood of having at least one mutant gene. Subjects who are identified as harboring two mutations can be followed closely for evidence of iron overload.

Molecular Detection of *HFE* Mutations. Both C282Y and H63D alter restriction enzyme sites. A common method for detection of these mutations is therefore polymerase chain reaction (PCR) amplification of portions of *HFE,* followed by restriction enzyme digestion of the PCR product. The G→A transition at nucleotide 845, which is responsible for the C282Y mutation, cre-

Table 6
Hereditary Risk Factors for Venous Thrombosis

	Carrier frequency in Caucasian general population (%)	Prevalence in venous thrombosis (%)
Factor V Leiden	3–7	20
Prothrombin G20210A	2	6
Protein C deficiency	0.2–0.4	4
Protein S deficiency	Unknown	2
Antithrombin deficiency	0.02–0.16	2

Data from refs. *42* and *98*.

ates a restriction site for the enzyme *Rsa*I. The C→G mutation at nucleotide 187 that gives rise to the H63D mutation destroys an *Mbo*I site. Figure 13 in chapter 4 illustrates the use of PCR/restriction enzyme digestion for detection of the C282Y mutation. Commercial systems to detect these mutations are also available.

INHERITED THROMBOPHILIA

Venous thrombosis is a significant cause of morbidity and mortality. Thrombosis has a multifactorial etiology, as was described by the 19th century German pathologist Virchow, who attributed thrombosis to three general factors: changes in the vessel wall, decreases in blood flow rate, and alterations in the composition of blood. The molecular bases of several inherited abnormalities that increase the risk of thrombosis have been identified in recent years. These include surprisingly common mutations such as factor V Leiden and the G20210A mutation in the 3′ untranslated region of the prothrombin (factor II) gene. The principal genetic factors that are associated with an increased thrombotic risk are shown in Table 6. As would be expected of a multifactorial process, genetic risk factors act in concert with each other and with environmental factors such as oral contraceptive use or immobilization in predisposing an individual to a thrombotic event.

Factor V Leiden

Activated factor V (Va) is part of the prothrombinase complex, which also includes activated factor X (Xa) and phospholipid (Fig. 2).

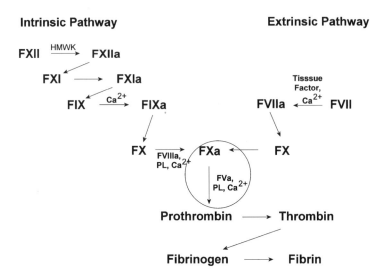

Fig. 2. The coagulation cascade. In the traditional model, the cascade is separated into the extrinsic and intrinsic pathways. Activated factor V is part of the pro-thrombinase complex that includes Xa, phospholipid (PL), and calcium (circled).

This complex is responsible for conversion of prothrombin to throm-bin, the enzyme that is responsible for conversion of fibrinogen to fib-rin. Factor Va functions by accelerating the reaction catalyzed by Xa. Once it has been activated, inactivation of factor Va is achieved by acti-vated protein C (APC), which is a serine protease that cleaves Va at three sites (Arg306, Arg506, and Arg679), bringing about its prote-olytic destruction. The first site to be cleaved is adjacent to Arg506. In factor V Leiden (FVL), a single point mutation in the factor V gene, G1691A, changes codon 506 from arginine to glutamine. The resulting protein, when activated, is resistant to proteolytic cleavage by APC, causing an increased thrombotic tendency. The relative risk of venous thrombosis has been estimated to be 3–7-fold greater than normal for heterozygous subjects and 80-fold greater for homozygotes *(42)*.

FVL is found in approx 5% of Caucasians and approximately 20% of Caucasian patients with deep venous thrombosis *(42)*. It is the most common mutation that predisposes to thrombosis in that ethnic group but is rarely found in African or Asian populations. In Caucasians, FVL is believed to be a founder mutation that appeared between 21,000 and 34,000 years ago *(43)*. The mutation occurred at a CpG dinucleotide, a hot spot for mutations *(see* Chap. 1).

CLINICAL MANIFESTATIONS

The presence of FVL alone predisposes to venous thrombosis and venous thromboembolism (VTE). Evidence that FVL causes arterial thrombosis is less clear. Characteristic sites for thrombosis are the deep veins of the lower limbs, but the risk of cerebral thrombosis is also significantly increased. FVL compounds the risk of VTE in patients who have other risk factors for VTE. For example, oral contraceptive use and pregnancy are each associated with a 4–6-fold increased risk of thrombosis, but combined oral contraceptive use and FVL are associated with a 35-fold increased risk, and combined pregnancy and FVL with a 7–16-fold increased risk of thrombosis (44). FVL is also associated with increased risk of recurrent pregnancy loss in the second and third trimesters, of placental abruption, and of preeclampsia. Just as combinations of FVL and estrogen exposure increase the risk of VTE, so too do combinations of FVL and other inherited thrombophilias, for example, heterozygosity for both FVL and prothrombin 20210A. In a large meta-analysis, this combination was associated with an odds ratio of 20 for VTE compared with 4.9 for FVL and 3.8 for prothrombin 202010A (45).

HR2 ALLELE

The HR2 allele of factor V is defined by six intragenic polymorphisms comprising a distinct haplotype. These include four amino acid substitutions, Met385Thr, His1299Arg, Met1736Val, and Asp2194Gly. This allele has been reported to be associated with lower normalized APC ratios measured in vitro (46). It appears to increase the risk of thrombosis in FVL heterozygous individuals, but whether it predisposes to thrombosis in subjects without FVL remains unclear, because of conflicting data from different studies (47–50).

DETECTION OF FVL BY MOLECULAR METHODS

Molecular testing for FVL provides definitive identification of this mutation in affected patients and can be performed on samples from patients who have been anticoagulated. Various molecular approaches have been used to characterize the mutation. The FVL mutation destroys a restriction site for *Mnl*I. This forms the basis of a convenient PCR/restriction enzyme digestion assay. Other methods in use in clinical laboratories in the United States include LightCycler® and Invader® (*see* Chap. 4).

DETECTION OF FVL BY ACTIVATED PROTEIN C RESISTANCE ASSAY

Approximately 5% of patients with APC resistance do not have FVL *(51,52)*. For this reason, DNA testing alone for the FVL may miss some patients who have APC caused by non-Leiden mutations in factor V, or by other etiologies. First-generation testing protocols for activated protein C resistance were based on measuring the activated partial thromboplastin time (aPTT) with and without addition of exogenous APC. Treatment of plasma with APC leads to breakdown of factor Va and factor VIIIa and so prolongs the aPTT. In normal subjects, the ratio of the aPTT in plasma that has been treated with APC to the aPTT in an untreated sample is >2.0. In subjects with FVL it is <2.0 *(53)*.

Second-generation assays involve predilution of the patient sample with factor V-deficient plasma *(54)*. This modification corrects for some other abnormalities such as factor VIII deficiency, and some lupus anticoagulants and may neutralize the effect of heparin *(55)*. This modification reportedly increases the sensitivity and specificity of the APC assay for identification of FVL to almost 100% *(56)*. Some authors recommend that the APC assay be used for screening in patients with thrombosis and that molecular testing for FVL be reserved for samples with borderline results, or for confirmation of positive results *(57)*.

Prothrombin G20210A

Prothrombin G20210A is found in approx 3% of Caucasians but rarely among African or Asian populations. This mutation in the prothrombin gene is in the 3′ untranslated region of the gene. Unlike FVL, the prothrombin 20210A mutation does not alter the sequence of the encoded protein but leads to increased plasma levels of prothrombin by a mechanism involving increased mRNA accumulation and protein synthesis *(58)*. Increased levels of prothrombin cause a thrombotic tendency, which has been estimated to be threefold greater among heterozygotes than among normal subjects *(59)*.

CLINICAL MANIFESTATIONS

Prothrombin 20210A is associated with an increased risk of VTE, including deep venous thrombosis and cerebral vein thrombosis, but the magnitude of these associations is less than that seen with FVL. The mutation is also found with increased frequency among women with spontaneous pregnancy losses and complications, and in women with thrombotic complications associated with oral contraceptive use. An increased risk of myocardial infarction in women aged 18–44 who had the G20210A mutation has been reported *(60)*. The mutation was of greatest significance in these women if they also had other major risk factors for myocardial infarction such as smoking, obesity, hypertension, diabetes mellitus, or hypercholesterolemia.

DETECTION

Prothrombin G20210A does not alter a restriction site. PCR-based methods to detect this mutation employ mutagenic primers that create a restriction site in the PCR product if the mutation is present (*see* Chap. 4). Commercial assays such as Invader are available, but these are not currently Food and Drug Administration (FDA)-approved. Because of the wide range in plasma prothrombin levels, measurement of these cannot be used to identify the mutation in individual patients, and so molecular approaches are used.

Recommendations for Genetic Testing for FVL and Prothrombin G20210A

A CAP consensus conference has produced recommendations for FVL and prothrombin G20210A testing *(44,61)*. These are shown in Table 7. The ACMG has produced similar guidelines *(62)*.

HUNTINGTON'S DISEASE

Huntington's disease (HD; OMIM 143100) is an autosomal dominant disorder characterized by neurological degeneration leading to progressive dementia and chorea. Clumsiness and subtle behavioral changes are common in the early stages of the disease. Symptoms usually begin in middle age, but the onset of symptoms can occur at much younger or older ages. Approximately 1 in 10,000 individuals has HD.

The HD gene, *IT15,* is located on chromosome 4p16.3. Exon 1 contains a CAG repeat encoding a polyglutamine tract. In normal subjects, the number of CAG repeats varies from 10 to 26, with most alleles having 15–20 repeats. In patients with HD, the number of repeats varies from 36 to 121 repeats *(63),* with most mutant alleles having 40–50 repeats. In subjects with alleles containing repeats in the range of 36–41, there is variable penetrance of clinical dis-

Table 7

College of American Pathologists Consensus Conference Recommendations for Factor V Leiden and Prothrombin 20210A Testing

---

Testing for factor V Leiden (FVL) or prothrombin 20210A is recommended in the following situations:

1. History of recurrent venous thromboembolism (VTE)
2. First VTE at younger than 50 yr of age
3. First unprovoked VTE at any age
4. First VTE at an unusual anatomic site (e.g., cerebral, mesenteric, portal, or hepatic veins)
5. First VTE at any age in a subject who has a first-degree relative who had a VTE at younger than 50 yr of age
6. First VTE related to pregnancy, puerperium, or oral contraceptive use
7. First VTE related to hormone replacement therapy
8. Women with unexplained pregnancy loss in 2nd or 3rd trimester

Testing for FVL or prothrombin 20210A is controversial in the following situations:

1. Women smokers with myocardial infarction at younger than 50 yr of age
2. Patients aged over 50 yr with first VTE in the absence of cancer or intravascular device
3. First VTE related to selective estrogen receptor modulators or tamoxifen
4. Selected cases of women with unexplained severe preeclampsia, placental abruption, or intrauterine growth retardation

Testing for FVL or prothrombin 20210A may be indicated in the following situations after appropriate genetic counseling:

1. Asymptomatic adult family members of probands with known FVL mutations, especially those with a strong family history of thrombosis at younger than 50 yr of age
2. Asymptomatic family members who are pregnant or are considering oral contraceptives or pregnancy

Testing for FVL or prothrombin 20210A is not recommended in the following situations:

1. General population screening
2. As a routine initial test during pregnancy
3. As a routine test prior to or during oral contraceptive use, hormone replacement therapy, or selective estrogen receptor modulator therapy
4. As a prenatal test, initial newborn test, or routine test in asymptomatic prepubescent children
5. As a routine initial test in patients with arterial thrombotic events; however, testing for FVL may be considered in certain unusual situations, such as in patients with unexplained arterial thrombosis without atherosclerosis, or in young patients who smoke

---

ease, with resulting uncertainty about the advice that should be given during genetic counseling. Alleles with 27–35 repeats represent "intermediate alleles" or "mutable normal alleles," which are not associated with HD but which may be at risk of undergoing expansion during transmission to offspring, particularly during father-child transmission. Contraction of the CAG repeats can also occur during transmission from parent to child. There is an inverse correlation between the number of repeats and the age of onset of symptoms *(64)*. Cases of juvenile HD are associated with expansions of over 60 repeats.

New mutations have been described, but their frequency is uncertain, with estimates ranging from approx 1–3% of all cases of HD to ≥10% *(64)*. This variation may be partly caused by ascertainment biases that favor detection of patients with larger repeats associated with more severe disease and stronger family histories of HD. Patients with shorter repeats *(36–40)* may not develop symptoms until old age and may have a mild phenotype, leading to failure to recognize the presence of the disease in this group. It has been suggested that such patients have a higher rate of new mutations than do more severely affected patients *(64)*.

The mechanism of neuronal death in HD is not clear, but it is generally assumed to represent a gain-of-function mutation. It is of interest that patients with Wolf-Hirschhorn syndrome (OMIM 194190) have a heterozygous deletion of 4p– that includes *IT15*. These patients do not display evidence of HD, suggesting that HD is not caused by haploinsufficiency of *IT15*. Current evidence implicates a toxic effect of the polyglutamine tract on cell function *(65)*.

Molecular Detection of IT15 Expansions

Recommended guidelines for laboratory testing for HD have been published *(66)*. It is important to note that the CAG repeat region is adjacent to a CCG repeat region that is also polymorphic, with a range of 7–12 repeats. The presence of the CCG repeat has implications for the selection of PCR primers for laboratory diagnosis to ensure that accurate sizing of the CAG repeat is obtained.

Phenocopies of HD

Rarely, patients with symptoms of HD have normal numbers of repeats, indicating that phenocopies of the disease exist *(67)*. One such phenocopy has been identified as arising from a 192-bp insertion in the prion protein (PrP) gene, *PRNP*, on chromosome 20p12 *(68)*. This insertion encodes an octapeptide repeat. The existence of phenocopies of HD is an important consideration in evaluating suspected HD patients who do not have a CAG expansion in *IT15*.

FRAGILE X SYNDROME

Fragile X syndrome is an X-linked familial disorder the most important characteristic of which is mental retardation. The disease is uncommon, with approx 1 in 4000 males and 1 in 8000 females being affected. The name of this disease comes from the associated cytogenetic abnormality, namely, the appearance of a break or fragile site in the X chromosome, which can be observed after cells are cultured in media with a low folate concentration. This fragile site is the most common of several fragile sites on the X chromosome. The responsible gene, *FMR1*, is located at Xq27.3, which corresponds to the location of the fragile site.

Males with fragile X syndrome have mental retardation associated with autistic behavior. Physical features include a prominent jaw, large ears, and, in adulthood, enlarged testicles. Females are affected less commonly than males. The penetrance in females is reported to be 30%.

Fragile X syndrome is caused by an unstable trinucleotide (CGG) repeat in the 5′ untranslated region of the FMR1 gene. Among normal individuals, the number of copies of this repeat ranges from approx 5 to approx 44, with a mode of 29 or 30 repeats. The region of CGG repeats is interrupted in normal alleles by two AGG triplets at approximately the 10th and 20th repeats. These appear to be important for maintenance of the normal number of copies of the CGG repeat. At the upper end of the normal range is a "gray zone," in which alleles have approx 45 to approx 54 repeats.

Individuals with fragile X syndrome have more than 230 copies of the repeat and often have repeats numbering in the thousands. This is known as a full mutation. Between the upper end of the normal range of repeat numbers and the beginning of the range that is associated with clinical disease is the premutation range. This is defined as approx 55 to approx 200 repeats. Subjects with a premutation size allele do not have clinical manifestations of the disease.

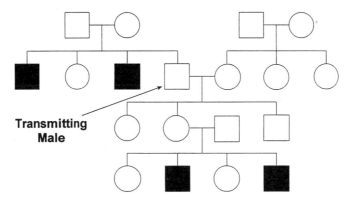

Fig. 3. Illustration of a transmitting male in a family with fragile X syndrome. The individual is implicated as having the abnormal chromosome, but because it does not carry a full expansion, he is asymptomatic. Both his brothers and his grandsons have full mutations.

However, alleles with repeat numbers that fall in the premutation range are at risk of undergoing expansion to a larger size, particularly during meiosis in females. The newly expanded allele can be either in the premutation range or in the full mutation range depending on the initial size of the repeat and the degree of expansion. Thus, a female with a premutation is at risk of having an offspring with a full mutation. The estimated risks of full expansion of a premutation allele are 13% for 56–59 repeats, 21% for 60–69 repeats, 58% for 70–79 repeats, 73% for 80–89 repeats, and 97% for 90–199 repeats *(69)*.

Because of the tendency toward expansion leading to a full mutation, pedigrees tend to show a higher percentage of affected individuals in successive generations. This observation was known as the *Sherman paradox* before the molecular basis of the disease was discovered. A second paradox was the existence of "transmitting males" in fragile X families. These are individuals who are carriers of the trait (as determined by analysis of the pedigree), but who do not manifest any clinical symptoms. In classical mendelian genetics, males who carry X-linked disease traits are affected. However, in the case of fragile X, it is possible that a male may be a premutation carrier and may transmit the disease allele but not be clinically affected. An illustration of this is shown in Fig. 3. The mechanism of the CGG expansion is unclear but is thought to be owing to slippage during DNA replication. The AGG triplets may be important in stabilizing the trinucleotide repeat region.

The large CGG expansion in full-mutation alleles induces methylation of the 5′ region of *FMR1,* including methylation of important regulatory elements such as the CpG island that are situated upstream of the gene. This methylation results in downregulation of *FMR1* transcription. In addition to potential direct effects of methylation on DNA transcription, methylation also leads to deacetylation of histone proteins that may also limit the ability of the transcription apparatus to produce *FMR1* transcripts. It is also known that translation of mRNA transcripts bearing a full CGG expansion is inefficient. Methylation therefore silences gene transcription, and the phenotype is believed to result from absence of production of the FMR1 protein (FMRP). Most patients with full mutations are somatic mosaics: different cells and tissues contain different numbers of copies of the repeat. This is presumably because of mitotic instability of the trinucleotide repeats. In addition to abnormal methylation as a cause of loss of FMRP, rare inactivating mutations in *FMR1* have been described including point mutations and deletions.

The function of FMRP is not yet well characterized, but the protein has been shown to be associated with polyribosomes, suggesting that it may be involved in translation of some mRNAs. Several RNA molecules have been identified that bind to FMRP and are involved in the formation of neuronal synapses *(70,71)*. RNA molecules that bind FMRP contain a *G-quartet*—a planar formation of four guanine residues. These findings suggest that disrupted translation of a few RNAs encoding proteins involved in synapse formation may underlie the mental retardation that is a hallmark of this disease.

Molecular Detection of Fragile X Syndrome

Molecular diagnosis of fragile X syndrome involves determination of the number of trinucleotide repeats and the methylation status of the gene. Southern analysis can be used for both purposes; however, PCR provides more accurate determination of the number of repeats in normal and smaller premutation alleles.

SOUTHERN BLOTTING

Southern analysis can be used to determine the number of CGG repeats and is particularly useful for this purpose in samples with full expansions. By using a methylation-sensitive restriction enzyme to digest genomic DNA, an assessment can also be made of the methylation status of *FMR1*.

The Southern blot approach is shown in Fig. 4. Genomic DNA is restricted with two enzymes, *Eco*RI and *Sac*II. The latter is a methylation-sensitive enzyme that will not cut if its target in genomic DNA is methylated. This enzyme is one of several that can be used to test for methylation at the CpG regulatory island upstream of *FMR1*. Depending on the gender of the subject and whether the CpG island is methylated, several different diagnostic patterns are seen (Fig. 4).

1. In DNA from normal males, the CpG island is not methylated—the gene must be transcribed—and so the restriction fragment detected by the probe is 2.8 kb in length.
2. In DNA from normal females, the CpG island is not methylated on active X chromosomes. This gives rise to the 2.8-kb fragment that is also seen in normal males. In X chromosomes that have been lyonized, the CpG island is methylated, and so *Sac*II fails to cut at this point. The resulting fragment is 5.2 kb in length, corresponding to the distance between the two *Eco*RI sites. A normal female DNA sample will therefore show two bands on Southern blot analysis.
3. DNA from a premutation male shows a small increase in size of the fragment between the *Eco*RI site and the *Sac*II site corresponding to the presence of a premutation. The *Sac*II site is not methylated in premutations.
4. DNA from a female carrying a single premutation shows a four-band pattern. The normal chromosome can be active or lyonized, and these give rise to the usual 2.8- and 5.2-kb fragments. The premutation chromosome can also be active or lyonized. Each of these gives rise to a fragment that is slightly longer than the normal 2.8 and 5.2 kb. The additional length is owing to the premutation.
5. DNA from an affected male shows a large increase in the length of the restriction fragment. This arises from two alterations. First, the large CGG expansion increases the fragment size. Second, abnormal methylation at the CpG island prevents *Sac*II cutting. The size of the expansion is indicative of the number of copies of the trinucleotide repeat. There is usually a range of fragment sizes, indicating mitotic instability.
6. DNA from an affected female shows the usual 2.8- and 5.2-kb fragments, corresponding to the normal X chromosome, which can be either active or lyonized. The chromosome carrying the full mutation shows a large expansion, as seen in an affected male.
7. Occasionally, some full-expansion alleles may not be completely methylated. These may appear as bands of <5.2 kb. In addition, mosaicism can be found in which alleles with different numbers of repeats are present.

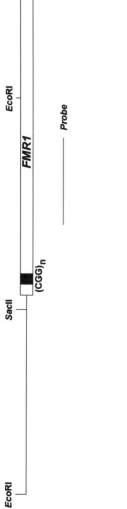

EcoRI

SacII

EcoRI

FMR1

(CGG)n

Probe

5.2 kb

2.8 kb

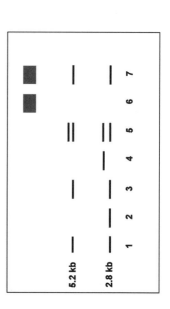

5.2 kb

2.8 kb

1 2 3 4 5 6 7

Fig. 4. Principle of Southern blot analysis of the *FMR1* gene. The positions of the restriction sites for *Eco*RI and *Sac*II are indicated. The CGG trinucleotide repeats are in the 5′ untranslated region of the gene. The typical position of the probe used for hybridization is indicated, as are the 5.2- and 2.8-kb restriction fragments to which the probe hybridizes. The patterns of possible hybridization are shown in the box and described in the text.

Suitable Tissues. Peripheral blood is the normal source of DNA used for fragile X analysis. Prenatal diagnosis can be performed on chorionic villus samples (CVS) or amniocytes; however, the methylation pattern of DNA in CVS is different from that of more mature tissues; in particular, the methylation associated with both normal lyonization and with full expansion of the CGG repeat may be absent. The ACMG has produced technical guidelines for laboratories that perform fragile X testing *(72)*.

POLYMERASE CHAIN REACTION

By selecting primers on either side of the trinucleotide repeat region, PCR can be performed across this region. The size of the resulting PCR product can be determined and depends on the number of copies of the CGG repeat. This approach is very convenient for producing accurate measurements of repeats that are numbered in the normal and lower premutation ranges. Because of the difficulties of performing PCR across larger numbers of CGG repeats, this technique is less commonly used in clinical laboratories for analysis of large premutations or full expansions, for which the number of CGG repeats can number in the thousands. DNA from males with a full expansion usually fails to produce an observable PCR product, a phenomenon that is not without diagnostic importance.

MITOCHONDRIAL DISORDERS

The mitochondrial genome is 16.6 kb in length and encodes 13 polypeptides that are components of mitochondrial respiratory chain complexes, 22 tRNAs, and 2 rRNAs. Each mitochondrion can contain 5–10 copies of the mitochondrial genome, and each somatic cell can contain hundreds of mitochondria. Mutations in polypeptides that are subunits of a respiratory chain enzyme are generally associated with a phenotype caused by deficiency of the enzyme in question, whereas mutations in a mitochondrial tRNA may be associated with a more extensive phenotype because of the more general impairment in protein synthesis.

Mitochondrial genetics show three features that differ from nuclear genetics. First, mitochondria are maternally transmitted. Each oocyte contains up to 100,000 mitochondria. Disease-causing mitochondrial mutations are therefore transmitted from mother to children but are not transmitted by fathers to their offspring. Second, all mitochondria do not necessarily have the same genome. In the case of disease-causing mutations, any cell may have a mixture of normal mitochondria and mutant mitochondria. This phenomenon is known as heteroplasmy. Third, in the case of heteroplasmy, the expression of a disease phenotype depends on the ratio of normal to mutant mitochondria. Although a deleterious mutation may be present, it may not manifest as a disease phenotype until a critical threshold of impaired biochemical function is reached. This threshold may vary according to a cell's energy requirements and the nature of the mutation itself. Most mitochondrial disorders manifest phenotypically principally in tissues that have a high metabolic activity including skeletal muscle, neurons, heart, and some endocrine tissues.

In addition to these differences in pattern of genetic inheritance between mitochondria and the nucleus, mitochondria also use a slightly different genetic code that is similar to that of prokaryotes. A commonly held theory of the origin of mitochondria is that these subcellular organelles are derived from a prokaryote. Of clinical importance in this regard is the association between aminoglycoside toxicity and a mutation, A1555G, in the mitochondrial 12S ribosomal subunit gene (*see* Chap. 10) *(73)*. Aminoglycosides exert their antibiotic effect by inhibiting prokaryotic ribosomes, and it is believed that the A1555G mutation renders cochlear mitochondria highly susceptible to aminoglycoside-induced toxicity.

It is also important to bear in mind that mitochondrial disorders may arise from mutations in nuclear genes that encode mitochondrial proteins. The majority of proteins that are present in mitochondria are encoded by nuclear genes. In the case of a mutation in a nuclear gene encoding a mitochondrial protein, the disease inheritance pattern is one of the classic mendelian patterns discussed in Chapter 2, and heteroplasmy is not seen.

Examples of Mitochondrial Disorders Caused by Mutations in MtDNA

LEBER'S HEREDITARY OPTIC NEUROPATHY

Leber's hereditary optic neuropathy (LHON; OMIM 535000) is characterized principally by deterioration or loss of central vision. Usually both eyes are affected within a few months, leading to severe visual impairment. The disease affects males more commonly than females, and onset is usually in adolescence or early adulthood, although it may become manifest at any age. Approximately 90% of patients harbor one of three mtDNA mutations (3460A, 11778A, and 14484C); however, other mutations have also been been reported to be associated with LHON. Of the three listed, 11778A is the most common, being found in approx 50% of patients, and is also associated with the worst prognosis. On the other hand, 14484C is associated with a relatively favorable prognosis.

A mitochondrial mutation is not by itself sufficient for development of LHON, although it is a requirement. Other factors that influence disease expression include age and gender. Variable penetrance has been observed even in families that are homoplasmic for a mtDNA mutation. Approximately 40% of patients do not have a family history of the disease.

KEARNS-SAYRE SYNDROME

Kearns-Sayre syndrome (KSS; OMIM 530000) is characterized by progressive external ophthalmoplegia (weakness of the external muscles of the eye), pigmentary retinopathy, age of onset under 20 yr, and one of the following: high cerebrospinal fluid protein concentration, cardiac conduction block, or ataxia *(74)*. Additional, variably present features include weakness of the skeletal muscles, deafness, short stature, and diabetes or other endocrine disorders such as diabetes, hypogonadism, hypoparathyroidism, and growth hormone deficiency. KSS has been found to be associated with both deletions and duplications of mtDNA .

MYOCLONIC EPILEPSY WITH RAGGED RED FIBERS

Myoclonic epilepsy with ragged red fibers (MERRF; OMIM 545000) is a mitochondrial encephalomyopathy characterized by a constellation of symptoms that includes myoclonic epilepsy, ataxia, deafness, and ragged red fibers. The latter are seen on muscle biopsies stained with Gomori's modified trichrome stain and represent subsarcolemmal aggregates of mitochondria. In up to 90% of patients, MERRF is caused by a point mutation, A8344G, in the mitochondrial tRNALys gene *(75,76)*.

MITOCHONDRIAL MYOPATHY, ENCEPHALOPATHY, LACTIC ACIDOSIS, AND STROKE-LIKE EPISODES

Mitochondrial myopathy, encephalopathy, lactic acidosis, and stroke-like episodes (MELAS; OMIM 540000) is characterized by episodic vomiting, developmental delay in children, headaches and seizures, metal retardation or dementia, and stroke-like episodes characterized by hemiparesis, hemianopia, cortical blindness, and sensorineural deafness. The stroke-like episodes usually have an acute onset and may be transient. The mean age of onset of symptoms is 10 yr, commonly with migraine-like headaches and vomiting. Exercise tolerance is reduced. Neurological function deteriorates with time, and death commonly occurs by the fourth decade. Seizures are common and may be exacerbated by valproate, a commonly used antiepileptic drug (77). Muscle biopsy shows ragged red fibers in most patients; however, this finding is not specific for MELAS . Eighty percent of patients carry a point mutation, A3243G, in the gene encoding mitochondrial tRNA[Leu] (78), and a further 8% have another point mutation, T3271C, in the same gene (79).

Example of Mitochondrial Disorders Caused by Mutations in Nuclear DNA

FRIEDREICH'S ATAXIA

Friedreich's ataxia is an autosomal recessive disease caused by mutations in *FRDA*. The disease, which has an incidence of 1 in 20,000, is characterized by a triad that includes preadolescent onset of symptoms, progressive cerebellar dysfunction, and hypoactive reflexes in the lower limbs. An axonal sensory neuropathy can be demonstrated by electrophysiological studies (80). Other symptoms may include cardiomyopathy, kyphoscoliosis, optic atrophy, hearing loss, and diabetes mellitus. The range and progression of symptoms can be variable, even between affected siblings.

FRDA is on chromosome 9q13. The gene is composed of seven exons spread over 95 kb and encodes a 1.3-kb transcript. The encoded protein is termed frataxin. Alternative splice products have been described, but their function is unknown. The most common mutation, found in approx 96–98% of mutant alleles, is an expansion of a GAA trinucleotide repeat in intron 1. Normal subjects have

≤40 repeats, and affected individuals have approx 66–1700 repeats *(80,81)*. Other mutations have also been described. In general, longer trinucleotide expansions are associated with earlier age of onset and with more severe disease. This is related to lower levels of production of the protein.

Decreased frataxin levels appear to result in accumulation of iron in mitochondria. This excess iron may lead to production of free radicals with resulting oxidative damage to mitochondria *(81)*.

INBORN ERRORS OF METABOLISM

In many countries, public health programs exist for early identification of newborns with certain congenital diseases. The rationale for widespread testing for these disorders in the newborn period is that appropriate intervention is available that can dramatically alter the outcome for affected patients if a diagnosis is made very early in life. The list of diseases that are included in newborn screening programs varies among jurisdictions; however, the following are nearly always included in such programs: hyperphenylalaninemias, galactosemia, sickle cell anemia, and hypothyroidism. Other disorders that are tested in some programs include maple syrup urine disease, congenital adrenal hyperplasia, biotinidase deficiency, homocystinuria, and medium chain acyl-CoA dehydrogenase (MCAD) deficiency (Table 8). With increasing use of tandem mass spectrometry for analysis of blood spots, a wider number of diseases, some of which are very rare, can be detected.

Phenylketonuria

Phenylketonuria (PKU; OMIM 261600) is an autosomal recessive disease usually caused by mutations in the phenylalanine hydroxylase gene, *PAH*, located on chromosome 12q22-q24.1. PKU results from decreases in activity of phenylalanine hydroxylase, the enzyme that catalyzes the conversion of the amino acid phenylalanine to tyrosine. In <3% of patients, the deficiency of PAH activity is caused by defects in the synthesis or recycling of tetrahydrobiopterin (BH_4), an essential cofactor of PAH. Expression of the clinical features of the disease requires both genetic and environmental factors, the latter being dietary exposure to phenylalanine, an essential amino acid.

Table 8
Tests Performed in Newborn Screening Programs

Disease	Clinical features	Genes
Phenylketonuria	Mental retardation, seizures, developmental delay, autistic behavior	Phenylalanine hydroxylase, dihydropteridine reductase
Galactosemia	Hepatomegaly, liver failure, cataracts, mental retardation, *E. coli* sepsis	Galactose-1-phosphate uridylyl transferase
	Cataracts in infancy	Galactokinase
Homocystinuria	Lens dislocation, thrombosis, mental retardation, seizures, developmental delay, marfanoid habitus, scoliosis, osteoporosis	Cystathionine β-synthetase
Maple syrup urine disease	Lethargy, irritability, ketoacidosis, metabolic coma	Branched chain ketoacid decarboxylase (not monogenic because of subunits)
Congenital adrenal hyperplasia	Salt-wasting crisis, virilization of affected females	Steroid 21-hydroxylase (*CYP21*)
	Virilization of affected females, hypertension	Steroid 11β-hydroxylase (*CYP11B*)
Congenital hypothyroidism	Cretinism	Usually non-genetic or complex genetic, but some genes identified (*see* text)
Biotinidase deficiency	Alopecia, seizures, skin rash hypotonia, developmental delay, metabolic coma	Biotinidase
Sickle cell anemia	Anemia, sickling crises, infections	β-Globin
Medium-chain acyl-CoA dehydrogenase deficiency (and other fatty acid oxidation defects caused by deficiencies of acyl-CoA dehydrogenases)	Hypoglycemia, hyperammonemia hepatomegaly, metabolic crisis, elevated acylcarnitine	MCAD, SCAD, LCAD

A variety of degrees of severity of enzyme impairment are recognized and are associated with severity of clinical disease. These conditions are collectively termed hyperphenylalaninemias, and the most severe form is classic PKU. Non-PKU hyperphenylalaninemias represent milder forms of the disease. Hyperphenylalaninemia is associated with a plasma phenylalanine level of >120 μM, whereas PKU is associated with plasma phenylalanine levels of >1000 μM. Classic PKU is associated with severe psychomotor retardation, autistic behavior, seizures, skin rash, microcephaly, and light pigmentation.

With the advent of successful dietary management of newborns with PKU, these patients can expect a normal life and reproductive potential. Mothers with PKU must adhere strictly to a low-phenylalanine diet and be carefully monitored to avoid the teratogenic effects of hyperphenylalaninemia in their fetuses. Maternal PKU is associated with psychomotor retardation, microcephaly, intrauterine growth retardation, and congenital heart defects in the offspring of PKU mothers who receive inadequate medical care during pregnancy.

CLINICAL FEATURES

Clinical features of classic PKU include mental retardation, psychosis, seizures, an eczema-like skin rash, and a "mousy" odor. Biochemical features include elevated levels of phenylalanine (>20 mg/dL) and accumulation and excretion of phenylketones. PKU has an incidence of approx 1 in 10,000 to 1 in 25,000 newborns in the United States. The disease is more common in Caucasians and Native Americans than in other ethnic groups.

SCREENING FOR AFFECTED NEWBORNS

A positive screening result for PKU is established by identification of elevated phenylalanine levels in blood spots collected on filter paper from newborns. The original Guthrie test is a semi-quantitative microbiological assay in which *Bacillus subtilus* spores are grown on an agar plate containing an inhibitor of L-phenylalanine. Discs from the filter paper are applied to the agar. Phenylalanine in the dried blood spot diffuses into the surrounding agar, allowing growth of the bacteria. The extent of the zone of growth around the disc indicates the amount of phenylalanine in the disc. In many centers, microbiological assays have been replaced by quantitative measurements of phenylalanine. Tandem mass spec-

Table 9
Common Mutations in the Phenylalanine Hydroxylase
Gene in Europeans

Mutation	Prevalence (%)[a]
R408W	31
IVS12nt+1g→a	11
IVS10nt-11g→a	6
I65T	5
Y414C	5
R261Q	4

[a] Prevalences are among affected patients.
Data from ref. 99.

trometry allows for rapid measurement of multiple amino acids and can be used to screen for several inborn errors of metabolism *(82)*.

MOLECULAR GENETICS

Approximately 400 *PAH* mutations have been identified to date; however, more than 60% of all mutations in Caucasians are accounted for by just six mutations, shown in Table 9. A listing of mutations and their phenotypic associations is maintained at http://data.mch.mcgill.ca/pahdb_new/.

Galactosemia

Galactosemia (OMIM 230400) is caused by an inability to metabolize galactose. The major dietary source of galactose is the milk sugar lactose, which is a disaccharide composed of glucose and galactose. Lactose is converted to these monosaccharides by lactase, an enzyme present in the small intestine. Conversion of galactose to glucose requires several enzyme-catalyzed reactions, shown in Fig. 5. Galactosemia can be caused by one of several enzymatic deficiencies, all of which are inherited as autosomal recessive disorders. The most common, and the one associated with classic galactosemia, is deficiency of galactose-1-phosphate uridylyltransferase (GALT).

GALACTOSE-1-PHOSPHATE URIDYLYLTRANSFERASE DEFICIENCY

Deficiency of GALT (OMIM 230400) is the mechanism underlying classic galactosemia. This is a severe metabolic disease characterized by cataract formation in infancy, mental retardation,

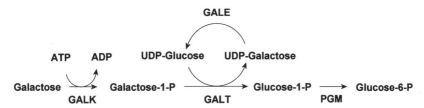

Fig. 5. The Leloir pathway of galactose metabolism. To convert galactose to glucose, a series of enzymatic steps is required. These include steps that are catalyzed by galactokinase (GALK), galactose-1-phosphate uridylyltransferase (GALT), and phosphoglucomutase (PGM). UDP-galactose-4-epimerase catalyzes the interconversion of UDP-galactose and UDP-glucose.

hepatomegaly, and a substantial risk of neonatal *E. coli* sepsis. Even with stringent avoidance of dairy products, there is a high frequency of ovarian failure in women with this disorder. The prevalence of GALT deficiency varies from approx 1 in 23,000 in Ireland to less than 1 in a million in Japan *(83,84)*. Based on population samples, it is estimated that the incidence in the Caucasian population is approx 1 in 47,000 to 1 in 80,000; in the African-American population, it is approx 1 in 25,000 *(85)*. Newborn screening for galactosemia is commonly performed by measurement of GALT activity in rehydrated blood spots from newborn filter cards.

Duarte and Los Angeles Alleles. The *GALT* gene is located on 9p13. Frequent mutations include Q188R, K285N, and S135L. The last of these is found in African Americans *(85)*. The Duarte allele, which is the most common deficiency allele, includes a missense mutation (N314D), a deletion of 4 bp in the promoter region, and several intron mutations. This variant is associated with approx 75% of normal activity in heterozygotes and 50% of normal activity in homozygotes. Patients who are compound heterozygotes for a classic galactosemia mutation and the Duarte allele (D/G compound heterozygotes) have approx 5–20% of normal enzyme activity. The Los Angeles allele, which has increased enzyme activity, is also characterized by N314D but does not have the promoter mutation or intron mutations. It also contains a silent codon polymorphism, C1721T (Leu218Leu). At the protein level, both the Duarte and Los Angeles variants are identical and differ from wild-type *GALT* only by the N314D substitution. The decreased activity of the Duarte allele appears to be primarily attributable to the 4-bp promoter deletion, which causes decreased gene transcription *(86)*. In a panethnic population in the United States, the Duarte and Los Angeles alleles were found to be present at frequencies of 5.1 and 2.7% *(85)*.

Galactokinase Deficiency

Deficiency of galactokinase (OMIM 230300) is caused by mutations in the *GALK* gene. The cardinal feature of galactokinase deficiency is cataract formation in the first few months of life, which has been attributed to accumulation of galactitol. The other features associated with classic galactosemia, notably mental retardation and hepatic toxicity, are not present. The disease is rare, with an incidence of 1 in 150,000 to 1 in 1,000,000 newborns *(87)*.

UDP-Galactose-4-Epimerase Deficiency

UDP-galactose-4-epimerase (epimerase) (OMIM 230350) deficiency exists in two forms: a more severe, generalized deficiency, and a milder form, sometimes called *peripheral,* that is restricted to epimerase deficiency in red cells. The generalized form is extremely rare and is characterized by features of classic galactosemia with long-term growth retardation and learning difficulties *(88)*. In understanding the varying clinical severity associated with epimerase deficiency, it should be noted that, in addition to catalyzing interconversion of UDP-galactose and UDP-glucose, this enzyme also catalyzes the interconversion of UDP-N-acetylglucosamine and UDP-N-acetylgalactosamine. These latter compounds are important in the synthesis of polysaccharides and glycosylated peptides, particularly in the central nervous system. Different mutations have variable effects on each reaction *(89)*. One mutation, V94M, has been observed in several patients with the severe, generalized form of the disease *(89)*.

Congenital Hypothyroidism

Congenital hypothyroidism (CH) affects approx 1 in 3000 to 1 in 4000 newborns in the Caucasian population but is much less common among African Americans (approx 1 in 30,000). Both transient and permanent forms of CH are recognized; this discussion pertains to permanent forms. Normal thyroid function is essential for mental and physical development in infancy and childhood, and insufficiency of thyroid hormones is associated with cretinism. The common etiologies of CH are thyroid dysgenesis and defects involving pathways of thyroid hormone synthesis.

Primary CH is characterized by increased levels of thyrotropin (TSH) and decreased levels of thyroxine. In more than 80% of patients, permanent congenital hypothyroidism is caused by failure of normal development of the thyroid gland (agenesis: 35–40%; ectopic location: 35–40%; or hypoplasia: 5%; OMIM 218700). The vast majority of these cases are sporadic, and the mechanisms underlying the developmental abnormality are generally unknown. Females are more commonly affected than males. In a few sporadic cases and familial cases, mutations involving specific genes have been identified. These include the *PAX8* gene, which encodes a transcription factor, and the thyroid transcription factor-1 and -2 genes, *TTF1* and *TTF2 (90–92).*

A few known defects in hypothalamic and pituitary function can lead to CH. These include mutations in the gene encoding the β-chain of thyrotropin and mutations in genes for transcription factors that are essential for normal pituitary development and function (*POU1F1, PROP1, LHX3,* and *HESX1*). Mutations in these genes give rise to deficiencies of several pituitary hormones, including thyrotropin. A few patients with CH have been reported to have mutations in the gene encoding the thyrotropin receptor, *TSHR (93).* These are associated with variable degrees of thyroid abnormality. With milder impairment of receptor function, increased levels of thyrotropin can overcome the receptor defect, leading to euthyroid hyperthyrotropinemia *(94).*

Finally, CH may also be caused by mutations in genes that encode enzymes involved in production of thyroid hormone. These include thyroid peroxidase *(TPO),* thyroglobulin *(TG),* and the sodium-iodide symporter (*NIS,* or *SLC5A5) (92).*

CARRIER SCREENING FOR AUTOSOMAL RECESSIVE DISEASES

Carrier screening is performed with different objectives than is screening for affected individuals in newborn programs. The purpose of carrier screening is to identify asymptomatic individuals who are at risk of having a child with an autosomal recessive disease. Carrier screening is performed for diseases such as CF before

Table 10
Disorders for Which Carrier Screening is Commonly Performed in Ashkenazi Jewish Subjects

	Carrier frequency[a]	Clinical features	Gene	Common mutations	Carrier test
Bloom's syndrome	1/80	Proportional dwarfism, skin sun sensitivity, increased cancer risk, decreased fertility, chromosomal instability	BLM (DNA helicase RecQ)	2281del6ins7	DNA analysis
Canavan's disease	1/58	Fatal progressive neurodegeneration, spongy degeneration on biopsy	Aspartoacylase	A854C	DNA analysis
Familial dysautonomia	1/30	Lack of tearing, erratic blood pressure, scoliosis, pain insensitivity, lack of fungiform papillae of tongue	IKBKAP	IVS20 splice	DNA analysis
Fanconi's anemia, group C	1/66	Short stature, anemia, pancytopenia, increased risk of malignancy	FANCC	IVS4+4A→T	DNA analysis
Gaucher's disease, type 1	1/14	Thrombocytopenia, hepatospleno-megaly, bone abnormalities	Glucocerebrosidase	Five mutations are responsible for >95% of cases	DNA analysis
Niemann-Pick disease	1/121	Fatal progressive neurodegeneration, hepatosplenomegaly, cherry red spot	Sphingomyelinase	Three mutations are responsible for >95% of cases	DNA analysis
Tay-Sachs disease	1/27	Fatal progressive neurodegeneration, prominent startle response	Hexosaminidase A	4-bp insertion	DNA analysis, enzyme assay
Torsion dystonia	1/40	Involuntary muscle contraction	DYT1	3-bp, in-frame deletion	DNA analysis

[a] Carrier frequencies are in the Ashkenazi Jewish population.

or during pregnancy, with the aim being to identify couples in which both partners are carriers of an autosomal recessive disease and who therefore have a one in four risk of having an affected child with each pregnancy. As discussed above, carrier screening for CF is recommended for Caucasian and Ashkenazi Jewish couples, even if there is no family history of the disease. Carrier screening for Tay-Sachs and Canavan's diseases is recommended by the American College of Obstetricians and Gynecologists for Ashkenazi Jewish individuals because of the relatively high frequency of those disorders in that population. In practice, screening among the Ashkenazi Jewish population commonly includes tests for carriers of several other diseases that are more prevalent among that population. These are outlined in Table 10.

REFERENCES

1. Hamosh A, Fitz-Simmons SC, Macek M Jr, Knowles MR, Rosenstein BJ, Cutting GR. Comparison of the clinical manifestations of cystic fibrosis in black and white patients. J Pediatr 1998;132:255–9.
2. Doull IJ. Recent advances in cystic fibrosis. Arch Dis Child 2001;85:62–6.
3. Bals R, Weiner DJ, Wilson JM. The innate immune system in cystic fibrosis lung disease. J Clin Invest 1999;103:303–7.
4. Webb AK, Egan J. Should patients with cystic fibrosis infected with *Burkholderia cepacia* undergo lung transplantation? Thorax 1997;52:671–3.
5. Tummler B, Kiewitz C. Cystic fibrosis: an inherited susceptibility to bacterial respiratory infections. Mol Med Today 1999;5:351–8.
6. Ramachandran C, Melnick SJ. Multidrug resistance in human tumors—molecular diagnosis and clinical significance. Mol Diagn 1999;4:81–94.
7. Ashcroft FM, Gribble FM. New windows on the mechanism of action of K(ATP) channel openers. Trends Pharmacol Sci 2000;21:439–45.
8. Wine JJ. The genesis of cystic fibrosis lung disease. J Clin Invest 1999;103:309–12.
9. Hanrahan JW. Airway plumbing. J Clin Invest 2000;105:1343–4.
10. Stern RC. The diagnosis of cystic fibrosis. N Engl J Med 1997;336:487–91.
11. Schwiebert EM, Benos DJ, Fuller CM. Cystic fibrosis: a multiple exocrinopathy caused by dysfunctions in a multifunctional transport protein. Am J Med 1998;104:576–90.
12. Zeitlin PL. Advances in the diagnosis of cystic fibrosis in infants. J Pediatr 2001;139:345–6.
13. Rosenstein BJ, Cutting GR. The diagnosis of cystic fibrosis: a consensus statement. Cystic Fibrosis Foundation Consensus Panel. J Pediatr 1998;132:589–95.
14. Farrell PM, Kosorok MR, Rock MJ, et al. Early diagnosis of cystic fibrosis through neonatal screening prevents severe malnutrition and improves long-term growth. Wisconsin Cystic Fibrosis Neonatal Screening Study Group. Pediatrics 2001;107:1–13.
15. http://www.genet.sickkids.on.ca/cftr/.

16. Abeliovich D, Lavon IP, Lerer I, et al. Screening for five mutations detects 97% of cystic fibrosis (CF) chromosomes and predicts a carrier frequency of 1:29 in the Jewish Ashkenazi population. Am J Hum Genet 1992;51:951–6.

17. Chillon M, Casals T, Mercier B, et al. Mutations in the cystic fibrosis gene in patients with congenital absence of the vas deferens. N Engl J Med 1995;332:1475–80.

18. Daudin M, Bieth E, Bujan L, Massat G, Pontonnier F, Mieusset R. Congenital bilateral absence of the vas deferens: clinical characteristics, biological parameters, cystic fibrosis transmembrane conductance regulator gene mutations, and implications for genetic counseling. Fertil Steril 2000;74:1164–74.

19. Kim ED, Bischoff FZ, Lipshultz LI, Lamb DJ. Genetic concerns for the subfertile male in the era of ICSI. Prenat Diagn 1998;18:1349–65.

20. Cohn JA, Friedman KJ, Noone PG, Knowles MR, Silverman LM, Jowell PS. Relation between mutations of the cystic fibrosis gene and idiopathic pancreatitis. N Engl J Med 1998;339:653–8.

21. Girodon E, Cazeneuve C, Lebargy F, et al. CFTR gene mutations in adults with disseminated bronchiectasis. Eur J Hum Genet 1997;5:149–55.

22. Miller PW, Hamosh A, Macek M Jr, et al. Cystic fibrosis transmembrane conductance regulator (CFTR) gene mutations in allergic bronchopulmonary aspergillosis. Am J Hum Genet 1996;59:45–51.

23. Mickle JE, Cutting GR. Genotype-phenotype relationships in cystic fibrosis. Med Clin North Am 2000;84:597–607.

24. LeGrys VA. Assessment of sweat-testing practices for the diagnosis of cystic fibrosis. Arch Pathol Lab Med 2001;125:1420–4.

25. Crossley JR, Elliott RB, Smith PA. Dried-blood spot screening for cystic fibrosis in the newborn. Lancet 1979;1:472–4.

26. Gregg RG, Simantel A, Farrell PM, et al. Newborn screening for cystic fibrosis in Wisconsin: comparison of biochemical and molecular methods. Pediatrics 1997;99:819–24.

27. Ranieri E, Lewis BD, Gerace RL, et al. Neonatal screening for cystic fibrosis using immunoreactive trypsinogen and direct gene analysis: four years' experience. BMJ 1994;308:1469–72.

28. Wilcken B, Wiley V, Sherry G, Bayliss U. Neonatal screening for cystic fibrosis: a comparison of two strategies for case detection in 1.2 million babies. J Pediatr 1995;127:965–70.

29. Lester LA, Kraut J, Lloyd-Still J, et al. Delta F508 genotype does not predict disease severity in an ethnically diverse cystic fibrosis population. Pediatrics 1994;93:114–8.

30. Spence JE, Perciaccante RG, Greig GM, et al. Uniparental disomy as a mechanism for human genetic disease. Am J Hum Genet 1988;42:217–26.

31. Grody WW, Cutting GR, Klinger KW, Richards CS, Watson MS, Desnick RJ. Laboratory standards and guidelines for population-based cystic fibrosis carrier screening. Genet Med 2001;3:149–54.

32. Andrews NC. Disorders of iron metabolism. N Engl J Med 1999;341:1986–95.

33. Feder JN, Gnirke A, Thomas W, et al. A novel MHC class I-like gene is mutated in patients with hereditary haemochromatosis. Nat Genet 1996;13:399–408.

34. Feder JN, Penny DM, Irrinki A, et al. The hemochromatosis gene product complexes with the transferrin receptor and lowers its affinity for ligand binding. Proc Natl Acad Sci USA 1998;95:1472–7.

35. Waheed A, Parkkila S, Zhou XY, et al. Hereditary hemochromatosis: effects of C282Y and H63D mutations on association with beta2-microglobulin, intracellular processing, and cell surface expression of the HFE protein in COS-7 cells. Proc Natl Acad Sci USA 1997;94:12384–9.

36. Ajioka RS, Jorde LB, Gruen JR, et al. Haplotype analysis of hemochromatosis: evaluation of different linkage-disequilibrium approaches and evolution of disease chromosomes. Am J Hum Genet 1997;60:1439–47.

37. Lyon E, Frank EL. Hereditary hemochromatosis since discovery of the HFE gene. Clin Chem 2001;47:1147–56.

38. Bacon BR, Sadiq SA. Hereditary hemochromatosis: presentation and diagnosis in the 1990s. Am J Gastroenterol 1997;92:784–9.

39. Witte DL, Crosby WH, Edwards CQ, Fairbanks VF, Mitros FA. Practice guideline development task force of the College of American Pathologists. Hereditary hemochromatosis. Clin Chim Acta 1996;245:139–200.

40. Reyes M, Blanck HM, Khoury MJ. Screening for iron overload due to hereditary hemochromatosis. 2002. http://www.cdc.gov/nccdphp/dnpa/hemochromatosis/screening.htm

41. American Hemochromatosis Society. Guidelines for screening, diagnosis, treatment and management of patients with hereditary hemochromatosis/iron overload. 2000. http://www.americanhs.org/2000guidelines.htm

42. Rosendaal FR. Venous thrombosis: a multicausal disease. Lancet 1999;353:1167–73.

43. Zivelin A, Griffin JH, Xu X, et al. A single genetic origin for a common Caucasian risk factor for venous thrombosis. Blood 1997;89:397–402.

44. Press RD, Bauer KA, Kujovich JL, Heit JA. Clinical utility of factor V leiden (R506Q) testing for the diagnosis and management of thromboembolic disorders. Arch Pathol Lab Med 2002;126:1304–18.

45. Emmerich J, Rosendaal FR, Cattaneo M, et al. Combined effect of factor V Leiden and prothrombin 20210A on the risk of venous thromboembolism—pooled analysis of 8 case-control studies including 2310 cases and 3204 controls. Study Group for Pooled-Analysis in Venous Thromboembolism. Thromb Haemost 2001;86:809–16.

46. Bernardi F, Faioni EM, Castoldi E, et al. A factor V genetic component differing from factor V R506Q contributes to the activated protein C resistance phenotype. Blood 1997;90:1552–7.

47. Alhenc-Gelas M, Nicaud V, Gandrille S, et al. The factor V gene A4070G mutation and the risk of venous thrombosis. Thromb Haemost 1999;81:193–7.

48. Faioni EM, Franchi F, Bucciarelli P, et al. Coinheritance of the HR2 haplotype in the factor V gene confers an increased risk of venous thromboembolism to carriers of factor V R506Q (factor V Leiden). Blood 1999;94:3062–6.

49. de Visser MC, Guasch JF, Kamphuisen PW, Vos HL, Rosendaal FR, Bertina RM. The HR2 haplotype of factor V: effects on factor V levels, normalized activated protein C sensitivity ratios and the risk of venous thrombosis. Thromb Haemost 2000;83:577–82.

50. Yamazaki T, Nicolaes GA, Sorensen KW, Dahlback B. Molecular basis of quantitative factor V deficiency associated with factor V R2 haplotype. Blood 2002;100:2515–21.

51. Zoller B, Svensson PJ, He X, Dahlback B. Identification of the same factor V gene mutation in 47 out of 50 thrombosis-prone families with inherited resistance to activated protein C. J Clin Invest 1994;94:2521–4.

52. Graf LL, Welsh CH, Qamar Z, Marlar RA. Activated protein C resistance assay detects thrombotic risk factors other than factor V Leiden. Am J Clin Pathol 2003;119:52–60.

53. Dahlback B, Carlsson M, Svensson PJ. Familial thrombophilia due to a previously unrecognized mechanism characterized by poor anticoagulant response to activated protein C: prediction of a cofactor to activated protein C. Proc Natl Acad Sci USA 1993;90:1004–8.

54. Jorquera JI, Montoro JM, Fernandez MA, Aznar JA, Aznar J. Modified test for activated protein C resistance. Lancet 1994;344:1162–3.

55. Trossaert M, Conard J, Horellou MH, et al. Modified APC resistance assay for patients on oral anticoagulants. Lancet 1994;344:1709.

56. Tripodi A, Negri B, Bertina RM, Mannucci PM. Screening for the FV:Q506 mutation—evaluation of thirteen plasma-based methods for their diagnostic efficacy in comparison with DNA analysis. Thromb Haemost 1997;77:436–9.

57. Tripodi A, Mannucci PM. Laboratory investigation of thrombophilia. Clin Chem 2001;47:1597–606.

58. Gehring NH, Frede U, Neu-Yilik G, et al. Increased efficiency of mRNA 3′ end formation: a new genetic mechanism contributing to hereditary thrombophilia. Nat Genet 2001;28:389–92.

59. Poort SR, Rosendaal FR, Reitsma PH, Bertina RM. A common genetic variation in the 3′-untranslated region of the prothrombin gene is associated with elevated plasma prothrombin levels and an increase in venous thrombosis. Blood 1996;88:3698–703.

60. Rosendaal FR, Siscovick DS, Schwartz SM, Psaty BM, Raghunathan TE, Vos HL. A common prothrombin variant (20210 G to A) increases the risk of myocardial infarction in young women. Blood 1997;90:1747–50.

61. McGlennen RC, Key NS. Clinical and laboratory management of the prothrombin G20210A mutation. Arch Pathol Lab Med 2002;126:1319–25.

62. Grody WW, Griffin JH, Taylor AK, Korf BR, Heit JA. American College of Medical Genetics consensus statement on factor V Leiden mutation testing. Genet Med 2001;3:139—48.

63. Kremer B, Goldberg P, Andrew SE, et al. A worldwide study of the Huntington's disease mutation. The sensitivity and specificity of measuring CAG repeats. N Engl J Med 1994;330:1401–6.

64. Falush D, Almqvist EW, Brinkmann RR, Iwasa Y, Hayden MR. Measurement of mutational flow implies both a high new-mutation rate for Huntington disease and substantial underascertainment of late-onset cases. Am J Hum Genet 2001;68:373–85.

65. Cummings CJ, Zoghbi HY. Fourteen and counting: unraveling trinucleotide repeat diseases. Hum Mol Genet 2000;9:909–16.

66. AnonymousACMG/ASHG statement. Laboratory guidelines for Huntington disease genetic testing. The American College of Medical Genetics/American Society of Human Genetics Huntington Disease Genetic Testing Working Group. Am J Hum Genet 1998;62:1243–7.

67. Andrew SE, Goldberg YP, Kremer B, et al. Huntington disease without CAG expansion: phenocopies or errors in assignment? Am J Hum Genet 1994;54:852–63.

68. Moore RC, Xiang F, Monaghan J, et al. Huntington disease phenocopy is a familial prion disease. Am J Hum Genet 2001;69:1385–8.

69. Nolin SL, Lewis FA 3rd, Ye LL, et al. Familial transmission of the FMR1 CGG repeat. Am J Hum Genet 1996;59:1252–61.

70. Darnell JC, Jensen KB, Jin P, Brown V, Warren ST, Darnell RB. Fragile X mental retardation protein targets G quartet mRNAs important for neuronal function. Cell 2001;107:489–99.
71. Brown V, Jin P, Ceman S, et al. Microarray identification of FMRP-associated brain mRNAs and altered mRNA translational profiles in fragile X syndrome. Cell 2001;107:477–87.
72. Maddalena A, Richards CS, McGinniss MJ, et al. Technical standards and guidelines for fragile X: the first of a series of disease-specific supplements to the Standards and Guidelines for Clinical Genetics Laboratories of the American College of Medical Genetics. Quality Assurance Subcommittee of the Laboratory Practice Committee. Genet Med 2001;3:200–5.
73. Prezant TR, Agapian JV, Bohlman MC, et al. Mitochondrial ribosomal RNA mutation associated with both antibiotic-induced and non-syndromic deafness. Nat Genet 1993;4:289–94.
74. Ashizawa T, Subramony SH. What is Kearns-Sayre syndrome after all? Arch Neurol 2001;58:1053–4.
75. Shoffner JM, Lott MT, Lezza AM, Seibel P, Ballinger SW, Wallace DC. Myoclonic epilepsy and ragged-red fiber disease (MERRF) is associated with a mitochondrial DNA tRNA(Lys) mutation. Cell 1990;61:931–7.
76. Shoffner JM, Wallace DC. Mitochondrial genetics: principles and practice. Am J Hum Genet 1992;51:1179–86.
77. Lam CW, Lau CH, Williams JC, Chan YW, Wong LJ. Mitochondrial myopathy, encephalopathy, lactic acidosis and stroke-like episodes (MELAS) triggered by valproate therapy. Eur J Pediatr 1997;156:562–4.
78. Goto Y, Nonaka I, Horai S. A mutation in the tRNA(Leu)(UUR) gene associated with the MELAS subgroup of mitochondrial encephalomyopathies. Nature 1990;348:651–3.
79. Goto Y, Nonaka I, Horai S. A new mtDNA mutation associated with mitochondrial myopathy, encephalopathy, lactic acidosis and stroke-like episodes (MELAS). Biochim Biophys Acta 1991;1097:238–40.
80. Evidente VG, Gwinn-Hardy KA, Caviness JN, Gilman S. Hereditary ataxias. Mayo Clin Proc 2000;75:475–90.
81. Pandolfo M. Molecular pathogenesis of Friedreich ataxia. Arch Neurol 1999;56:1201–8.
82. Levy HL. Newborn screening by tandem mass spectrometry: a new era. Clin Chem 1998;44:2401–2.
83. Murphy M, McHugh B, Tighe O, et al. Genetic basis of transferase-deficient galactosaemia in Ireland and the population history of the Irish Travellers. Eur J Hum Genet 1999;7:549–54.
84. Aoki K, Wada Y. Outcome of the patients detected by newborn screening in Japan. Acta Paediatr Jpn 1988;30:429–34.
85. Suzuki M, West C, Beutler E. Large-scale molecular screening for galactosemia alleles in a pan-ethnic population. Hum Genet 2001;109:210–5.
86. Elsas LJ, Lai K, Saunders CJ, Langley SD. Functional analysis of the human galactose-1-phosphate uridyltransferase promoter in Duarte and LA variant galactosemia. Mol Genet Metab 2001;72:297–305.
87. Hunter M, Angelicheva D, Levy HL, Pueschel SM, Kalaydjieva L. Novel mutations in the GALK1 gene in patients with galactokinase deficiency. Hum Mutat 2001;17:77–8.

88. Walter JH, Roberts RE, Besley GT, et al. Generalised uridine diphosphate galactose-4-epimerase deficiency. Arch Dis Child 1999;80:374–6.
89. Wohlers TM, Christacos NC, Harreman MT, Fridovich-Keil JL. Identification and characterization of a mutation, in the human UDP-galactose-4-epimerase gene, associated with generalized epimerase-deficiency galactosemia. Am J Hum Genet 1999;64:462–70.
90. Macchia PE, Lapi P, Krude H, et al. PAX8 mutations associated with congenital hypothyroidism caused by thyroid dysgenesis. Nat Genet 1998;19:83–6.
91. Macchia PE. Recent advances in understanding the molecular basis of primary congenital hypothyroidism. Mol Med Today 2000;6:36–42.
92. Kopp P. Perspective: genetic defects in the etiology of congenital hypothyroidism. Endocrinology 2002;143:2019–24.
93. Utiger RD. Thyrotropin-receptor mutations and thyroid dysfunction. N Engl J Med 1995;332:183–5.
94. Sunthornthepvarakui T, Gottschalk ME, Hayashi Y, Refetoff S. Brief report: resistance to thyrotropin caused by mutations in the thyrotropin-receptor gene. N Engl J Med 1995;332:155–60.
95. Anonymous. Population variation of common cystic fibrosis mutations. The Cystic Fibrosis Genetic Analysis Consortium. Hum Mutat 1994;4:167–77.
96. Merryweather-Clarke AT, Pointon JJ, Shearman JD, Robson KJ. Global prevalence of putative haemochromatosis mutations. J Med Genet 1997;34:275–8.
97. Steinberg KK, Cogswell ME, Chang JC, et al. Prevalence of C282Y and H63D mutations in the hemochromatosis (HFE) gene in the United States. JAMA 2001;285:2216–22.
98. Seligsohn U, Lubetsky A. Genetic susceptibility to venous thrombosis. N Engl J Med 2001;344:1222–31.
99. Nowacki PM, Byck S, Prevost L, Scriver CR. PAH Mutation Analysis Consortium Database: 1997. Prototype for relational locus-specific mutation databases. Nucleic Acids Res 1998;26:220–5.

6   Molecular Origins of Cancer

Cancer is caused by genetic mutations. In most patients with cancer, these mutations are acquired, but some patients inherit a germline tumor-predisposing mutation. Although the specific genetic abnormalities in cancers can be extremely complex, most mutations involve a few general cellular functions: impairment of the control of cell division (tumor suppressor genes and their proteins), aberrant activation of pathways that stimulate cell proliferation (oncogenes and their proteins), and inactivation of pathways that lead to cell death (apoptosis). The relative importance of these types of mutation varies among tumors. For example, retinoblastoma is caused by loss of activity of the pRB tumor suppressor protein, chronic myeloid leukemia is caused by activation of the Abelson proto-oncogene, and follicular cell lymphoma is commonly associated with activation of pathways that inhibit bcl-2-mediated apoptosis. By the time tumors come to clinical attention they may have acquired very complex genetic disturbances involving multiple pathways that regulate cell proliferation, stimulate angiogenesis, and confer metastatic capability. Thus, although the principles discussed below form a useful framework for studying the molecular basis of cancer, the complete profile of molecular abnormalities in any tumor is likely to be very complex.

TUMOR SUPPRESSOR GENES

Tumor suppressor genes encode proteins that regulate normal cell proliferation. The products of these genes therefore act like brakes on cell division, and mutations in theses genes are manifested by deregulation of the cell cycle control mechanisms. In general, loss of function of both alleles of an autosomal tumor suppressor gene is needed for a malignant phenotype to manifest. The usual requirement that both alleles be mutated by separate mutational events ("two hits") was originally proposed by Knudson in 1971 (1) in a

From: *Principles of Molecular Pathology*
Edited by: A. A. Killeen © Humana Press Inc., Totowa, NJ

study of patterns of development of sporadic and familial retinoblastoma. The two hits can occur as two independent mutations in a somatic cell, or, in the case of many familial cancer syndromes, an individual may inherit a germline mutation that inactivates one allele of a tumor suppressor. Loss of function of the remaining wild-type allele through a second, acquired mutation in a cell of such an individual would further reduce activity of the tumor suppressor gene product in that cell and its progeny. Depending on the relative importance of the tumor suppressor gene in a given tissue, the loss of both alleles may confer a malignant phenotype.

Mutations in Tumor Suppressor Genes

Mutations that inactivate tumor suppressor genes are, in general, no different from those that may be found at any genetic locus. However, acquired epigenetic alterations, particularly silencing of promoter regions by methylation of cytosine residues, is increasingly recognized as a mechanism of inactivation of some tumor suppressor genes. Methylation of promoter sequences might cause inhibition of gene expression through three possible mechanisms (2). First, binding of transcription factors to DNA may be directly inhibited by methylation itself. Second, transcriptional repressors might bind to methylated DNA and prevent binding of transcriptional activators. Two proteins with such an ability to bind to methylated DNA are the methylcytosine binding proteins, MeCP-1 and MeCP-2. Third, methylation may induce alterations in the structure of chromatin that may prevent gene transcription.

An example of a tumor suppressor gene that can be inactivated by aberrant methylation is *APC*. *APC* is mutated in >90% of patients with familial adenomatous polyposis coli, a familial cancer syndrome discussed in Chapter 7. *APC*-inactivating mutations can also be demonstrated in 80% of sporadic colorectal cancers, and mutation of this gene is believed to be an early event in the natural history of colorectal cancers. Eighteen percent of primary sporadic colorectal cancers show hypermethylation of the *APC* promoter region (3). This hypermethylation is nearly always found on the allele that does not contain an inactivating mutation, i.e., in this situation one allele is inactivated by DNA mutation, and the other is silenced through hypermethylation. These abnormalities prevent the expression of functional APC protein. Other tumor suppressor genes known to be inactivated by hypermethylation include *BRCA1, MLH1, FHIT, p14, p15,* and *p16 (4).*

Loss of Heterozygosity

A common finding that suggests a region of a chromosome contains a tumor suppressor gene is loss of heterozygosity (LOH). The existence of naturally occurring polymorphisms means that pairs of homologous chromosomes have genetic variations throughout much of their sequences. These include differences in polymorphic elements such as variable number tandem repeats and single-nucleotide polymorphisms. Such polymorphisms are very useful as experimental markers for confirming the presence of both copies of a chromosome, or region of chromosome, in a tissue sample. Conversely, if a region of two homologous chromosomes contains polymorphic markers in germline DNA, but frequently loses one set of markers in tumor samples in different patients, then this finding suggests that the region contains a tumor suppressor gene. In addition to arising from deletions of one chromosome, LOH can also arise by replacement of DNA in a region of a chromosome by the corresponding DNA from the homologous chromosome during a recombination event. This renders genes in the replaced region homozygous, and therefore homozygous for any recessive mutations, such as inactivating mutations in tumor suppressor genes.

Examples of Tumor Suppressor Genes

Several dozen genes are known or putative tumor suppressor genes (*see* Table 1 for examples). Of these, two play critical roles in the development of a wide range of tumors. These are the retinoblastoma gene *(RB1)* and the p53 gene *(TP53).* Mutations in each of these are associated with both familial and sporadic forms of cancer.

RETINOBLASTOMA AND THE *RB1* GENE

The prototypic disease caused by loss of activity of a tumor suppressor gene is retinoblastoma. Retinoblastoma is a malignant tumor of the developing retina that has an incidence of approx 1 in 20,000. Once the retina has fully developed, usually by 5 yr of age, the risk of developing this tumor is greatly reduced, although not eliminated *(5).* The tumor is therefore primarily one of childhood, and most cases are diagnosed before 5 yr of age.

Table 1
Examples of Tumor Suppressor Genes

Gene	Chromosomal location	Inherited tumor	Sporadic tumor
RB1	13q14	Retinoblastoma	Retinoblastoma, sarcomas, bladder, breast, esophageal, lung
TP53	17p13	(Li-Fraumeni)	Bladder, breast, colorectal, esophageal, liver, lung, ovarian, brain, sarcomas, lymphomas, leukemias
DCC	18q21		Colorectal cancer
MCC	5q21		Colorectal cancer
APC	5q21	Colon (FAP)	Colorectal, stomach, pancreas
WT1	11p13	Wilms tumor	Wilms tumor
WT2	11p15	Weidemann-Beckwith syndrome	Renal rhabdoid tumors, embryonal rhabdomyosarcoma
NF1	17q11	Neurofibromatosis I	Colon, astrocytoma
NF2	22q11	Neurofibromatosis II	Schwannoma, meningioma
VHL	3p25	von Hippel-Lindau	Renal cell carcinoma syndrome
MEN1	11q23	Multiple endocrine neoplasia, type I	Parathyroid, pancreaticoduodenal neuroendocrine tumors (PNTs), and pituitary tumors
NM23	17q21		Melanoma, breast, colorectal, prostate, meningioma, others
CDKN2	9p21	Melanoma	Melanoma, brain tumors, leukemias, sarcomas, bladder, breast, kidney, lung, ovarian

Modified from ref. 54.

Approximately 30–40% of patients with retinoblastoma have inherited a germline mutation in *RB1*. These patients therefore have only a single wild-type allele, and a deleterious mutation in this may eliminate functional pRb activity in a cell and its progeny. Why retinal cells are chiefly at risk for tumor development in patients with germline mutations is unknown. Patients who inherit a *RB1* mutation have an 80–90% risk of developing retinoblastoma, develop a tumor at an earlier age, and have a tendency to develop bilateral retinoblastomas as well as an increased risk of developing certain other tumors later in life, notably osteosarcomas and melanomas. The rate of development of second tumors is highly dependent on the use and dosage of radiation to treat the primary tumor *(6)*. Nearly all patients with bilateral retinoblastomas have a germline mutation. Of patients with germline mutations, approx 10% develop "trilateral" retinoblastoma, i.e., unilateral or bilateral retinoblastoma, and an intracranial neuroblastic tumor.

Mutations in RB1. The *RB1* gene is located on chromosome 13q14 and is composed of 27 exons. The most common germline mutations (66%) in patients with hereditary retinoblastoma are single nucleotide mutations and small insertions or deletions. Approximately 10% of patients with hereditary retinoblastoma have deletions of *RB1* that are detectable by Southern blot analysis. In 8%, there is a deletion or rearrangement of 13q14 that is visible by cytogenetic study. In the remaining patients, no mutation is identified, possibly because of limitations of current mutation detection systems. The majority (65%) of somatic mutations are associated with LOH *(7)*.

pRb and Cell Cycle Control. The protein encoded by *RB1,* pRb, plays a critical role in the regulation of the cell cycle. The cell replication cycle is divided into four phases, G_1 (gap 1), S (synthesis of DNA), G_2 (gap 2), and M (mitosis) (Fig. 1). Cells that are not actively replicating are said to be in G_0. The boundary between G_1 and S is an important checkpoint for regulation of cell division. This is called the *restriction point* (or *start* in yeast experiments) and is important because cells that pass through the restriction point will normally complete a cell division. The restriction point is therefore a critical point at which cell division is controlled.

Formation of proteins that are required for DNA replication is essential for successful cell replication. These proteins include

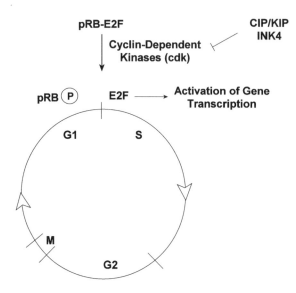

Fig. 1. Control of the G1/S restriction point by pRb. pRb inhibits the transcription factor, E2F, by binding to it. During the end of G1, levels of cyclin-dependent kinases, particularly cyclin D-cdk 4 (or 6), and cyclin E-cdk2 increase. These lead to phosphorylation of pRb, which decreases its binding to E2F. The latter molecule is then able to activate transcription of genes that are essential for DNA replication to occur, and the cell cycle can progress. Mutations that eliminate pRb activity remove control at this checkpoint.

DNA polymerase α, proliferating cell nuclear antigen, thymidine kinase, thymidylate synthase, ribonucleotide reductase, and DNA repair proteins such as RAD51 *(8)*. Transcription of all of these is stimulated by a group of transcriptional regulatory proteins known as E2F. pRb binds to E2F and blocks its ability to stimulate the transcription of genes necessary for DNA replication. In addition to inhibiting E2F-mediated transcription, the pRB-E2F complex can recruit histone deacetylase activity that causes local chromatin condensation and downregulates transcription of target genes. In the absence of pRb activity, e.g., because of mutations on both alleles, this important control mechanism at the G_1/S cell cycle checkpoint is impaired and the regulation of the cell cycle is disrupted.

During normal cell division, pRb must release E2F so that the latter molecule can function as a transcriptional activator. This release is accomplished by phosphorylation of pRb by cyclin-dependent kinases (cdks). pRb that is phosphorylated binds E2F less strongly.

Active cdks include a catalytic (kinase) subunit and a cyclin subunit that functions as a regulator. Other proteins may be involved in the formation of the cdk holoenzymes *(9)*.

Several different catalytic and cyclin subunits exist. The D- and E-type cyclins are involved in cell cycle control at the restriction point. The D-type cyclins are expressed in quiescent cells exposed to mitogenic stimuli, and they form active cdks with two different catalytic subunits, cdk4 and cdk6. Both cyclin D-cdk4 and cyclin D-cdk6 are capable of phosphorylating pRb, leading to release of E2F and progression of the cell through the restriction point. Cyclin E forms a functional cdk with the catalytic subunit, cdk2, which leads to further phosphorylation (hyperphosphorylation) of pRb. Transcription of cyclin E is activated by E2F1, which means that the mitogen-dependent production of cyclin D is replaced by a mitogen-independent activation of cdks as the cell passes through the restriction point. As cells pass through the S, G_2, and M phases of cell cycle, phosphorylation of pRb is maintained by complexes that include cyclin A-cdk and cyclin B-cdk.

Normal control of production of D cyclins is regulated by mitogenic stimuli. Pathologic overexpression of cyclin D is observed in a wide variety of tumors (10) and may arise from at least two mechanisms, translocations, such as t(11;14)(q13;q32), and gene amplification. In t(11;14)(q13;q32), which is present in nearly all cases of mantle cell lymphoma and in some other lymphoid malignancies, the cyclin D1 gene,*CCND1* (which is also known as *BCL-1* and *PRAD1*) on chromosome 11 is juxtaposed to the *IgH* locus on chromosome 14. The strong promoter function of the *IgH* locus leads to overexpression of *CCND1* (*see* Chapt. 8).

Inhibitors of Cyclin-Dependent Kinases. The cdks are regulated by inhibitory proteins of two general classes, the CIP/KIP family and the INK family. The CIP/KIP family of proteins, which includes p21, p27, and p57 regulates the activity of cyclin/cdk complexes. p27 is a general inhibitor of these complexes. As the cell progresses through G_1 to the restriction point, the level of cyclin D rises, whereas the level of p27, which is high in resting cells, decreases as it forms complexes with cyclin D/cdk. This fall in p27 level tends to relieve the negative effect of p27 on cell cycle progression. Cyclin E/cdk2 can also phosphorylate p27, which leads to accelerated destruction of the latter molecule. Thus, transition through G_1 and beyond the restriction point is associated with increased levels of cyclin/cdk complexes and declining levels of the cell cycle inhibitor, p27.

It might be expected that pathologically decreased levels of p27 would lead to increased progression through the restriction point, and, indeed, the importance of this marker as a prognostic marker in certain cancers has been demonstrated. Loss of p27 is an adverse prognostic factor in a wide variety of tumors, but especially breast cancer *(11)*. Interestingly, loss of just one of the two *p27* alleles is an adverse prognostic marker and appears to be an exception to the general principle that loss of both copies of a tumor suppressor gene are needed for a malignant phenotype to manifest *(12)*.

The cdk inhibitor, p21, rises during G_1. In cooperation with proliferating cell nuclear antigen (PCNA), it can inhibit cdk2 and is believed to play a role in checking the cell cycle while DNA damage is repaired. Its transcription is regulated by p53. p21 is also believed to be involved in cell differentiation processes and in apoptosis.

The cyclin D-dependent kinases, cdk4 and cdk6, are also inhibited by a group of proteins called INK4 that bind to the cdks and release bound CIP/KIP proteins. The effect of this is to cause inhibition of cdk2 because of binding of the inhibitory CIP/KIP proteins to this kinase. This results in blocking of the cell cycle at the restriction point because cyclin E/cdk2 is inhibited. The INK4 proteins include p16, p15, p18, and p19. These are also known as INK4a, INK4b, INK4c, and INK4d, respectively. *p16/INK4α* (also known as *MTS1* and *CDKN2*) is mutated in some forms of familial melanoma, in most cases of pancreatic cancer, and in many other tumors, demonstrating the importance of these important checks on cell cycle progression.

TP53

The tumor suppressor gene, *TP53,* which encodes the protein p53, plays an important role in cancer development. It is mutated in most cancers and is probably the most commonly mutated tumor suppressor gene. *TP53* is located on chromosome 17p13.1, and the encoded protein consists of 393 amino acids. It is composed of three regions: a central DNA binding core (including amino acids 100–300), the amino-terminal domain, which is involved in activation of gene transcription, and the carboxy-terminal region (including amino acids 300–393), which has several functions including formation of p53 tetramers. Expression of p53 is induced by damage to DNA; in response to such damage, the protein can lead to arrest of the cell cycle in G_1 or G_2, or to apoptosis. Because it protects against accumulations of potentially oncogenic DNA mutations, p53 is known as the "guardian of the genome."

p53 is a transactivator of gene expression. Target genes contain the p53 DNA binding site, a 10-bp sequence, in their promoter regions. It can also function as a repressor of expression of some genes that lack this sequence. Binding to DNA is through the central region of the protein. The N-terminal transactivating domain facilitates binding to the promoter of genes involved in transcription such as TATA box-binding protein *(13,14)*.

Targets of p53 transcriptional activation include p21, which, as discussed above, is an inhibitor of cdk2 *(15)*. The effect of this inhibition is to block passage of the cell through the G_1/S restriction point, which allows time for damaged cells to repair DNA before it is replicated. Other gene targets of p53 activation include the human homolog of the mouse double minute gene, *HDM2,* which encodes a protein that can remove p53 (thereby creating a negative feedback loop that may regulate p53 activity), and several proapoptotic members of the Bcl-2 family (*see* Apoptosis section below) *(16)*.

p53-mediated arrest of the cell cycle in G2 is mediated by at least two mechanisms, and probably by others. The first involves inhibition of expression of cyclin B1, an activator of the kinase cdk1, which is essential for mitosis *(17)*. The second involves induction of p21, Gadd45, and 14-3-3σ protein, which can all inactivate Cdc25C, a phosphatase that activates cdk1 by dephosphorylating it *(18)*. Both of these mechanisms lead to reduction in cdk1 activity and checking of the cell cycle.

Mechanisms of p53 Inactivation. p53 can be inactivated by several mechanisms including mutation and increased degradation of the protein. Most mutations in p53 that are associated with cancers arise in one of a few codons in the central core region including codons 175, 245, 248, and 273 (germline mutations) or 278 (acquired mutations). A database of mutations is maintained at www.iarc.fr/p53/. Three mechanisms of tumorigenesis have been proposed in connection with p53 mutations. First, because tetramers appear to be the functional form of the wild-type protein, mutations in one allele can exert a "dominant-negative" phenotype by reducing the formation of tetramers composed only of wild-type p53 (*see* Chapt. 3). Mutant p53 may bind less strongly to hdm2 (binding is normally followed by pro-teasomal degradation of p53), thereby prolonging the half-life relative of p53. Second, in addition to a dominant-negative effect of p53 mutations, it appears that certain mutations are oncogenic indepen-dent of any association with wild-type p53, i.e., they behave as gain-of-function mutations more typically associated with activation of an oncogene. The mechanisms for this effect are not fully understood but may involve transactivation of other genes involved in tumorigenesis such as c-*myc* and the multidrug resistance gene, *MDR1*. As a third mechanism of tumorigenesis, absence of all p53 activity is associated with a markedly increased rate of tumor formation in mice, a typical characteristic of a tumor suppressor gene. Families with Li-Fraumeni syndrome carry germline mutations in *TP53* (*see* Chap. 7).

In addition to mutations to *TP53* itself, p53 can be inactivated by formation of complexes with other proteins. Among these are several proteins produced by oncogenic viruses including adenovirus E1B protein and the E6 protein of oncogenic human papillomavirus (HPV). Binding of viral proteins to p53 blocks its transactivation function and appears to play an important role in the tumorigenicity of these viruses. As mentioned previously, p53 can form an inactivat-ing complex with mdm-2, which results in p53 translocation from the nucleus to the cytoplasm, where it is degraded by the proteasome *(19)*. Mdm-2 is encoded by the human homolog of the mouse double minute-2 gene, *HDM2,* on chromosome 12q *(20)*. This oncogene is commonly amplified in sarcomas from different tissues, and the resulting high levels of mdm-2 lead to p53 inactivation *(20)*.

Oncogenic Mechanisms of Human Papillomavirus

Cancer of the cervix is induced, in almost every case, by HPV, a double-stranded DNA virus that is spread by sexual contact. In the United States, an estimated 15,000 women are diagnosed with cer-vical cancer each year, and 5000 die from this disease. Various HPV types are recognized, some of which are strongly associated with cancer, the most common of these being types 16 and 18 (Table 2). Study of the oncogenic mechanisms of HPV has provided important insights into basic cancer mechanisms.

HPV infects basal epithelial cells that are capable of replication *(21)*. Cell replication leads to lateral spread and migration of

Table 2
Human Papillomavirus Types

Risk of cervical cancer	Type
High	16, 18, 31, 33, 35, 39, 45, 51, 52, 56, 58, 59, 68
Low	6, 11, 42, 43, 44

infected cells toward the surface epithelium and is associated with viral replication and release of new virus. The oncogenic ability of HPV is directly related to the roles of the viral proteins E5, E6, and E7. E5 binds to several membrane receptors that stimulate cell division including epidermal growth factor receptor, platelet-derived growth factor receptor, colony-stimulating factor-1 receptor, and p185neu *(22)*. E6 protein can form a complex with p53, leading to its destruction by the ubiquitin-proteasome system *(23,24)*. Destruction of p53 leads to impairment of the important cell cycle checkpoint control and apoptosis-inducing functions of the protein. E6 also leads to inactivation of the proapoptotic factor BAK and to activation of telomerase and stabilization of several kinases that stimulate growth *(25)*. E7 can form a complex with pRB, leading to its destruction *(26)*. E7 also stimulates the S-phase cyclins A and E and blocks the cdk inhibitor p21 *(25)*. E6 and E7 appear to act synergistically in cell transformation.

ONCOGENES

Oncogenes represent activated forms of proto-oncogenes—normal genes encoding proteins that are involved in stimulating cell division. If the normal flow of mitogenic stimuli is thought of as a series of stages proceeding from mitogens acting on membrane receptors, to signaling by cytoplasmic intermediaries, to activation of a variety of nuclear factors, then oncogene function can be conceptualized as acting at one of these stages. In most instances, proto-oncogenes acquire a gain of function with resulting upregulation of activity of the encoded protein. This differs from the tumorigenic mechanism of tumor suppressor genes, which tends to involve loss-of-function of genes that are essential for cell cycle regulation. Oncogenes can exert their phenotype if just one of the two alleles is activated (i.e., they have a dominant phenotype at the cellular level). By contrast, both alleles of a tumor suppressor gene generally must

Table 3
Examples of Oncogenes

Gene	Chromosomal location	Inherited tumor	Sporadic tumor
ABL	9q34.1		Chronic myeloid leukemia (BCR-ABL); (see Chap. 8)
BCL2	18q21		Follicular cell lymphoma, chronic lymphocytic leukemia (see Chap. 8)
CCND1	11q13.3		Parathyroid adenoma, mantle cell lymphoma, breast (also known as cyclin D1)
ERBB2	17q21.1		Breast, ovarian, lung (also known as HER-2/neu)
HRAS	11p15.5-p15.1		Breast, lung, kidney, bladder, colon
MYC	8q24.13-q24.13		Burkitt's lymphoma, breast, lung, ovarian
MYCN	2p24.1		Neuroblastoma (also known as N-myc)
NF1	17q11.2	Neurofibromatosis	
RET	10q11.2	MEN II syndromes	Medullary thyroid cancer (see Chap. 7)

be inactivated by two separate "hits" before the abnormal phenotype manifests. Like mutant tumor suppressor genes, mutations in some oncogenes are transmitted from one generation to another and are associated with familial cancer syndromes that show a dominant mode of inheritance. Examples of oncogenes are shown in Table 3.

Oncogenes are commonly activated through one of the following general mechanisms: chromosomal translocation, gene amplification, insertion near a strong promoter, and activating mutations.

Chromosomal Translocation

Chromosomal translocations involve breakage of two or more chromosomes and fusion of the pieces to form new chromosomes. Depending on the specific breakpoints and fusions, a proto-oncogene may be fused to a gene that is actively transcribed in the cell, leading to overexpression of the oncogene. The classic example of this phenomenon is fusion of the *BCR* gene on chromosome 22 with the *ABL* proto-oncogene on chromosome 9. *ABL* encodes a protein with tyrosine kinase activity that is involved in stimulating cell division. The fusion protein retains the functional domain of the normal ABL enzyme, but the activity of this enzyme is increased, and the activity has a different subcellular localization than normal (*see* Chap. 8). As a result of BCR-ABL expression, cells are stimulated to divide. This fusion is seen in essentially all patients with the adult form of chronic myeloid leukemia (*see* Chap. 8).

Numerous other examples of fusion genes that have oncogenic activity are known. Many of these involve malignancies of the hematopoietic or lymphoid systems and are discussed in Chapter 8. Among solid tumors, some translocations are particularly common. Ewing's sarcoma (ES) and primitive neuroectodermal tumor (PNET) form an overlapping diagnostic entity with similar small round cell tumors: Askin's tumor (located in the thorax), paravertebral small cell tumor, and extraosseous ES. These poorly differentiated tumors express high levels of CD99. Approximately 85% of patients with ES have a fusion involving the *EWS* gene on chromosome 22q12 with the *FLI1* gene on chromosome 11q24 [t(11;22)(q24;q12)], and a further 10% have a fusion between *EWS* and the *ERG* gene on chromosome 21 [t(21;22q12)]. Other partner genes of *EWS* in translocations that are seen infrequently in ES/PNET include *ETV1* (7q22), *E1AF* (17q12), and *FEV* (2q33). Detection of these chromosomal translocations is very helpful in classifying tumors if the morphology and other findings are inconclusive. EWS partner genes are members of the *ETS* gene family, named because they encode a common domain that results in binding of the protein to specific DNA sequences, the *e*rythroblastosis virus *t*ransforming *s*equence domain. In these translocations, the N-terminal portion of EWS is fused with the C-terminal portion of the translocation partner to form a transcription factor. In the case of the usual ES translocation, *EWS-FLI1*, the ETS domains of *FLI1* may result in abnormal expression of *FLI1* target genes, or, because of properties unique to the fusion protein, may activate or repress other genes. The exact mechanisms of tumor development are not known, but other mutations may also be involved: mutations in *TP53* and *INK4* are present in 20–30% of ES/PNET tumors. The *EWS-FLI1* translocation can be demonstrated by Southern blot, fluorescence *in situ* hybridization (FISH), or reverse transcription polymerase chain reaction (RT-PCR). In addition to ES, *EWS* translocations are also seen in some other mesenchymal tumors.

Gene Amplification

Gene amplification is a frequent mechanism of overexpression of the proto-oncogenes *HER-2* and *MYCN* (also known as N-myc). *HER-2* is also known as *neu, HER-2/neu,* and *c-erb*B-2. The HER-2/neu locus is on chromosome 17q11-q12. The protein is a cell membrane receptor with an intracellular protein kinase domain and belongs to a family of such membrane-bound protein kinases that includes epidermal growth factor receptor (EGFR). HER-2/neu is overexpressed in a wide variety of tumors including breast, ovarian, endometrial, prostate, pancreatic, and salivary gland *(27)*. HER-2/neu overexpression is found in approx 30% of breast cancers, and its overexpression is an adverse prognostic feature associated with other adverse markers such as lack of expression of estrogen and progesterone receptors.

HER-2/neu is a target for an immune-based therapy for breast cancers that overexpress this receptor. A "humanized" murine monoclonal antibody (i.e., engineered to contain a human Fc region) directed against HER-2/neu has been shown to be active against breast cancer cells both in vitro and in vivo. This antibody is available under the generic name trastuzumab (commercial name, Herceptin). Administration of this antibody to breast cancer patients with evidence of HER-2/neu overexpression has been shown to have a beneficial therapeutic effect *(28)*.

Detection of HER-2/neu overexpression can be performed by immunohistochemistry, FISH, Southern blot, Northern blot, or measurement of shed HER-2/neu by immunoassay performed on serum samples. Food and Drug Administration (FDA)-approved kits for FISH and immunohistochemistry are available for clinical use.

Amplification of *MYCN,* the gene encoding N-myc, is associated with neuroblastomas, being amplified in approximately one-third of cases *(29)*. The degree of amplification is usually in the range of 50- to 100-fold but may be up to 500-fold. The amplified *MYCN* gene may be present in homogeneously staining regions of chromosomes—but usually not situated at the gene's native locus at 2p24.1—or in double minutes. The mechanisms by which the gene are amplified remain uncertain. Identification of *MYCN* amplification in neuroblastomas is associated with an adverse prognosis. Amplification of *MYCN* has also been reported in cases of small cell lung cancer, medullary thyroid carcinoma, retinoblastoma, and breast cancer; however, the significance of these observations is limited by the small number of cases reported to date *(30)*.

Insertion Near a Strong Promoter

In addition to fusing two genes, translocations can bring a gene into a region of the genome that is actively transcribed. This can lead to overexpression of a structurally normal protein. An example of this is myc overexpression that results from the t(8;14) translocation found in 80% of cases of Burkitt's lymphoma (*see* Chap. 8). The immunoglobulin heavy chain *(IgH)* contains strong Ig enhancer elements that can stimulate transcription of nearby genes. The t(8;14) translocation brings the *MYC* gene in proximity to *IgH* and its Ig enhancers, leading to overexpression of the former gene. The myc protein produced in this translocation is normal but is produced in excessive amounts. The same general mechanism leads to overexpression of myc in Burkitt's lymphomas with the t(2;8) (kappa locus) or t(8;22) (lambda locus) translocations. Myc has multiple cellular roles, some of which are implicated in its oncogenic abilities. Overexpression is associated with disturbances in cell cycle regulation, destabilization of genomic integrity, inhibition of cell differentiation, induction of apoptosis, and activation of telomerase *(31)*.

Activating Mutations

Several proto-oncogenes are activated by mutations in their sequences. These represent gain-of-function mutations. Examples of such proto-oncogenes include *Ras, Ret,* and *Myc.* Activating mutations in *RET* are the basis of multiple endocrine neoplasia, type 2, and are discussed in Chapter 7.

ACTIVATING MUTATIONS IN *RAS*

The Ras family includes a number of proteins that have structural and functional similarities. Members of the family include K-ras, H-ras, and N-ras. The Ras proteins are membrane receptors that are members of a larger family of proteins known as G proteins. In contrast to the G proteins, which are composed of trimers of G_α, G_β,

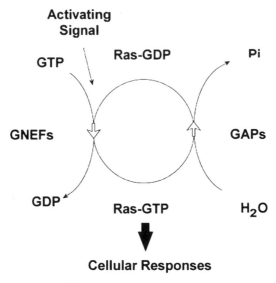

Fig. 2. The ras-GTP protein cycle. Ras proteins are members of the G family of signaling molecules that stimulate diverse cellular processes including cell division. In its resting state, ras is bound to GDP. Activation of the protein, e.g., by binding of a ligand, leads to dimerization and autophosphorylation of certain tyrosine residues. This allows adaptor proteins and guanine nucleotide exchange factors (GNEFs) to bind. These cause dissociation of GDP from ras and allow GTP to bind, thus forming the active form of the ras protein, which acts as a signaling molecule. Inactivation of ras by hydrolysis of bound GTP requires guanine triphosphatase-activating proteins (GAPs) such as the NF1 protein. Mutations in the ras protein that prevent hydrolysis of bound GTP result in continual signaling. A similar result can be caused by mutations in GAPs that disable the GTPase function of ras.

and G_γ subunits, the Ras proteins are monomers that are most closely related to the G_α subunit of the trimeric members of the G protein family.

G proteins cycle between a resting state in which guanosine diphosphate (GDP) is bound to the protein and an active state in which guanosine triphosphate (GTP) is bound (Fig. 2). On binding the ligand, the receptor forms dimers, which results in autophosphorylation of certain tyrosine residues on the cytoplasmic portion of the protein. This leads to recruitment of adaptor proteins such as Grb2, which, in turn, leads to binding of guanine nucleotide exchange factors (GNEFs) such as son of sevenless (SOS). GNEFs stimulate the release of bound GDP from the G protein, and this enables GTP to bind, which generates the active form of the G protein. The G protein-GTP complex activates downstream signaling pathways that are involved in cellular functions including cell proliferation and differentiation, cell cycle regulation, apoptosis, and angiogenesis *(32)*.

Hydrolysis of bound GTP by the GTPase activity of the G protein leads to signal diminution. The GTPase activity is greatly augmented by binding of cytoplasmic GTPase-activating proteins (GAPs) such as NF1. Binding of such factors accelerates the hydrolysis of GTP to GDP, thereby returning the G protein to its quiescent state.

Ras mutations that are associated with tumorigenesis are characterized by persistence of the active G protein-GTP complex, which consistently stimulates one of the Ras signaling pathways. Different Ras proteins are implicated in tumorigenesis in different tissues and with different frequencies. Mutations in *K-ras* are present in approx 90% of pancreatic cancers, 50% of colorectal cancers, and 30% of adenocarcinomas of the lung. *N-ras* is mutated in 30% of acute myeloid leukemias. *H-ras* is mutated in 10% of bladder cancers. Follicular and undifferentiated papillary thyroid cancers are associated with mutations in *H-, N-,* or *K-ras* in 50–60% of cases. It is estimated that up to 30% of all cancers are associated with a mutation in one of the *Ras* genes.

An interesting observation, with potential therapeutic implications, is that binding of Ras proteins to the cell membrane requires the presence of a farnesyl (C15) group at the carboxy end of the protein. Farnesyl pyrophosphate (FPP) is an intermediary in the biosynthetic pathway of cholesterol. Farnesyl transferase (FT) catalyzes the addition of the farnesyl group from FPP to a "CAAX" motif in the carboxy region of a target protein. Here, "C" is the cysteine to which the farnesyl group is added, "A" is an aliphatic amino acid (i.e., leucine valine, or isoleucine), and "X" is methionine, leucine, glutamine, or serine. After addition of the farnesyl group, an endopeptidase removes the three amino acids ("AAX") on the carboxy side of the farnesylation site, and the end of the protein is O-methylated. Inhibitors of FT are currently undergoing evaluation as possible anticancer agents that might be of value in treating tumors in which a Ras protein is activated by a mutation.

In addition to activating mutations in Ras proteins themselves, mutations in GAP proteins can also lead to increased activity of Ras signaling by slowing hydrolysis of bound GTP. This is the molecular basis of type 1 neurofibromatosis (NF1), which is caused by mutation in a GAP protein. NF1 (also known as von Recklinghausen's syndrome) is a highly penetrant autosomal dominant disorder with a prevalence of approx 1 in 3000, although the rate varies among different populations, being higher in some north African and Asian groups than among Caucasians *(33,34)*. Approximately 50% of cases represent new mutations *(33)*. Clinically, it is characterized by peripheral neurofibromas. The plexiform variant of these tumors is associated with an increased risk of developing malignant peripheral nerve sheath tumors. Other clinical features include café-au-lait spots, freckling of the intertriginous regions of the axillae and groin, benign hamartomas of the irises known as Lisch nodules, and increased frequencies of malignant glioma, pheochromocytoma, and juvenile myelomonocytic leukemia (JMML). Up to 10% of cases of JMML occur in patients with NF1 *(35,36)*.

The gene responsible for NF1, neurofibromin, is located on chromosome 17q11.2. It spans 350 kb of DNA, includes at least 59 exons, and generates alternatively spliced products. Neurofibromin protein contains 2818 amino acids *(37)*. Approximately 80% of mutations cause protein truncation; thus protein truncation assays are of use in laboratory diagnosis (*see* Chap. 4).

APOPTOSIS

Apoptosis, also called programmed cell death, is a physiological mechanism whereby metazoans can shape the architecture of tissues by removal of healthy but unwanted cells and by removal of damaged cells. Apoptosis is essential for processes as seemingly diverse as formation of the digits and elimination of cancerous cells. Apoptosis is a normal process that is distinguished from necrosis, which is an unintended death of cells arising from irreversible injury such as ischemia or trauma. Each cell carries the seeds of its own destruction in the form of genes that are proapoptotic. The effects of these are opposed by antiapoptotic genes. It is the balance between these opposing forces that determines whether a cell will live or activate the apoptotic pathway leading to its self-destruction. Apoptosis can be thought of as occurring in four stages: an initiating event, a cytoplasmic response, apoptosis itself, and removal of cellular debris by phagocytes.

Initiation of Apoptosis

A variety of factors external or internal to the cell can initiate apoptosis. Withdrawal of external survival signals alone can be sufficient to initiate apoptosis *(38).* Apoptosis can be actively induced by other cells, particularly by activated T-lymphocytes. One of the best characterized extracellular factors that leads to apoptosis is Fas ligand (FasL). FasL is produced by cytotoxic T-lymphocytes and natural killer (NK) cells. A wide variety of cells, but particularly lymphocytes, express a membrane-bound receptor, Fas (also known as CD95 or APO-1), which can bind FasL and initiate apoptosis. Fas and FasL are members of superfamilies of tumor necrosis factor (TNF) receptors and their cognate ligands. This family of receptors has an extracellular region composed of three to six cysteine-rich domains and an intracellular cytoplasmic tail that is required for signal transduction and is known as the death domain. Binding of the ligand to its receptor leads to formation of a trimeric complex that includes three receptor molecules and three ligands *(39).* Formation of the trimeric complex is probably essential for transmission of a death signal to the interior of the cell. Crosslinking of Fas receptors by antibodies can also trigger apoptosis.

Once a Fas/FasL trimer has formed, its cytoplasmic tail, which contains homophilic death domains, can bind an adaptor molecule, Fas-associated death domain protein (FADD) *(40).* This binding involves homophilic interaction between death domains on both Fas and FADD. FADD, in turn, can bind pro-caspase 8 (also known as FLICE) via homophilic interaction between death effector domains on both proteins. Binding of pro-caspase 8 by FADD leads to generation of the active form of the enzyme, caspase 8. This initiates the apoptotic trigger. The complex of Fas, FADD, and pro-caspase 8 is known as the death-inducing signaling complex (DISC).

Similar pathways for external death signaling via related ligands and receptors have been described. These include TNF, which binds to TNF receptor 1 (TNFR1), and TNF-related apoptosis-inducing ligand (TRAIL), which binds to the death receptors (DR), DR4 and DR5. The death domains of these proteins can bind different molecules: TNFR1 binds TNFR-associated death domain (TRADD) protein, which leads to activation of the c-Jun N-terminal kinase (JNK) pathway. Alternatively, TRADD can bind FADD and initiate apoptosis via activation of caspase 8.

Cytotoxic T-lymphocytes have an alternative mechanism for inducing apoptosis in target cells: delivery of perforin and granzyme B to the membranes of cells to be destroyed. Perforin forms channels in membranes through which granzyme B can enter the target cell. Granzyme B is an enzyme capable of activating caspase 3 *(41)*. This perforin/granzyme B apoptosis pathway bypasses the Fas "death receptor" mechanism.

A third mechanism for initiating apoptosis involves the release of cytochrome c from mitochondria. This mechanism is implicated in apoptosis induced by cellular injuries caused by agents such as ionizing radiation and cytotoxic drugs. Through incompletely understood mechanisms, such injury leads to release of cytochrome c which can bind a cytoplasmic molecule known as Apaf-1, and dATP. This complex, which is known as the apoptosome, can recruit and convert pro-caspase 9 to caspase 9, which can initiate the caspase cascade. Control of cytochrome c release is determined by members of the Bcl-2 family of proteins, which consists of at least 15 members that play critical roles in cell survival or cell death by apoptosis. The *BCL2* gene itself was identified as being overexpressed in B-cell lymphomas that have the t(14;18) translocation *(42)*. This protein promotes tumorigenesis by inhibiting apoptosis, a mechanism that is distinct from that of either tumor suppressor genes or other oncogenes. Proapoptotic members of the Bcl-2 family include Bax, Bak, and Bok. Prosurvival members include Bcl-2 and Bcl-x_L. The net effect of these proteins may be determined by the relative ratios of prosurvival and proapoptotic members. These can form heterodimers, thereby potentially inactivating each other's effects *(43,44)*. If the ratio favors proapoptotic members, they may be able to titrate out the antiapoptotic members. Bcl-2 is found on the cytoplasmic side of the mitochondrial membrane and also on the endoplasmic reticulum and nuclear membrane. It appears to function, at least in part, by inhibiting the apoptosome. Bcl-2 may also stabilize the mitochondrial membrane, thereby inhibiting release of cytochrome c.

Changes Associated with Apoptosis

Once a cell has committed to execution of the apoptotic pathway, a series of morphological and biochemical changes is initiated. Apoptosis is characterized by distinctive changes in the morphology of cells including shrinkage, blebbing of the external membrane, condensation of the nucleus, and fragmentation of DNA. Production of an endonuclease that cleaves DNA into 50-kb fragments is highly characteristic of apoptosis. Biochemical changes include expression of phosphatidylserine on the exterior face of the cell membrane (normally it is on the interior side of the membrane) and expression of the cell membrane intracellular adhesion molecule-3 (ICAM-3). These cell surface changes may be critical for phagocytic removal of apoptosed cells. Apoptosis does not illicit an inflammatory response.

Caspases

The destruction of cells undergoing apoptosis is brought about, in most cases, by activation of a cascade of proteases known as caspases (for *c*ysteinyl *asp*artate-specific protein*ases*). These enzymes contain cysteine at their active sites and cleave substrate peptides on the carboxy side of certain aspartic acid residues. Caspases are synthesized as pro-enzymes that are activated by proteolytic cleavage. Activated caspases, in turn, can cleave other pro-caspases in a cascade that resembles the complement or coagulation pathways. Once activated, certain caspases, known as effector caspases, are responsible for the destruction of the cell. These include caspases 6 and 7 and especially caspase 3, which is essential for caspase-mediated apoptosis *(45,46)*. Activation of the caspase cascade is by initiator caspases. These include caspase 8 and caspase 9. As discussed above, caspase 8 is activated by DISC. Caspase 9 is activated by the apoptosome.

Mutations in Genes Involved in Apoptosis

Several diseases have been shown to arise from mutations in genes that play important roles in apoptosis. As mentioned above and in Chapter 8, most cases of follicular lymphoma are associated with overexpression of *BCL2* as a result of the 14;18 translocation that brings the *BCL2* gene on chromosome 18 in proximity to the *IgH* gene on chromosome 14. Mutations in the TNF-R1 receptor gene cause familial periodic fever *(47)*, whereas mutations in the Fas receptor gene cause type I autoimmune lymphoproliferative syndrome *(48)*. Type II autoimmune lymphoproliferative syndrome is caused by mutations in caspase 10 *(49)*. Mutations in perforin are

associated with some cases of familial hemophagocytic lymphohistiocytosis *(50)*.

TELOMERASE

During cell division, DNA is replicated by DNA polymerase α.
This enzyme requires a short RNA primer that hybridizes to the 5'
region of the DNA to be replicated. However, this RNA primer is
then hydrolyzed and so the 5' end of a DNA fragment is not replicated, leading to shortening with each cycle of cell division. This
replication mechanism prevents complete replication of the ends of
chromosomes, the telomeres; at each cell division, chromosomes
would be expected to lose approx 50–200 bp *(51)*. The consequences of loss of telomere sequence are cellular senescence, apoptosis, or chromosomal instability with formation of fusions
involving the uncapped chromosome ends.

Beginning at the single-celled zygote stage, a human may have as
many as 10^{15} cell divisions in a lifetime. Clearly, even with a genome
of approx 10^9 bp, cells could not sustain the loss of even a single base
pair during each cell division. This loss of chromosome ends, which
is known as the *end-replication problem,* is rectified in some cells,
including at least 85% of malignancies, by expression of telomerase,
an enzyme that increases the number of copies of the telomere repeat.
Telomeres are made up of repeats of the sequence TTAGGG. Telomerase is a reverse transcriptase composed of a DNA polymerase and a
bound RNA template containing the complement of the telomere
sequence. The polymerase is known as hTERT and the RNA as hTR.
Enzyme activity can be detected using methods that either detect
telomerase (hTERT) by its activity, by immunohistochemical staining, or by RT-PCR to detect its mRNA. hTR can be detected by RT-
PCR, by Northern blotting, or by *in situ* hybridization.

As mentioned, most tumors re-express telomerase, and this
appears to be a critical factor for survival of tumor cells. This observation was initially greeted with optimism: telomerase might prove
to be a generic cancer marker. Although telomerase has been shown
to be a useful marker in some studies, its broader diagnostic application is limited by the recognition that some normal cells, including stem cells, epithelial basal cells, and activated lymphocytes
express telomerase activity. It is also reactivated in conditions such
as follicular thyroid adenomas, Graves' disease, and Hashimoto's

thyroiditis *(52)*. Thus, detection of telomerase is not completely specific for cancer. However, it may be an important target for novel anticancer pharmaceuticals.

Mutations in hTR and Aplastic Anemia

Inherited mutations in the gene encoding dyskerin, *DKC1,* have been described in patients with X-linked dyskeratosis congenita, a rare disease characterized by abnormal skin pigmentation, nail dystrophy, leukoplakia, and bone marrow failure leading to aplastic anemia. This protein associates with certain small nucleolar RNAs including hTR RNA. In addition, mutations in *hTR* have been reported in patients with an autosomal dominant form of this disorder. Recently, approx 10% of patients with idiopathic aplastic anemia have been shown to harbor mutations in *hTR (53)*.

REFERENCES

1. Knudson AG Jr. Mutation and cancer: statistical study of retinoblastoma. Proc Natl Acad Sci USA 1971;68:820–3.
2. Singal R, Ginder GD. DNA methylation. Blood 1999;93:4059–70.
3. Esteller M, Sparks A, Toyota M, et al. Analysis of adenomatous polyposis coli promoter hypermethylation in human cancer. Cancer Res 2000;60:4366–71.
4. Garinis GA, Patrinos GP, Spanakis NE, Menounos PG. DNA hypermethylation: when tumour suppressor genes go silent. Hum Genet 2002;111:115–27.
5. Shields CL, Shields JA, Shah P. Retinoblastoma in older children. Ophthalmology 1991;98:395–9.
6. Wong FL, Boice JD Jr, Abramson DH, et al. Cancer incidence after retinoblastoma. Radiation dose and sarcoma risk. JAMA 1997;278:1262–7.
7. Lohmann DR. RB1 gene mutations in retinoblastoma. Hum Mutat 1999;14:283–8.
8. Nevins JR. The Rb/E2F pathway and cancer. Hum Mol Genet 2001;10:699–703.
9. Sherr CJ. The Pezcoller lecture: cancer cell cycles revisited. Cancer Res 2000;60:3689–95.
10. Donnellan R, Chetty R. Cyclin D1 and human neoplasia. Mol Pathol 1998;51:1–7.
11. Tsihlias J, Kapusta L, Slingerland J. The prognostic significance of altered cyclin-dependent kinase inhibitors in human cancer. Annu Rev Med 1999;50:401–23.
12. Pietenpol JA, Bohlander SK, Sato Y, et al. Assignment of the human p27Kip1 gene to 12p13 and its analysis in leukemias. Cancer Res 1995;55:1206–10.
13. Chen X, Farmer G, Zhu H, Prywes R, Prives C. Cooperative DNA binding of p53 with TFIID (TBP): a possible mechanism for transcriptional activation. Genes Dev 1993;7:1837–49.
14. Horikoshi N, Usheva A, Chen J, Levine AJ, Weinmann R, Shenk T. Two domains of p53 interact with the TATA-binding protein, and the adenovirus 13S E1A protein disrupts the association, relieving p53-mediated transcriptional repression. Mol Cell Biol 1995;15:227–34.
15. Bunz F, Dutriaux A, Lengauer C, et al. Requirement for p53 and p21 to sustain G2 arrest after DNA damage. Science 1998;282:1497–501.
16. Vousden KH. p53: death star. Cell 2000;103:691–4.

17. Innocente SA, Abrahamson JL, Cogswell JP, Lee JM. p53 regulates a G2 check-point through cyclin B1. Proc Natl Acad Sci USA 1999;96:2147–52.

18. Hermeking H, Lengauer C, Polyak K, et al. 14-3-3 sigma is a p53-regulated inhibitor of G2/M progression. Mol Cell 1997;1:3–11.

19. Inoue T, Geyer RK, Howard D, Yu ZK, Maki CG. MDM2 can promote the ubiqui-tination, nuclear export, and degradation of p53 in the absence of direct binding. J Biol Chem 2001;276:45255–60.

20. Oliner JD, Kinzler KW, Meltzer PS, George DL, Vogelstein B. Amplification of a gene encoding a p53-associated protein in human sarcomas. Nature 1992;358:80–3.

21. zur Hausen H. Papillomavirus infections—a major cause of human cancers. Biochim Biophys Acta 1996;1288:F55–78.

22. Hwang ES, Nottoli T, Dimaio D. The HPV16 E5 protein: expression, detection, and stable complex formation with transmembrane proteins in COS cells. Virology 1995;211:227–33.

23. Scheffner M, Werness BA, Huibregtse JM, Levine AJ, Howley PM. The E6 onco-protein encoded by human papillomavirus types 16 and 18 promotes the degrada-tion of p53. Cell 1990;63:1129–36.

24. Werness BA, Levine AJ, Howley PM. Association of human papillomavirus types 16 and 18 E6 proteins with p53. Science 1990;248:76–9.

25. zur Hausen H. Papillomaviruses and cancer: from basic studies to clinical applica-tion. Nat Rev Cancer 2002;2:342–50.

26. Dyson N, Howley PM, Munger K, Harlow E. The human papilloma virus-16 E7 oncoprotein is able to bind to the retinoblastoma gene product. Science 1989;243:934–7.

27. Hynes NE, Stern DF. The biology of erbB-2/neu/HER-2 and its role in cancer. Biochim Biophys Acta 1994;1198:165–84.

28. Yamauchi H, Stearns V, Hayes DF. When is a tumor marker ready for prime time? A case study of c-erbB-2 as a predictive factor in breast cancer. J Clin Oncol 2001;19:2334–56.

29. Westermann F, Schwab M. Genetic parameters of neuroblastomas. Cancer Lett 2002;184:127–47.

30. Nesbit CE, Tersak JM, Prochownik EV. MYC oncogenes and human neoplastic disease. Oncogene 1999;18:3004–16.

31. Hecht JL, Aster JC. Molecular biology of Burkitt's lymphoma. J Clin Oncol 2000;18:3707–21.

32. Adjei AA. Blocking oncogenic Ras signaling for cancer therapy. J Natl Cancer Inst 2001;93:1062–74.

33. Littler M, Morton NE. Segregation analysis of peripheral neurofibromatosis (NF1). J Med Genet 1990;27:307–10.

34. Garty BZ, Laor A, Danon YL. Neurofibromatosis type 1 in Israel: survey of young adults. J Med Genet 1994;31:853–7.

35. Castro-Malaspina H, Schaison G, Passe S, et al. Subacute and chronic myelomonocytic leukemia in children (juvenile CML). Clinical and hematologic observations, and identification of prognostic factors. Cancer 1984;54:675–86.

36. Luna-Fineman S, Shannon KM, Atwater SK, et al. Myelodysplastic and myelopro-liferative disorders of childhood: a study of 167 patients. Blood 1999;93:459–66.

37. Shen MH, Harper PS, Upadhyaya M. Molecular genetics of neurofibromatosis type 1 (NF1). J Med Genet 1996;33:2–17.

38. Raff MC, Barres BA, Burne JF, Coles HS, Ishizaki Y, Jacobson MD. Programmed cell death and the control of cell survival: lessons from the nervous system. Sci-ence 1993;262:695–700.

39. Banner DW, D'Arcy A, Janes W, et al. Crystal structure of the soluble human 55 kd TNF receptor-human TNF beta complex: implications for TNF receptor activation. Cell 1993;73:431–45.

40. Chinnaiyan AM, O'Rourke K, Tewari M, Dixit VM. FADD, a novel death domain-containing protein, interacts with the death domain of Fas and initiates apoptosis. Cell 1995;81:505–12.

41. Atkinson EA, Barry M, Darmon AJ, et al. Cytotoxic T lymphocyte-assisted suicide. Caspase 3 activation is primarily the result of the direct action of granzyme B. J Biol Chem 1998;273:21261–6.

42. Ngan BY, Chen-Levy Z, Weiss LM, Warnke RA, Cleary ML. Expression in non-Hodgkin's lymphoma of the bcl-2 protein associated with the t(14;18) chromosomal translocation. N Engl J Med 1988;318:1638–44.

43. Korsmeyer SJ, Shutter JR, Veis DJ, Merry DE, Oltvai ZN. Bcl-2/Bax: a rheostat that regulates an anti-oxidant pathway and cell death. Semin Cancer Biol 1993;4:327–32.

44. Oltvai ZN, Milliman CL, Korsmeyer SJ. Bcl-2 heterodimerizes in vivo with a conserved homolog, Bax, that accelerates programmed cell death. Cell 1993;74:609–19.

45. Woo M, Hakem R, Soengas MS, et al. Essential contribution of caspase 3/CPP32 to apoptosis and its associated nuclear changes. Genes Dev 1998;12:806–19.

46. Janicke RU, Sprengart ML, Wati MR, Porter AG. Caspase-3 is required for DNA fragmentation and morphological changes associated with apoptosis. J Biol Chem 1998;273:9357–60.

47. Drenth JP, van der Meer JW. Hereditary periodic fever. N Engl J Med 2001;345:1748–57.

48. Straus SE, Jaffe ES, Puck JM, et al. The development of lymphomas in families with autoimmune lymphoproliferative syndrome with germline Fas mutations and defective lymphocyte apoptosis. Blood 2001;98:194–200.

49. Wang J, Zheng L, Lobito A, et al. Inherited human Caspase 10 mutations underlie defective lymphocyte and dendritic cell apoptosis in autoimmune lymphoproliferative syndrome type II. Cell 1999;98:47–58.

50. Stepp SE, Dufourcq-Lagelouse R, Le Deist F, et al. Perforin gene defects in familial hemophagocytic lymphohistiocytosis. Science 1999;286:1957–9.

51. Huffman KE, Levene SD, Tesmer VM, Shay JW, Wright WE. Telomere shortening is proportional to the size of the G-rich telomeric 3'-overhang. J Biol Chem 2000;275:19719–22.

52. Hiyama E, Hiyama K. Clinical utility of telomerase in cancer. Oncogene 2002;21:643–9.

53. Vulliamy T, Marrone A, Dokal I, Mason PJ. Association between aplastic anaemia and mutations in telomerase RNA. Lancet 2002;359:2168–70.

54. Reinartz J. Cancer genes. In: Coleman WB, Tsongalis GJ, eds. The Molecular Basis of Human Cancer. Totowa, NJ: Humana, 2002:45–64.

7   Familial Cancer Syndromes

Familial cancer syndromes represent a small proportion of the overall number of cancers that are diagnosed each year. However, given the high incidence of some cancers (such as breast and colorectal), the absolute number of patients with hereditary cancer syndromes is quite large, and many cancer patients may be unaware that they have a hereditary cancer syndrome. The study of familial cancer syndromes has led to discovery of genes that also play a significant role in the development of nonfamilial, sporadic cancers. In addition, genetic cancer syndromes can offer opportunities for early cancer diagnosis and treatment in subjects at high risk because of identification of inherited mutations. For these reasons, familial cancer syndromes form an important area for both basic research and clinical practice. In this chapter, the molecular aspects of selected hereditary cancer syndromes are reviewed.

HEREDITARY BREAST AND OVARIAN CANCER

Breast cancer is one of the most common forms of cancer in women. Approximately 1 in 10 women in the United States will develop breast cancer during her lifetime. Of all breast cancers, the great majority are sporadic, but approx 5–10% are owing to inherited mutations; of these, mutations in two genes, *BRCA1* and *BRCA2,* account for 15–20% of hereditary breast cancers and 60–80% of cases of hereditary breast and ovarian cancer *(1).* Breast cancer associated with mutations in *BRCA1* or *BRCA2* is characterized by autosomal dominant inheritance, which means that in 50% of cases, the mutant gene in an affected woman was inherited from her father. Other familial syndromes with significant breast cancer risks include Cowden's syndrome, Li-Fraumeni syndrome, and ataxia-telangiectasia. The last of these is an autosomal recessive disease in which cells are unusually sensitive to ionizing radiation. Carriers of mutations in the gene that causes ataxia-telangiectasia,

From: *Principles of Molecular Pathology*
Edited by: A. A. Killeen © Humana Press Inc., Totowa, NJ

ATM, also appear to be at increased risk of developing breast cancer *(2).* A mutation in the *CHEK2* gene, 1100de1C, which is present in 0.3–1.4% of Caucasian populations tested to date is associated with a 1.4–4.7-fold increased risk of breast cancer *(3,4).*

BRCA1

BRCA1 was the first breast cancer gene to be identified. Linkage analysis revealed the existence of a locus on chromosome 17q21 in families with multiple cases of breast cancer and early-onset breast cancer *(5).* The gene was cloned in 1994 *(6,7).* *BRCA1* is believed to function as a tumor suppressor gene: subjects who develop *BRCA1*-related breast cancer inherit one mutant copy of *BRCA1* and later develop a somatic inactivating mutation in the remaining wild-type allele, thus eliminating the expression of functional BRCA1 protein in malignant cells. The lifetime risk of developing breast cancer in *BRCA1* mutation carriers is estimated to be 60–80%, and the lifetime risk of developing ovarian cancer is 20–40% *(1).*

The *BRCA1* gene contains 24 exons, of which 22 encode the protein. Exon 11 is unusually long and encodes 60% of the protein, which has a molecular mass of 220 kDa. Several distinct regions with differing functions have been identified in the protein. The N-terminal region contains a zinc-binding RING finger domain that may be involved in interactions with other proteins. There are binding domains for p53 and Rad 51 that are separated by a nuclear localization signal. BRCA2 binds toward the carboxy-terminus region. The BRCA1 carboxy-terminus (BRCT) domain also contains binding sites for proteins involved in transcription, and similar domains are present in many other genes that are involved in the cellular response to DNA damage. BRCA1 appears to have several functions including repair of DNA damage, control of the cell cycle, and control of transcription *(8).*

Mutations have been described throughout the gene. Among Ashkenazi Jewish patients with breast cancer, two *BRCA1* mutations, 185delAG and 5382insC, are relatively common and represent founder mutations. However, in most populations, the diversity of mutations is such that common mutations are not present. Most germline mutations in *BRCA1* cause protein truncation or loss of function of the BRCT domain involved in regulating gene transcription. Several genes that are regulated by BRCA1 have been identified including *MYC,* cyclin D1, and certain proteins involved in cytokine signaling pathways *(9).*

BRCA2

BRCA2 was the second breast cancer gene to be identified. Approximately 5–15% of familial breast cancer is attributable to mutations in this gene; the percentage varies among different ethnic populations. *BRCA2* is located on chromosome 13q12-13, contains 27 exons, and encodes a 384-kDa nuclear protein *(10).* The gene has little homology to any other mammalian gene. Exons 10 and 11 are large. The latter encodes multiple copies of a repetitive BCR unit that are involved in binding the protein to RAD51, a protein that is involved in repair of some types of DNA damage. This suggests that *BRCA2* is also involved in DNA repair.

As with *BRCA1,* founder mutations in *BRCA2* are present in certain populations. Among Ashkenazi Jewish subjects, 6174delT is found in 1.5% of the population and accounts for up to 8% of cases of familial breast cancer. In Iceland, a 5-bp deletion, 999del5, is present in 0.4% of the population and 8.5% of patients with breast cancer *(11).* Mutations in *BRCA2* are also associated with increased risk of male breast cancer and with increased risk of other cancers including prostate, gallbladder, bile duct, stomach, and melanoma *(12).*

Mutation Screening for BRCA1 *and* BRCA2

Guidelines have been produced by the National Comprehensive Cancer Network for identification of individuals and families with familial breast/ovarian cancer (Table 1). Because of the high prevalence of 185delAG and 5382insC *(BRCA1)* and 6174delT *(BRCA2)* mutations among Ashkenazi Jews, these mutations are sometimes offered as an initial screening panel in this population. However, for the general population, screening for unknown mutations in *BRCA1* and *BRCA2* in suspected hereditary breast/ovarian cancer families involves comprehensive sequencing of the coding regions and exon/intron boundaries. Even sequencing may not detect all mutations: large deletions on one allele and exon duplications are not easily demonstrated by sequencing, and some splice mutations may also be undetectable. The estimated rate of failure to detect a mutation on routine testing is approx 5–15% *(13).* In a small proportion of high-risk cases (i.e., those individuals with multiple affected relatives, a

Table 1
National Comprehensive Cancer Network Practice Guideline for Identification of Hereditary Breast and /or Ovarian Cancer (HBOC)

Criteria [a,b]

- Member of known *BRCA1/BRCA2* kindred
- Personal history of breast cancer + one or more of the following:
  - Diagnosed age ≤ 40 yr[c] with or without a family history
  - Diagnosed age ≤ 50 yr or bilateral, with ≥ 1 close blood relative with breast cancer ≤ 50 yr or ≥ 1 close blood relative with ovarian cancer
  - Diagnosed at any age, with ≥ 2 close blood relatives with ovarian cancer at any age.
  - Diagnosed at any age with breast cancer, especially if ≥ 1 woman is diagnosed before age 50 yr or has bilateral disease
  - Close male blood relative has breast cancer
  - Personal history of ovarian cancer
  - If of Ashkenazi Jewish descent and diagnosed age ≤ 50 yr, no additional family history is required, or at any age if history of breast and/or ovarian cancer in close blood relative
- Personal history of ovarian cancer + one or more of the following:
  - ≥ 1 close blood relative with ovarian cancer
  - ≥ 1 close female blood relative with beast cancer at age ≤ 50 yr or bilateral breast cancer
  - ≥ 2 close blod relatives with breast cancer
  - ≥ 1 close male blood relative with breast cancer
  - If of Ashkenazi Jewish discent, no additional family history is required
- Personal history of male breast cancer + one or more of the following:
  - ≥ 1 close male blood relative with breast cancer
  - ≥ 1 close female blood relative with breast or ovarian cancer
  - If of Ashkenazi Jewish descent, no aditional family history is required
- Family history only 1/M close family member meeting any the above criteria

a. Criteria suggestive of hereditary breast/ovarian cancer syndrome that warrant further professinal evaluation.

b. When investigating family histories for HBOC, all close relatives on the same side of the family should be included. Close relatives include first-, second-, and third-degree relatives.

c. May consider age range between ≤ 40 yr and ≤ 50 yr if clinical situation warrants.

family history that includes ovarian cancer, and early age of onset), a missense mutation will be identified, the functional significance of which may be uncertain. No functional assays for BRCA1 or BRCA2 are available to examine the effects of a missense mutation, and in the absence of more definitive data, it may be impossible to determine the significance of a missense mutation. Factors suggesting that a missense mutation may be a benign polymorphism include its presence in controls without a family history of breast/ovarian cancer, segregation in families independently of cancer development, and encoding of a conservative amino acid substitution. Factors suggesting that a missense mutation is a deleterious mutation include its absence from control samples, presence in multiple families with breast/ovarian cancer, and encoding a nonconservative amino acid substitution.

Because mutation testing for hereditary breast cancer syndromes involves complex issues and may not yield a definitive answer, testing should be performed in the context of genetic counseling. Asymptomatic subjects who are identified as having a *BRCA1* or *BRCA2* mutation should be screened carefully and regularly for early cancer. Prophylactic mastectomy and oophorectomy may be an option for some women to decrease the risk of developing cancer.

COLORECTAL CANCER

Colorectal cancer is among the most common type of nonskin tumors in Western populations. Approximately 5% of all colorectal cancers are owing to familial cancer syndromes. These can be grouped into cancers associated with polyposis syndromes and those that are not associated with polyposis syndromes. The most common of the polyposis syndromes is familial adenomatous polyposis (FAP), which is caused by mutations in the adenomatous polyposis coli *(APC)* gene on 5q21. This is a relatively rare disorder, with a frequency of <1% of all colorectal cancers. Hereditary nonpolyposis colorectal cancer (HNPCC) is caused by mutations in one of a number of mismatch repair genes, including *MSH2* (2p22), *MLH1* (3p21), *PMS1* (2q31), *PMS2* (7p22), and *MSH6* (2p16), and accounts for most inherited colorectal cancer syndromes.

Familial Polyposis Syndromes
FAMILIAL ADENOMATOUS POLYPOSIS

FAP is a rare autosomal dominant disorder with an incidence of approx 1 in 5000 to 1 in 13,500 *(14,15)*. The disease is characterized by the presence of multiple (hundreds to thousands) adenomatous polyps of the colon and rectum and carries a high risk of development of cancer. Most patients with FAP develop colorectal cancer by age 40 if untreated. In addition to colorectal cancer, patients with FAP also have a high risk of developing upper gastrointestinal tumors, particularly carcinoma at the ampulla of Vater *(16)*. Additional features of FAP include congenital hypertrophy of the retinal pigment epithelium (CHRPE), a condition present in up to 90% of patients in some family studies *(17)*. This abnormality can be observed by fundoscopy, even in infants, and is useful in identifying at-risk individuals in families with FAP. Patients with FAP have an increased frequency of desmoid tumors, hepatoblastomas, medulloblastomas (Turcot's syndrome), and dental abnormalities including supernumerary or missing teeth *(18–21)*.

Gardner's syndrome, which includes, in addition to colonic polyps, osteoid tumors of the mandible and long bones, as well as epidermoid cysts, is a variant form of FAP. An attenuated form of FAP with fewer (<100) polyps but also a high risk of cancer development is also recognized *(22)*.

Hereditary Mutations in *APC*. FAP is caused by mutations in the *APC* tumor suppressor gene on chromosome 5q21. The main gene transcript includes 15 exons that encode a large protein of 312 kDa, comprised of 2843 amino acids. Alternatively spliced transcripts have been described.

Approximately one-third of all germline mutations occur at codons 1061 and 1309, and 80% of mutations cause premature chain termination. These are detectable by a protein truncation assay. Germline mutations in *APC* are associated with a high degree of penetrance: most patients with germline mutations develop colorectal cancer by age 40. Approximately 25% of all patients have a new germline mutation *(23)*.

I1307K. A missense mutation in *APC*, I1307K, that is present in approx 6–8% of Ashkenazi Jewish individuals, but that is rarely seen in other populations, is associated with an increased risk of colon cancer. This mutation is a T→A transversion at nucleotide 3920; it creates an uninterrupted series of eight adenine residues and renders DNA around this position unusually susceptible to additional, somatic mutations *(24)*. Although the I1307K mutation does not by itself lead to cancer, it is significant because it increases the risk of developing additional, cancer-causing mutations in *APC*.

Somatic Mutations in *APC*. Somatic mutations in *APC* are present in 75% of sporadic colorectal cancers and appear to be an early event in tumorigenesis. Mutations fall into three general classes: loss of heterozygosity, sequence mutations, and promoter hypermethylation that silences gene transcription. Most sequence mutations are located in a region of exon 15 called the mutation cluster region (MCR). Codons 1309, 1450, and 1554 are frequently mutated *(25)*. In families with FAP, a germline mutation is inherited on one allele, and a "second hit" on the other allele leads to mutation of the remaining gene.

Effects of *APC* Mutations. APC protein is involved in regulating the activity of the Wg/Wnt pathway of cell signaling. Wingless (Wg) is named from a cell-cell signaling pathway in *Drosophila* that involves a protein known as armadillo, the human homolog of which is β-catenin. β-Catenin functions as an activator of transcription factors including T-cell factor/lymphoid enhancer factor (Tcf/lef). In this role, β-catenin is involved in upregulation of several genes involved in cell proliferation including *c-myc,* cyclin D1, and inhibition of apoptosis *(25)*.

Cellular levels of β-catenin are controlled by a degradation system that involves formation of a complex including β-catenin, APC, a serine threonine glycogen synthase kinase (GSK-3β), and axin (Fig. 1). This complex phosphorylates β-catenin at serine and threonine residues, which is a prelude to its ubiquination and removal by the ubiquitin-proteasome system *(26,27)*.

In the Wnt signaling pathway, binding of a Wnt ligand to the receptor, which is known as frizzled, leads to activation of another protein, disheveled. The names of these proteins come from work in *Drosophila.* Disheveled binds axin and leads to inhibition of phosphorylation of β-catenin by the axin/GSK-3β/APC complex. This allows free β-catenin to accumulate and enter the nucleus, where it functions to stimulate transcription. Mutations in APC that destroy the ability of the axin/GSK-3β/APC complex to phosphorylate β-catenin also lead to higher intracellular levels of free β-catenin with the same effects on gene transcription as occur during Wnt stimulation. These effects tend to confer a growth and survival advantage for cells harboring *APC* mutations. The importance of β-catenin in tumorigenesis is also shown by the observation that mutations in β-catenin preventing its phosphorylation and subsequent ubiquination have been found in some colorectal tumors in which the *APC* gene is still functional *(26)*.

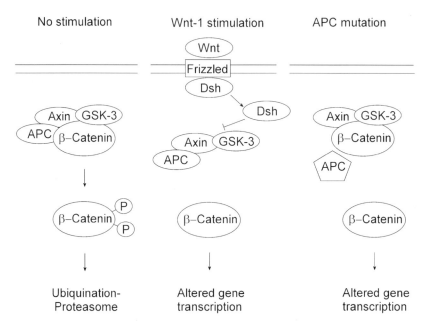

Fig. 1. The Wnt-1 signaling pathway and APC. β-Catenin is phosphorylated by a complex that includes APC, axin, and glycogen synthase kinase-3′ β (GSK-3). Phosphorylation leads to removal of β-catenin by the proteasome. In the Wnt-1 pathway, binding of a Wnt ligand to the membrane receptor frizzled leads to activation of the protein disheveled. This inhibits phosphorylation of β-catenin, which can then activate a transcriptional factor, TCF4/Lef, of several target genes that include cyclin D, cdk1, myc, and the multidrug transpoter, mdr1. Mutations in *APC* can also inhibit phosphorylation of β-catenin by preventing normal interaction of the phosphorylating complex.

More recently, a role for APC in assembly of the mitotic spindle has been described *(28,29)*. During cell division, the chromosomes are attached to microtubules responsible for ensuring that each daughter cell inherits a full complement of chromosomes. APC is involved with a protein known as EB1 in binding the microtubules to the kinetochores, the structures on the chromosomes to which the microtubules attach. This observation suggests that APC mutations may contribute to the chromosomal instability observed in many colorectal tumors by disrupting the normal pattern of chromosome segregation during mitosis *(30)*. However, this has not been firmly established *(31)*.

PEUTZ-JEGHERS SYNDROME

Peutz-Jeghers syndrome (PJS; OMIM 175200) is an autosomal dominant disorder characterized by pigmentation of the skin and mucous membranes, particularly in the perioral region, and by gastrointestinal hamartomatous polyps. The disease prevalence is approx 1 in 25,000. PJS patients are at risk of developing bleeding and intussusception associated with the polyps. In addition, there is an increased risk of development of malignancies including gastrointestinal, testicular, breast, ovarian, and sex cord tumors with annular tubules. The lifetime risk of developing cancer in PJS is over 90% *(32)*.

In most families, PJS is caused by mutations in the gene *LKB1* (also known as *STK11*) on chromosome 19p13.3, which encodes a serine/threonine protein kinase enzyme. The gene is believed to function as a tumor suppressor gene *(33)*. At least one other PJS gene exists because up to 30% of patients do not harbor germline *LKB1* mutations.

JUVENILE POLYPOSIS

Juvenile polyposis (JP; OMIM 174900) is characterized by development of hamartomatous gastrointestinal polyps and an increased risk of developing gastrointestinal cancer. Mutations in the *SMAD4/DPC4* gene on chromosome 18q21.1 have been demonstrated in some families with JP *(34,35)*. Other loci may also be responsible for this disease. In JP, the hamartomatous polyps are not premalignant, but the surrounding stromal tissue has been suggested to predispose to cancer formation *(36)*.

The SMAD proteins are involved in a signaling pathway of transforming growth factor-β (TGF-β). In addition to associations with JP, *SMAD4* mutations are strongly associated with pancreatic cancer. The gene is inactivated in approximately one-half of pancreatic cancers *(37)*.

Hereditary Nonpolyposis Colorectal Cancer

HNPCC (OMIM 120436) has an incidence of approx 1 in 1000 individuals and approx 3% of all patients with colorectal cancer. This disease is also known as Lynch's syndrome. HNPCC is inherited as an autosomal dominant trait and is caused by mutations in genes involved in mismatch repair, *MLH1, MSH2, MSH6,* and *PMS2*. Patients with HNPCC carry germline mutations in one of these genes. Ninety percent of patients with HNPCC have germline mutations in *MLH1* or *MSH2*.

CLINICAL FEATURES OF HNPCC

HNPCC is characterized by a high risk—estimated to be 80% over a lifetime—of developing colorectal cancer. The mean age of tumor presentation is 44 yr. Colonic tumors that arise in patients with HNPCC have several characteristic pathologic features including a tendency to develop in the proximal colon, production of mucin, elicitation of a lymphocytic inflammatory response, development of more than one tumor in a metachronous (i.e., different time of onset) or synchronous (i.e., simultaneous time of onset) manner, lower degree of differentiation, and fewer lymph node metastases *(38)*. HNPCC patients generally have a better prognosis than do patients with sporadic colorectal cancer. In addition to a high risk of colorectal cancer, patients with HNPCC are at increased risk of developing other tumors: endometrial cancer, stomach cancer, ovarian cancer, transitional cell carcinoma of the ureters and renal pelvis, small bowel cancer, and bile duct cancer. The risk of developing endometrial cancer is women with HNPCC mutations is slightly higher than the risk of developing colorectal cancer *(39)*.

HNPCC is suggested by a strong family history of colorectal cancer, particularly if there is early age of onset, and by a family or personal history of development of other characteristic tumors. Formal criteria have been established by different groups. These are the Amsterdam criteria and the Bethesda criteria (Tables 2 and 3). The Amsterdam criteria are stricter than the Bethesda criteria, and if they are used to select families for molecular genetic testing for HNPCC, a mutation will be identified in a higher proportion of patients who are tested than if the Bethesda criteria are used to select patients for testing. However, because fewer patients meet the Amsterdam criteria, some patients with germline mutations will not be selected for testing who would qualify for testing if the Bethesda criteria were applied. By not testing these families, opportunities for mutation identification in patients and presymptomatic family members are lost *(40)*.

DEFECTIVE MISMATCH REPAIR/MICROSATELLITE INSTABILITY

The molecular abnormality in HNPCC is defective DNA mismatch repair. A mismatch can involve base-base mispairing on complementary strands of DNA or an insertion-deletion loop

Table 2

Amsterdam Criteria for Clinical Diagnosis of Hereditary Nonpolyposis
Colon Cancer (HNPCC)

A. Original International Collaborative Group Criteria (Amsterdam I), 1991
  1. Three relatives with histologically verified colon cancer should be
     identified
     a. One should be a first-degree relative of the other two
     b. At least two successive generations in the family should be affected
     c. At least one individual should be diagnosed with colorectal cancer
        before age 50
  2. Familial adenomatous polyposis should be excluded
B. Revised International Collaborative Group Criteria (Amsterdam II), 1999
  1. Three relatives with a histologically verified HNPCC-associated cancer
     (i.e., colorectum, endometrium, small bowel, ureter, or renal pelvis)
     a. One should be a first-degree relative of the other two
     b. At least two successive generations should be affected
     c. At least one should be diagnosed before age 50
  2. Familial adenomatous polyposis should be excluded in the colorectal
     cancer cases

Table 3

Bethesda Criteria for Hereditary Nonpolyposis Colon Cancer (HNPCC)

- Individuals with cancer in families that meet the Amsterdam criteria
- Individuals with two HNPCC-related cancers including synchronous or
  metachronous colorectal tumors
- Individuals with colorectal cancer and a first-degree relative with colorectal
  cancer and/or HNPCC-related extracolonic cancer and/or a colorectal adenoma: one of the cancers diagnosed by age 45, and the adenoma diagnosed
  by age 40
- Individuals with colorectal cancer or endometrial cancer diagnosed before
  age 45
- Individuals with right-sided colorectal cancer with an undifferentiated
  histopathologic pattern (solid/cribriform), diagnosed by age 45
- Individuals with signet-ring cell-type colorectal cancer diagnosed by age 45
- Individuals with adenomas diagnosed by age 40

(Fig. 2). The latter may arise in a region containing repetitive
DNA segments (i.e., microsatellites) as a result of slippage of
DNA polymerase during DNA replication. Repair of such mismatches is a complex process that involves several proteins,
including those implicated in HNPCC. Mismatch repair can be

A **Mismatched basepair**

ACCT ^{T}GCGCG
TGGA $_G$CGCGC

B **Microsatellite slippage**

TGGGCACACACACACACACAGGTCCA
ACCCGTGTGT GTGTGTGTGTCCAGGT
GTGT

Fig. 2. Examples of DNA mismatches. **(A)** A mismatched base pair. **(B),** Slippage at a microsatellite repeat leads to one strand having extra base pairs.

demonstrated in vitro as microsatellite instability (MSI) in tumor samples. Approximately 10–15% of all colon cancers have MSI, but >95% of HNPCC-associated tumors have MSI.

MSI is detected by analyzing the size of certain microsatellite repeats in tumor samples. Because of mismatch repair defects, microsatellites show alterations in the number of copies of the repeating unit in the microsatellite relative to the number of copies present in the patient's germline DNA. These alterations can be either increases or decreases in the number of copies of the repeat, and these originate as insertions or deletions that occur during DNA replication that have not been correctly repaired by the mismatch repair process (Fig. 3).

Guidelines for standardization of laboratory assays to detect MSI have been published by the National Cancer Institute *(41)*. These

Fig. 3. (A) Autoradiograph of BAT25 amplified from a tumor bearing a defect in a mismatch repair gene, *hMSH2*. The normal sample is derived from transformed lymphoblasts (L670) from this patient, and the tumor sample is a cell line (Vaco 670) derived from the patient's tumor. Samples 2N and 2T from the second patient consist of normal colonic epithelium (2N) and colonic adenocarcinoma (2T). **(B)** Electropherograms of amplicons of BAT25 amplified from cell lines 1N and 1T as shown in **(A).** The sharp peaks (no arrow) are size markers of 75, 100, 139, 150, and 160 bp. Peak heights are quantified as random fluorescent units (RFUs) on the *y*-axis. The peaks at and around 120 and 116 bp (indicated by arrows) represent the BAT25 amplicons. These are shifted downward in size in the tumor (bottom) compared with normal tissue (top). (Reproduced with permission from ref. *(71)*.)

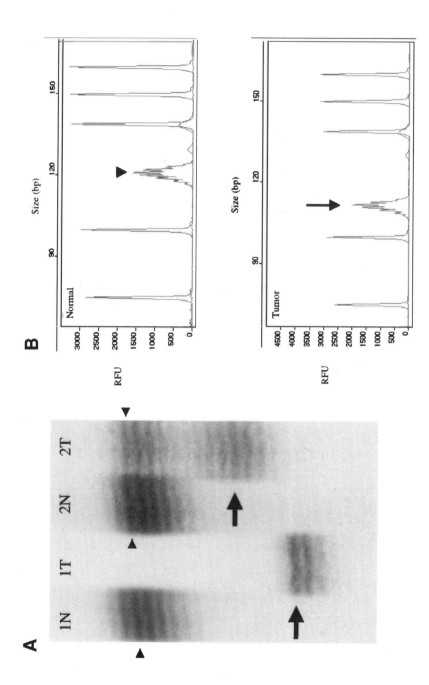

Table 4
International Guidelines for Evaluation of Microsatellite Instability (MSI)
in Colorectal Cancer

Marker	Repeating unit	GenBank accession No.
Reference Panel		
BAT25	Mononucleotide	9834508
BAT26	Mononucleotide	9834505
D5S346	Dinucleotide	181171
D2S123	Dinucleotide	187953
D17S250	Dinucleotide	177030

	No. of markers exhibiting instability length changes		
	5 Loci Analyzed	>5 Loci Analyzed	Interpretation
Criteria for interpretation			
	≥2	≥30–40%	MSI-H
	1	<30–40%	MSI-L
	0	0	MSS or MSI-L

Alternative loci	
BAT40	D8S87
BAT34C4	D18S69
TGF-B-RII	ACTC (635/636)
D18S55	D18S64
D18S58	D17S588
D18S61	D13S153
D3S1029	D17S787
D10S197	D7S519
D13S175	D20S100
D5S107	

Reproduced with permission from ref. 39.

guidelines define the microsatellite loci to be tested, the criteria for diagnosis of MSI, and criteria for classification of high- and low-frequency MSI (MSI-H and MSI-L) (Table 4).

Mutations That Cause Mismatch Repair. A database of mutations associated with mismatch repair is maintained at http:// www.nfdht.nl/database/mdbchoice.htm. Most patients with HNPCC have mutations in either *MLH1* or *MSH2*. Various mutations in *MLH1* have been reported with some clustering in exons 15 and 16 *(42)*. The gene includes 19 exons spread over approx 100 kb of genomic DNA *(43)*. In some populations, founder mutations account for a substantial proportion of known mutations *(44)*. HNPCC patients with *MLH1* germline mutations also have an increased risk of breast cancer *(40)*. In most patients with sporadic colorectal cancers with microsatellite instability, the tumors show hypermethylation of the *MLH1* promoter. This epigenetic modification is believed to lead to decreased expression of the protein *(45)*. *MSH2* contains 16 exons spread over 73 kb of genomic DNA *(46)*. Various mutations have been reported without evidence of clustering at any nucleotide.

Testing Strategies for HNPCC. HNPCC should be suspected in patients with a family history of colorectal cancer or one of the other HNPCC-associated tumors. Tumor samples from patients with colorectal cancer who meet the established criteria for HNPCC should be considered for microsatellite analysis. If this is positive, then mutational analysis in the genes that are known to cause HNPCC can be considered. If a mutation is identified, then testing can be offered to other family members. All testing should follow norms of informed consent. Several professional organizations in the United States have published recommendations for screening patients for hereditary colorectal cancer *(47–50)*.

Genetic Instabilities and the Development of Colorectal Cancer

Analyses of the histological stages of development and of genetic mutations in tumors at different stages of tumor progression have led to a general model that colorectal cancer begins as an adenoma and progresses through stages of increasing dysplasia leading to invasive cancer. Corresponding to this morphologic progression are progressive accumulations of genetic mutations *(51)*. A common view of specific genes that are mutated and the approximate order of their mutation is shown in Fig. 4. Among the earliest genes to be mutated in colorectal cancer is *APC*. Loss of heterozygosity of 8p, 17p, 18q, and 22q and mutations in k-ras are frequent. Inactivation of p53 appears to be involved in later stages of this progression.

Two major molecular pathways for development of colorectal cancer have been described. These are the mutator pathway (also known as the microsatellite instability pathway) and the tumor suppressor pathway (also known as the chromosomal instability pathway). These

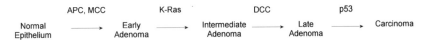

Fig. 4. Widely held model of progressive development of mutations in colonic epithelium leading to invasive colon cancer. Early lesions are associated with mutations in the adenomatous polyposis coli *(APC)* gene and the mutated in colon cancer *(MCC)* gene. These are followed by mutations in *K-ras* and the deleted in colon cancer *(DCC)* gene. Mutations in *p53* are believed to be a late event.

represent two different forms of genetic instability. To some extent, these pathways appear to be mutually exclusive, i.e., colorectal tumors tend to display either MSI or chromosomal instability (CIN).

The MSI pathway arises from mutations in mismatch repair enzymes. HNPCC is the prototype of abnormalities that involve this pathway, but the pathway can also arise in individuals who do not inherit a germline mutation in one of the mismatch repair enzymes. Nonhereditary mutations are commonly owing to hypermethylation of mismatch repair genes that decreases the expression of these genes. The MSI phenotype is most easily recognized (and defined) by the presence of MSI, but the spectrum of acquired mutations is broader than the simple presence of alterations in the number of copies of microsatellite repeats. For example, nucleotide mutation rates are several orders of magnitude more common in MSI than in normal cells *(52)*. Tumors that show MSI generally have a normal diploid karyotype.

The CIN pathway is characterized by gross chromosomal instability with gains and losses of chromosomes, chromosome fusions, and other cytogenetic abnormalities. Whereas the molecular basis of the MSI phenotype is known to involve mutations in mismatch repair genes, the underlying molecular basis of CIN is largely unknown *(30)*. In yeast experiments, mutations in >100 genes can give rise to CIN. These include genes involved in various aspects of the cell cycle.

MULTIPLE ENDOCRINE NEOPLASIA

The multiple endocrine neoplasias (MENs) are a group of heterogeneous familial diseases caused by mutations in the *MEN1* or *RET* genes. These diseases, summarized in Table 5, are characterized by development of tumors involving endocrine glands.

Table 5
Summary of Multiple Endocrine Neoplasia (MEN) Syndromes

Parameter	Characteristics
MEN1	
Clinical features:	Hyperparathyroidism, pancreaticoduodenal neuroendocrine tumors, pituitary tumors
Gene/protein	*MEN1*/menin; interacts with JunD; tumor suppressor gene.
Locus	11q13
Mutations	Various
MEN2A (Sipple's syndrome)	
Clinical features:	Medullary thyroid cancer (MTC) pheochromocytoma, hyperparathyroidism
Gene/Protein	RET/ret; tyrosine kinase; proto-oncogene
Locus	10q11
Mutations	Various, but cluster of five extracellular cysteines commonly mutated
MEN2B	Medullary thyroid cancer, pheochromocytoma, neural gangliomas
Gene/Protein	RET/ret; tyrosine kinase; proto-oncogene
Locus	10q11
Mutations	Nearly all patients have M918T
Familial medullary thyroid cancer	
Clinical features	MTC, often at a later age than MEN 2A or MEN 2B
Gene/Protein	RET/ret; tyrosine kinase; proto-oncogene
Locus	10q11
Mutations	Extracellular cluster of cysteines and several intracellular amino acids

Multiple Endocrine Neoplasia, Type 1

Multiple endocrine neoplasia, type 1 (MEN 1; OMIM 131100) is an autosomal dominant disorder characterized by hyperparathyroidism, pancreaticoduodenal neuroendocrine tumors (PNTs), and pituitary tumors. The responsible gene, *MEN1,* is located on chromosome 11q13 *(53).* Mutations in this gene that cause MEN 1 syndrome result in loss of function and have been described throughout the gene. Such loss-of-function mutations are characteristic of tumor suppressor genes *(54).* These mutations do not show a clear genotype-phenotype correspondence. The encoded protein, which is termed menin, is a nuclear protein of 610 amino acids that interacts with several transcription factors *(55)*. Defects in menin are therefore associated with loss of regulation of expression of other genes.

The most common finding in patients with MEN 1 is primary hyperparathyroidism caused by hyperplasia of the parathyroid glands. This affects up to 95% of individuals carrying a MEN 1 mutation. Following surgical resection of the hyperplastic glands, recurrence is more common than after resection of a solitary parathyroid adenoma. Supernumerary parathyroid glands are also found with increased frequency in MEN 1 patients.

Nonfunctioning PNTs or PNTs secreting pancreatic polypeptide are the most common type of PNT in MEN 1 patients. Among those with functional PNTs, gastrinomas and insulinomas are the most common type of tumor. Gastrinomas produce gastrin, which stimulates production of hydrochloric acid by the parietal cells of the stomach. This tumor may present as Zollinger-Ellison syndrome. From 15 to 50% of patients with MEN 1-related gastrinomas have liver metastases at diagnosis. Insulinomas produce insulin, even in the presence of hypoglycemia. Characteristic features include symptomatic hypoglycemia (glucose under 40 mg/dL) with a serum insulin of >5 μU/mL.

Pituitary tumors develop in 16–65% of patients with MEN 1. A variety of cell types can be involved, giving rise to prolactinomas (the most common type) or tumors secreting growth hormone, insulin-like growth factor 1, or corticotrophin.

Multiple Endocrine Neoplasia, Type 2

The multiple endocrine neoplasias, type 2 (MEN 2; OMIM 171400) are a group of diseases with autosomal dominant inheritance. They include MEN 2A, MEN 2B, and familial medullary thyroid cancer (MTC). These diseases are caused by gain-of-function mutations involving the *RET* proto-oncogene, which is located on chromosome 10q11. In all of these diseases, MTC, which is usually bilateral or multifocal, is the most common finding. In addition, Hirschsprung's disease, caused by congenital absence of autonomic ganglia in portions of the large bowel, has been associated with mutations in *RET,* although mutations in other genes can contribute to this disorder *(56)*.

The *RET* proto-oncogene encodes a cell membrane receptor tyrosine kinase. The extracellular portion of the receptor contains a cysteine-rich domain that is responsible for ligand binding. Identified ligands include glial-derived growth factor (GDNF) and neurturin. Ligand binding to the extracellular domain results in dimerization of the receptor and activation of tyrosine kinase.

MEN 2A (also known as Sipple's syndrome) is the most common type of MEN 2 syndrome. It is characterized by MTC, pheochromocytomas, and hyperparathyroidism resulting from parathyroid hyperplasia. Most patients are under 30. Common *RET* mutations in MEN 2A are found at a closely spaced group of five cysteine residues at amino acids 609, 611, 618, 620, and 634 *(57)*. These are located in the extracellular region of the molecule.

MEN 2B is characterized by MTC, pheochromocytomas, and neural gangliomas. Additional features include hyperflexible joints and marfanoid habitus. Unlike MEN 2A, hyperparathyroidism is not a feature of MEN 2B. Most patients with MEN 2B are younger than MEN 2A patients. At least 95% of MEN 2B patients have a common mutation, M918T, which is located in the tyrosine kinase domain. This is caused by a single nucleotide substitution, ATG→ACG at codon 918 *(57)*.

Familial MTC without other endocrine or neurological lesions appears at a later age. Mutations in familial MTC have been reported in the extracellular cluster of cysteines, at two amino acids, 768 and 804, and in the intracellular domain.

Mutation Screening in Multiple Endocrine Neoplasia

Guidelines for screening for germline mutations in MEN families have been produced *(57)*. For MEN 1, these guidelines recommend mutation testing for index cases, unaffected relatives, and some patients with atypical features of MEN 1. The estimated false-negative rate for genetic testing in MEN 1 is 10–20%. For MEN 2 families, prophylactic thyroidectomy (to avoid MTC) should be recommended for carriers identified through genetic testing. This surgery should be performed in infancy or early childhood. At least 95% of *RET* mutation carriers can be identified through molecular testing.

VON HIPPEL-LINDAU DISEASE

von Hippel-Lindau disease (VHL; MIM 193300) is a rare autosomal dominant disorder that affects approximately 1 in 30,000 to 1 in

40,000 individuals *(58,59)*. It is characterized by the presence of hemangioblastomas of the central nervous system, especially of the cerebellum and spinal cord, retinal hemangioblastomas, renal cell carcinoma (RCC), renal and pancreatic cysts, pheochromocytomas, hemangiomas of the adrenal glands, liver, and lungs, and papillary cystadenoma of the epididymis or broad ligament of the uterus. Ten percent of VHL patients have endolymphatic sac papillary adenocarcinomas that can lead to deafness in the affected ear. The most common presentation is with manifestations of cerebellar hemangioblastoma, and the mean age at the time of diagnosis is approx 30 yr. The lifetime risk of developing a cerebellar or retinal hemangioblastoma or RCC is at least 70%.

VHL is caused by mutations in the *VHL* gene, located on chromosome 3p25 *(60)*. This is a tumor suppressor gene consisting of three exons spread over 712 bp. Alternative splicing gives rise to two transcripts, one containing exon 2 and the other lacking that exon. An alternative translation start codon gives rise to a shorter form of the protein. Both the longer and shorter forms are believed to function as tumor suppressor genes. The encoded protein, pVHL, blocks transcriptional elongation by binding to two proteins involved in transcriptional elongation, elongin B and elongin C. Thus, VHL represents a disease caused by failure of regulation of gene transcription *(61)*.

One effect of *VHL* mutations is overproduction of vascular endothelial growth factor (VEGF). This factor stimulates production of blood vessels and may be an essential component in the development of some of the pathologic features of VHL. Normally, VEGF is produced, along with other proteins, in response to hypoxia. RCC cell lines with *VHL* mutations produce VEGF even in the presence of a normal pO_2. Transfection of a wild-type *VHL* gene into *VHL* (–/–) RCC cells restores the normal VEGF production in response to hypoxia *(62)*.

A database of mutations observed in VHL is maintained at http://www.umd.necker.fr:2005/. Mutations that have been identified include gene deletions detectable by Southern blot analysis, nonsense mutations, and other non-missense mutations. These more severe mutations tend to be associated with VHL type 1, which is not characterized by pheochromocytomas. By contrast, missense mutations tend to be associated with VHL type 2, which is characterized by pheochromocytomas. With comprehensive screening, mutations can be identified in essentially all VHL patients. Commonly, the wild-type allele is inactivated by hyper-methylation *(63)*.

HEREDITARY MELANOMA

Hereditary melanomas (OMIM 155600) account for approx 10% of all malignant melanomas; the remainder of cases are sporadic tumors. Among families with hereditary melanoma, approx 50% show linkage to 9p21, and within these families, mutations in the *CDKN2A* gene (also known as *p16, INK4A, CDK4I,* and *MTS1*) are found in approx 50% of affected patients. A few melanoma families worldwide have been identified who have a mutation in the *CDK4* gene.

As discussed in Chapter 1, *CDKN2A* encodes two proteins involved in cell cycle regulation: p16 and p14[ARF] protein. p16 functions as a tumor suppressor gene by inhibiting the activity of cyclin D/cdk4. This cyclin-dependent kinase plays an important role in the cell cycle checkpoint at the G_1/S boundary, known as the restriction point (*see* Chap. 6). cdk4 phosphorylates the retinoblastoma protein, pRb, which allows for release of the pRb-bound transcription activator, E2F. E2F is capable of activating transcription of a large number of genes involved in cell cycle progression. In the absence of inhibition by p16, an important negative regulator of cell cycle is removed, thereby facilitating both passage of cells through the checkpoint and cell division.

In addition to inhibiting the cell cycle at G_1/S, p16 is involved in retarding the cell cycle at the G_2 phase following exposure of cells to nonlethal doses of ultraviolet irradiation. This effect also appears to be mediated through inhibition of cdk4 activity. It has been proposed that the p16-dependent retardation of the cell cycle affords UV-irradiated cells time to repair DNA damage *(64)*.

p14[ARF], the other product of the *CDKN2A* locus, can interact with both pRb and p53, leading to cell cycle arrest at either G_1 or G_2. It can also prevent p53 destruction by binding mdm2. mdm2 is involved in the transport of p53 from the nucleus to the cytoplasm, where it is degraded in the proteasome *(65)*. Loss of p14[ARF] as a result of mutation would allow for increased rate of elimination of p53 and its downstream targets including the cyclin-dependent kinase inhibitor p21 and the proapoptotic protein bax.

In addition to the two proteins encoded by the *CDKN2A* gene, a third tumor suppressor gene, p15 (also known as *CDKN2B*), is located within the region of 9p21 that has been implicated in familial melanoma families by linkage analysis. Because mutations in *CDKN2A* account for only 25% of familial melanoma, other loci exist and await identification.

COWDEN'S SYNDROME

Cowden's syndrome (OMIM 158350) is a rare autosomal dominant disease associated with development of multiple hamartomas and an increased risk of breast, endometrial, and nonmedullary thyroid cancer. The prevalence of the disease is about 1 in 200,000. The risk of breast cancer in female patients with Cowden's syndrome is estimated to be 30%. The most common signs of the disease include mucocutaneous lesions: facial trichilemmomas, acral keratosis, oral papillomas, and scrotal tongue. Approximately one-third of patients have macrocephaly, and mental retardation affects approx 10%. Cowden's syndrome has some phenotypic overlap with other polyposis syndromes including juvenile polyposis and Bannayan-Zonana syndrome.

Cowden's syndrome is caused by mutations in the phosphatase and tensin homolog gene *(PTEN)* on chromosome 10q23.3 *(66)*. This is a tumor suppressor gene that contains 9 exons, gives rise to an mRNA of 5.5 kb, and encodes a protein of 403 amino acids with a molecular weight of 47 kDa. The protein is a dual-specificity phosphatase that can dephosphorylate tyrosine and serine/threonine residues in proteins. It can also convert phosphatidylinositol-3,4,5,-triphosphate (PIP_3) to PIP_2, an intermediate in a growth signaling pathway *(66)*. In addition to familial cancers associated with inherited mutations, *PTEN* is commonly mutated in many sporadic cancers including brain, breast, endometrium, kidney, and prostate *(67)*.

LI-FRAUMENI SYNDROME

Li-Fraumeni syndrome is a rare autosomal dominant disorder associated with development of multiple types of malignant tumor. The gene responsible for the disease in approx 50–70% of families is

Table 6
Criteria for Diagnosis of Li-Fraumeni Syndrome

Proband <45 yr of age diagnosed with sarcoma

First-degree relative of proband with a Li-Fraumeni tumor (sarcoma breast, brain, adrenal) diagnosed at <45 yr of age

Another first- or second-degree relative of proband with any cancer diagnosed at <45 yr of age or a sarcoma diagnosed at any age

TP53, located on chromosome 17p13.1 *(68).* A second gene mutated in Li-Fraumeni syndrome families is *hCHK2 (69).* The role of p53 is described in Chapter 6. This protein plays essential roles in regulation of the cell cycle, maintenance of genomic stability, regulation of apoptosis, and DNA repair. Patients with familial Li-Fraumeni syndrome have a germline mutation of one *TP53* allele. Tumor development follows somatic mutation of the remaining wild-type allele.

Li-Fraumeni syndrome is defined according to the criteria shown in Table 6. A wide variety of tumors are seen, including sarcoma, breast cancer, adrenal cancer, leukemia, and brain cancer. Many other common cancers are also seen with increased frequency in Li-Fraumeni families. Families that do not meet the strict criteria shown in Table 6 are referred to as Li-Fraumeni-like (LFL).

A database of mutations that have been found in *TP53* is maintained at http://www.iarc.fr/p53/. Most mutations in classic Li-Fraumeni families have been found in exons 5–8; however, these exons have been analyzed more frequently than other exons in mutation studies, possibly giving rise to a bias in favor of finding mutations in these exons *(70).* The majority of mutations are missense.

The National Comprehensive Cancer Network has produced guidelines for the management of families with Li-Fraumeni syndrome (http://www.nccn.org/physician_gls/index.html). Early detection of cancer development through annual physical examinations is emphasized.

REFERENCES

1. Nathanson KN, Wooster R, Weber BL. Breast cancer genetics: what we know and what we need. Nat Med 2001;7:552–6.
2. Easton DF. Cancer risks in A-T heterozygotes. Int J Radiat Biol 1994;66:S177–82.
3. Vahteristo P, Bartkova J, Eerola H, et al. A CHEK2 genetic variant contributing to a substantial fraction of familial breast cancer. Am J Hum Genet 2002;71:432–8.

4. Schutte M, Seal S, Barfoot R, et al. Variants in CHEK2 Other than 1100delC Do Not Make a Major Contribution to Breast Cancer Susceptibility. Am J Hum Genet 2003;72:1023–8.

5. Hall JM, Lee MK, Newman B, et al. Linkage of early-onset familial breast cancer to chromosome 17q21. Science 1990;250:1684–9.

6. Miki Y, Swensen J, Shattuck-Eidens D, et al. A strong candidate for the breast and ovarian cancer susceptibility gene BRCA1. Science 1994;266:66–71.

7. Futreal PA, Liu Q, Shattuck-Eidens D, et al. BRCA1 mutations in primary breast and ovarian carcinomas. Science 1994;266:120–2.

8. Venkitaraman AR. Cancer susceptibility and the functions of BRCA1 and BRCA2. Cell 2002;108:171–82.

9. Welcsh PL, Lee MK, Gonzalez-Hernandez RM, et al. BRCA1 transcriptionally regulates genes involved in breast tumorigenesis. Proc Natl Acad Sci USA 2002;99:7560–5.

10. Tavtigian SV, Simard J, Rommens J, et al. The complete BRCA2 gene and mutations in chromosome 13q-linked kindreds. Nat Genet 1996;12:333–7.

11. Johannesdottir G, Gudmundsson J, Bergthorsson JT, et al. High prevalence of the 999del5 mutation in Icelandic breast and ovarian cancer patients. Cancer Res 1996;56:3663–5.

12. Anonymous. Cancer risks in BRCA2 mutation carriers. The Breast Cancer Linkage Consortium. J Natl Cancer Inst 1999;91:1310–6.

13. Unger MA, Nathanson KL, Calzone K, et al. Screening for genomic rearrangements in families with breast and ovarian cancer identifies BRCA1 mutations previously missed by conformation-sensitive gel electrophoresis or sequencing. Am J Hum Genet 2000;67:841–50.

14. Burn J, Chapman P, Delhanty J, et al. The UK Northern region genetic register for familial adenomatous polyposis coli: use of age of onset, congenital hypertrophy of the retinal pigment epithelium, and DNA markers in risk calculations. J Med Genet 1991;28:289–96.

15. Bisgaard ML, Fenger K, Bulow S, Niebuhr E, Mohr J. Familial adenomatous polyposis (FAP): frequency, penetrance, and mutation rate. Hum Mutat 1994;3:121–5.

16. Bjork J, Akerbrant H, Iselius L, et al. Periampullary adenomas and adenocarcinomas in familial adenomatous polyposis: cumulative risks and APC gene mutations. Gastroenterology 2001;121:1127–35.

17. Traboulsi EI, Krush AJ, Gardner EJ, et al. Prevalence and importance of pigmented ocular fundus lesions in Gardner's syndrome. N Engl J Med 1987;316:661–7.

18. Clark SK, Neale KF, Landgrebe JC, Phillips RK. Desmoid tumours complicating familial adenomatous polyposis. Br J Surg 1999;86:1185–9.

19. Garber JE, Li FP, Kingston JE, et al. Hepatoblastoma and familial adenomatous polyposis. J Natl Cancer Inst 1988;80:1626–8.

20. Hamilton SR, Liu B, Parsons RE, et al. The molecular basis of Turcot's syndrome. N Engl J Med 1995;332:839–47.

21. Carl W, Sullivan MA. Dental abnormalities and bone lesions associated with familial adenomatous polyposis: report of cases. J Am Dent Assoc 1989;119:137–9.

22. Spirio L, Olschwang S, Groden J, et al. Alleles of the APC gene: an attenuated form of familial polyposis. Cell 1993;75:951–7.

23. Jass JR. Familial colorectal cancer: pathology and molecular characteristics. Lancet Oncol 2000;1:220–6.

24. Laken SJ, Petersen GM, Gruber SB, et al. Familial colorectal cancer in Ashke-
    nazim due to a hypermutable tract in APC. Nat Genet 1997;17:79–83.
25. Sieber OM, Tomlinson IP, Lamlum H. The adenomatous polyposis coli (APC)
    tumour suppressor—genetics, function and disease. Mol Med Today
    2000;6:462–9.
26. Morin PJ, Sparks AB, Korinek V, et al. Activation of beta-catenin-Tcf signaling in
    colon cancer by mutations in beta-catenin or APC. Science 1997;275:1787–90.
27. Korinek V, Barker N, Morin PJ, et al. Constitutive transcriptional activation by a
    beta-catenin-Tcf complex in APC-/- colon carcinoma. Science 1997;275:1784–7.
28. Fodde R, Kuipers J, Rosenberg C, et al. Mutations in the APC tumour suppressor
    gene cause chromosomal instability. Nat Cell Biol 2001;3:433–8.
29. Kaplan KB, Burds AA, Swedlow JR, Bekir SS, Sorger PK, Nathke IS. A role for
    the adenomatous polyposis coli protein in chromosome segregation. Nat Cell Biol
    2001;3:429–32.
30. Jallepalli PV, Lengauer C. Chromosome segregation and cancer: cutting through
    the mystery. Nat Rev Cancer 2001;1:109–17.
31. Sieber OM, Heinimann K, Gorman P, et al. Analysis of chromosomal instability in
    human colorectal adenomas with two mutational hits at APC. Proc Natl Acad Sci
    USA 2002;99:16910–5.
32. Giardiello FM, Brensinger JD, Tersmette AC, et al. Very high risk of cancer in
    familial Peutz-Jeghers syndrome. Gastroenterology 2000;119:1447–53.
33. Yoo LI, Chung DC, Yuan J. LKB1—a master tumour suppressor of the small intes-
    tine and beyond. Nat Rev Cancer 2002;2:529–35.
34. Howe JR, Roth S, Ringold JC, et al. Mutations in the SMAD4/DPC4 gene in juve-
    nile polyposis. Science 1998;280:1086–8.
35. Howe JR, Ringold JC, Summers RW, Mitros FA, Nishimura DY, Stone EM. A
    gene for familial juvenile polyposis maps to chromosome 18q21.1. Am J Hum
    Genet 1998;62:1129–36.
36. Kinzler KW, Vogelstein B. Landscaping the cancer terrain. Science
    1998;280:1036–7.
37. Schutte M, Hruban RH, Hedrick L, et al. DPC4 gene in various tumor types. Can-
    cer Res 1996;56:2527–30.
38. Haydon AM, Jass JR. Emerging pathways in colorectal-cancer development.
    Lancet Oncol 2002;3:83–8.
39. Aarnio M, Sankila R, Pukkala E, et al. Cancer risk in mutation carriers of DNA-
    mismatch-repair genes. Int J Cancer 1999;81:214–8.
40. Scott RJ, McPhillips M, Meldrum CJ, et al. Hereditary nonpolyposis colorectal
    cancer in 95 families: differences and similarities between mutation-positive and
    mutation-negative kindreds. Am J Hum Genet 2001;68:118–27.
41. Boland CR, Thibodeau SN, Hamilton SR, et al. A National Cancer Institute Work-
    shop on Microsatellite Instability for cancer detection and familial predisposition:
    development of international criteria for the determination of microsatellite insta-
    bility in colorectal cancer. Cancer Res 1998;58:5248–57.
42. Wijnen J, Khan PM, Vasen H, et al. Majority of hMLH1 mutations responsible for
    hereditary nonpolyposis colorectal cancer cluster at the exonic region 15–16. Am J
    Hum Genet 1996;58:300–7.
43. Han HJ, Maruyama M, Baba S, Park JG, Nakamura Y. Genomic structure of
    human mismatch repair gene, hMLH1, and its mutation analysis in patients with
    hereditary non-polyposis colorectal cancer (HNPCC). Hum Mol Genet
    1995;4:237–42.

44. Nystrom-Lahti M, Wu Y, Moisio AL, et al. DNA mismatch repair gene mutations in 55 kindreds with verified or putative hereditary non-polyposis colorectal cancer. Hum Mol Genet 1996;5:763–9.

45. Kuismanen SA, Holmberg MT, Salovaara R, et al. Epigenetic phenotypes distinguish microsatellite-stable and -unstable colorectal cancers. Proc Natl Acad Sci USA 1999;96:12661–6.

46. Kolodner RD, Hall NR, Lipford J, et al. Structure of the human MSH2 locus and analysis of two Muir-Torre kindreds for msh2 mutations. Genomics 1994;24:516–26.

47. Winawer SJ, Fletcher RH, Miller L, et al. Colorectal cancer screening: clinical guidelines and rationale. Gastroenterology 1997;112:594–642.

48. Anonymous. NCCN colorectal cancer screening practice guidelines. National Comprehensive Cancer Network. Oncology (Huntingt) 1999;13(5A):152–79.

49. Anonymous. Genetic testing for colon cancer: joint statement of the American College of Medical Genetics and American Society of Human Genetics. Joint Test and Technology Transfer Committee Working Group. Genet Med 2000;2:362–6. *Corporate name:* Joint Test and Technology Transfer Committee Working Group, American College of Medical Genetics, 9650 Rockville Pike, Bethesda, MD 20814-3998.

50. Anonymous. American Gastroenterological Association medical position statement: hereditary colorectal cancer and genetic testing. Gastroenterology 2001;121:195–7.

51. Vogelstein B, Fearon ER, Hamilton SR, et al. Genetic alterations during colorectal-tumor development. N Engl J Med 1988;319:525–32.

52. Cahill DP, Kinzler KW, Vogelstein B, Lengauer C. Genetic instability and darwinian selection in tumours. Trends Cell Biol 1999;9:M57–60.

53. Chandrasekharappa SC, Guru SC, Manickam P, et al. Positional cloning of the gene for multiple endocrine neoplasia-type 1. Science 1997;276:404–7.

54. Thakker RV. Multiple endocrine neoplasia. Horm Res 2001;56(suppl 1):67–72.

55. Wautot V, Vercherat C, Lespinasse J, et al. Germline mutation profile of MEN1 in multiple endocrine neoplasia type 1: search for correlation between phenotype and the functional domains of the MEN1 protein. Hum Mutat 2002;20:35–47.

56. Fitze G, Cramer J, Ziegler A, et al. Association between c135G/A genotype and RET proto-oncogene germline mutations and phenotype of Hirschsprung's disease. Lancet2002;359:1200–5.

57. Brandi ML, Gagel RF, Angeli A, et al. Guidelines for diagnosis and therapy of MEN type 1 and type 2. J Clin Endocrinol Metab 2001;86:5658–71.

58. Couch V, Lindor NM, Karnes PS, Michels VV. von Hippel-Lindau disease. Mayo Clin Proc 2000;75:265–72.

59. Sims KB. von Hippel-Lindau disease: gene to bedside. Curr Opin Neurol 2001;14:695–703.

60. Latif F, Tory K, Gnarra J, et al. Identification of the von Hippel-Lindau disease tumor suppressor gene. Science 1993;260:1317–20.

61. Friedrich CA. Genotype-phenotype correlation in von Hippel-Lindau syndrome. Hum Mol Genet 2001;10:763–7.

62. Iliopoulos O, Levy AP, Jiang C, Kaelin WG Jr, Goldberg MA. Negative regulation of hypoxia-inducible genes by the von Hippel-Lindau protein. Proc Natl Acad Sci USA 1996;93:10595–9.

63. Prowse AH, Webster AR, Richards FM, et al. Somatic inactivation of the VHL gene in von Hippel-Lindau disease tumors. Am J Hum Genet 1997;60:765–71.

64. Gabrielli BG, Sarcevic B, Sinnamon J, et al. A cyclin D-cdk4 activity required for G2 phase cell cycle progression is inhibited in ultraviolet radiation-induced G2 phase delay. J Biol Chem 1999;274:13961–9.

65. Zhang Y, Xiong Y, Yarbrough WG. ARF promotes MDM2 degradation and stabilizes p53: ARF-INK4a locus deletion impairs both the Rb and p53 tumor suppression pathways. Cell 1998;92:725–34.

66. Ali IU, Schriml LM, Dean M. Mutational spectra of PTEN/MMAC1 gene: a tumor suppressor with lipid phosphatase activity. J Natl Cancer Inst 1999;91:1922–32.

67. Li J, Yen C, Liaw D, et al. PTEN, a putative protein tyrosine phosphatase gene mutated in human brain, breast, and prostate cancer. Science 1997;275:1943–7.

68. Malkin D, Li FP, Strong LC, et al. Germ line p53 mutations in a familial syndrome of breast cancer, sarcomas, and other neoplasms. Science 1990;250:1233–8.

69. Bell DW, Varley JM, Szydlo TE, et al. Heterozygous germ line hCHK2 mutations in Li-Fraumeni syndrome. Science 1999;286:2528–31.

70. Varley JM, Evans DG, Birch JM. Li-Fraumeni syndrome—a molecular and clinical review. Br J Cancer 1997;76:1–14.

71. Berg KD, Griffin CA, Eshleman JR. Detection of microsatellite instability. In: Killeen AA., ed. Molecular Pathology Protocols. Totowa, NJ: Humana, 2000:59–71.

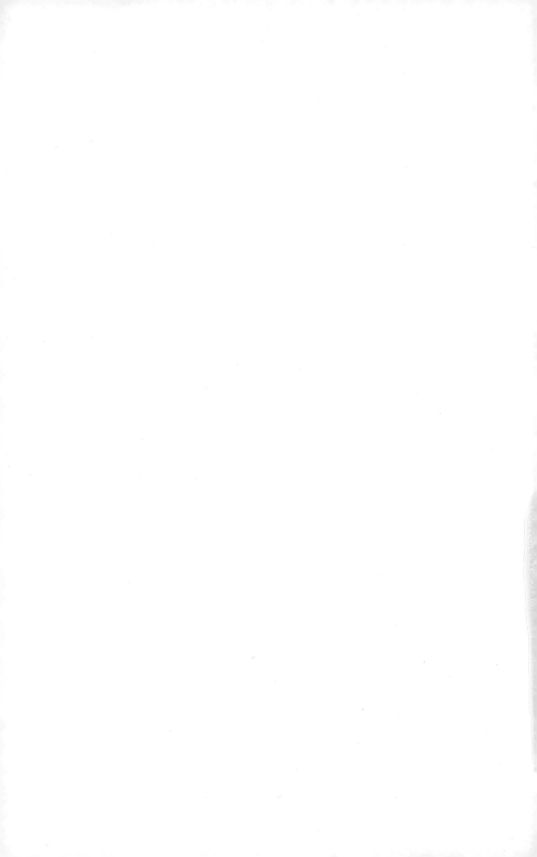

8 Molecular Pathology of Hematological Malignancies

Hematological malignancies are a heterogeneous group of disorders characterized by malignant expansion of hematopoietic cells. Our knowledge of the molecular etiology of these diseases has advanced significantly in recent years, and our understanding of the genetics of these disorders is among the most comprehensive of all tumors. Increasingly, this understanding of the molecular underpinnings of hematological malignancies is leading to development of classification systems that are based on demonstration of cytogenetic or molecular abnormalities, or on the pattern of genes expressed in these tumors. This represents a significant departure from older classification schemes.

In this chapter, the associations between various hematological neoplasms and recurring genetic abnormalities are described. Although the primary focus is on common, recurring genetic abnormalities, it should be emphasized that many hematological malignancies show complex molecular and cytogenetic abnormalities, and the specific abnormalities discussed here represent only a small fraction of the total spectrum of reported genetic abnormalities. For example, over 300 different chromosomal translocations have been reported in leukemias; the genes located at the chromosomal breakpoints have been characterized in approx 100 of them *(1)*.

GENETIC ABNORMALITIES IN MYELOID LEUKEMIAS

Chronic Myeloid Leukemia

Chronic myeloid leukemia (CML) is associated with a highly characteristic molecular abnormality in hematopoietic stem cells, the *BCR-ABL* fusion gene. This fusion arises from a reciprocal translocation, t(9;22)(q34;q11.2), that involves the breakpoint cluster region *(BCR)* gene on chromosome 22 and the Abelson *(ABL)* proto-onco-

From: *Principles of Molecular Pathology*
Edited by: A. A. Killeen © Humana Press Inc., Totowa, NJ

gene on chromosome 9. This translocation leads to formation of the Philadelphia chromosome, which was initially thought to be a deletion of 22q *(2)*. Later, with the development of chromosomal banding techniques, the Philadelphia chromosome was shown to be formed from a reciprocal translocation between 9q and 22q *(3)*. Historically, it was the first cytogenetic abnormality to be associated with a specific malignancy, and, more recently, the BCR-ABL fusion protein has become the first oncoprotein for which a specific pharmacological inhibitor based on rational drug design is available *(4,5)*.

The translocation is visible by conventional cytogenetic study (G-banding) in approx 95% of patients and is detectable by molecular techniques [Southern blot analysis or reverse transcription-polymerase chain reaction (RT-PCR)] in nearly all patients with CML *(6)*. The translocation is present in all myeloid lineages and in B-lymphocytes, indicating that the mutation arises in hematopoietic stem cells *(6)*. The translocation brings *ABL* in juxtaposition to *BCR,* resulting in the formation of a fusion gene composed of a 5′ sequence from the *BCR* region and 3′ sequence from *ABL.* The protein encoded by *BCR-ABL* has tyrosine kinase activity—a normal enzymatic property of the ABL protein but one that is present with increased activity in the *BCR-ABL* gene product—and is sufficient for the transformation of hematopoietic stem cells to a malignant phenotype *(7)*. Whereas normal ABL tyrosine kinase shuttles between the nucleus and the cytoplasm, BCR-ABL is essentially confined to the cytoplasm *(8)*

CML is characterized by distinct clinical phases that have characteristic cytogenetic and molecular correlates. The stable, chronic phase is associated with the presence of the Ph chromosome and *BCR-ABL* transcripts. With progression to the accelerated phase and eventually the blast phase, additional molecular and cytogenetic abnormalities appear. These include mutations in *TP53, p16 , RB, Ras,* and *EVI1.* In addition, nonrandom, secondary chromosomal abnormalities appear including duplication of the Ph chromosome, trisomy 8, trisomy 9, isochromosome 17q, trisomy 19, and loss of the Y chromosome *(9–11)*. In two-thirds of cases the acute leukemia that develops in the blastic phase is myeloid [acute myeloid leukemia (AML)] or undifferentiated [acute undifferentiated leukemia (AUL)], and in one-third of cases it is lymphoid [acute lymphoblastic leukemia (ALL)] *(11)*.

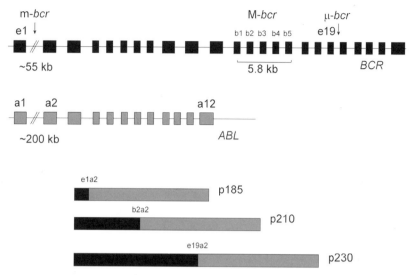

Fig. 1. The locations of the breakpoints in *BCR* and *ABL* determine the structure of the *BCR-ABL* fusion protein. Breakpoints in *BCR* occur in the m-bcr, M-bcr, or μ-bcr. Breakpoints in *ABL* nearly always occur 5′ of exon 2 (a2). These breakpoints give rise to fusion proteins of different lengths: 185, 210, and 230 kDa. Exons in *BCR* and *ABL* are shown by shaded boxes.

LOCATION AND SIGNIFICANCE OF BREAKPOINTS IN *BCR-ABL*

The locations of the breakpoints in both *BCR* and *ABL* determine the structure of the fusion mRNA and the resulting encoded protein (Fig. 1). Most breakpoints in *BCR* occur in a 5.8-kb region known as the major breakpoint cluster region (M-bcr) and result in joining of exon b2 or b3 of *BCR* to exon a2 of *ABL*. These fusions are known as b2a2 or b3a2 and result in production of a protein of approximately 210 kDa. A breakpoint in the minor breakpoint cluster region (m-bcr) includes only exon 1 of *BCR* and thus leads to production of a shorter protein of 185 kDa (sometimes reported as 190 kDa). A breakpoint in the micro-breakpoint cluster region, μ-bcr, leads to production of a 230-kDa protein.

These different breakpoints in *BCR* are associated with different forms of leukemia. In >90% of adults with CML, the breakpoint occurs in M-bcr, usually between exons b2 and b4, and usually within the introns. In Ph-positive ALL the breakpoint is in M-bcr in 20–30% of adult cases but in only approx 10% of childhood cases. Breakpoints in m-bcr occur in 50–77% of adults and up to 90% of children with Ph-positive ALL, but rarely in adults with CML. In CML, when the breakpoint is in m-bcr, the disease has some features in common with chronic myelomonocytic leukemia including monocytosis *(12)*. A breakpoint in μ-bcr is rare and is associated with chronic neutrophilic leukemia, a relatively indolent form of leukemia that is less likely than CML to progress to acute leukemia.

Breakpoints in *ABL* almost always occur 5′ to exon II. If exons Ia or Ib are included in the translocation, they are removed during mRNA processing. The region of *ABL* that is included in the *BCR-ABL* mRNA therefore includes exon II and exons further downstream encoding the tyrosine kinase activity. All three BCR-ABL proteins (p185, p210, and p230) have tyrosine kinase activity, and this activity appears to be essential for oncogenesis.

The reciprocal product of t(9;22) is a hybrid *ABL-BCR* fusion that does not encode a protein. This fusion is present on the derivative chromosome 9 [der(9)]. Recent observations indicate that the der(9) product is more complex than was initially thought. In particular, it has been observed that deletions on der(9) can be detected in approx 15% of patients with CML *(13,14)*. These deletions, which can be up to several megabases in length, usually involve loss of sequences derived from both chromosomes 9 and 22, and they appear to arise at the time of the initial translocation. The presence of such deletions is strongly associated with clinical outcome: in one retrospective study, the median survival of patients with der(9) deletions was 38 mo compared with 88 mo for patients who did not have a detectable deletion *(14)*. These observations indicate that additional sequences near the *BCR* and *ABL* genes are disrupted to varying extents among patients, suggesting that these additional sequences may play a role in the biology of CML.

DETECTION OF *BCR-ABL*

Either fluorescence *in situ* hybridization (FISH) or Southern blotting techniques can detect the *BCR-ABL* fusion gene in DNA. A conventional G-banded karyotype that demonstrates t(9;22), in the setting of characteristic clinical and laboratory findings, is sufficient to infer the presence of the *BCR-ABL* fusion gene. A cytogenetic evaluation is of value because it also reveals other cytogenetic abnormalities that may be present, provides an estimate of the percentage of cytogenetically abnormal cells, and provides a baseline to which additional abnormalities may be compared as the disease progresses. Detection of the *BCR-ABL* fusion gene is generally not possible using PCR-based analysis of genomic DNA because of the variable location of the breakpoints and the presence of introns that make the target too large to be amplified by standard PCR techniques.

Detection of *BCR-ABL* transcripts can be performed with RT-PCR, and this approach can be used to identify the location of the breakpoints of the fusion gene (e.g., as b2a3). In general, PCR methods are more sensitive than conventional cytogenetics or FISH for monitoring response to treatment *(15)*. Increasing levels of *BCR-ABL* transcript are associated with increased risk of disease relapse in patients who have achieved a clinical remission *(16)*.

IMATINIB MESYLATE (GLEEVEC)

An inhibitor of the Abelson tyrosine kinase, imatinib mesylate (STI-571/Gleevec, Novartis Pharmaceuticals), has been shown to have dramatic benefit in patients with chronic-phase CML, Ph-positive ALL, and CML in blast crisis *(4,5)*. Imatinib is a competitive inhibitor of the tyrosine kinase activities of ABL, the platelet-derived growth factor receptor, and c-kit. Blockade of the ATP binding site of ABL by imatinib has an antileukemic effect that has been demonstrated both in cell lines and in clinical studies. It is believed that inhibition of the tyrosine kinase activity of ABL prevents transduction of the BCR-ABL signal by inhibiting phosphorylation of tyrosine residues in target proteins. The specific pathways of signal transduction in CML involve erk1/2, Jun, PI3, STAT5, and NF-κB *(17)*. Unfortunately, resistance to imatinib develops rapidly in patients with advanced CML and Ph-positive ALL. The mechanisms of resistance include amplification of *BCR-ABL,* mutations in the tyrosine kinase that block the effect of the drug, increased expression of the multidrug resistance P-glycoprotein (which removes the drug from cells), and activation of non-BCR-ABL signaling pathways *(17)*.

In addition to inhibiting the BCR-ABL tyrosine kinase, imatinib also inhibits the cell surface growth factor receptor, c-kit, which is activated by mutations that result in constitutive tyrosine kinase activity in some gastrointestinal stromal tumors (GISTs). A favorable response of this kind of tumor to therapy with imatinib has been reported *(18)*.

Myelodysplastic Syndromes

The myelodysplastic syndromes (MDS) are defined according to the World Health Organization (WHO) classification as refractory anemia, refractory anemia with ringed sideroblasts, refractory cytopenia with multilineage dysplasia, refractory anemia with excess blasts, myelodysplastic syndrome (unclassifiable), and myelodysplastic syndrome associated with isolated del(5q). The MDS are clonal disorders characterized by ineffective hematopoiesis, and they progress to AML in up to 40% of cases. Patients commonly present with symptoms related to one or more cytopenias such as bruising, anemia, or infections. MDS can arise *de novo* (primary MDS) or in patients who have been previously treated with chemotherapeutic drugs or radiation (secondary MDS). The prognosis for patients with secondary MDS is generally worse than for patients with primary MDS. Most patients with MDS are elderly, although these diseases can arise at any age.

MDS are associated with relatively frequent chromosomal abnormalities including del(5q), monosomy 7, del(7q), trisomy 8, del(17p), and del(20q). Up to 50% of patients with primary myelodysplastic syndrome and up to 80% of patients with secondary myelodysplastic syndrome have a detectable chromosomal abnormality. A cytogenetic study at the time of diagnosis is valuable because demonstration of a chromosomal abnormality confirms the presence of a clonal process, offers prognostic information, and is a baseline to which cytogenetic analyses performed later in the course of disease can be compared. The International Myelodysplastic Syndrome Risk Analysis Workshop examined cytogenetic, morphological, and clinical data from patients in several large studies *(19)*. Analysis of data indicated that favorable cytogenetic findings in MDS are a normal karyotype or the following as the *sole* cytogenetic abnormality: -Y, del(5q), or del(20q). Unfavorable karyotypes are those that have complex (defined as ≥3) chromosomal abnormalities or abnormalities involving chromosome 7, such as 7q- or monosomy 7. Other cytogenetic findings were associated with an intermediate outcome.

It should be noted that loss of the Y chromosome can be seen in bone marrow from healthy elderly men, so this finding does not necessarily indicate a malignant clonal process *(20)*. In addition, isolated del(5q) (the 5q-syndrome), which is classified as a separate entity in the WHO classification, deserves comment. It is associated with refractory macrocytic anemia and with other variable hematological findings that include leukopenia, thrombocytosis, and hypolobulated megakaryocytes. There is a female/male ratio of 3:1, with a median age of approx 60 yr at presentation. The presence of del(5q) in this setting has a favorable prognosis, but in the presence of other cytogenetic abnormalities it confers a poor prognosis *(19)*.

Acute Myeloid Leukemias

CLASSIFICATION

The most common classification of AMLs in current use is the French-American-British (FAB) scheme that classifies these leukemias as M0–M7, as shown in Table 1. The FAB classification is based on morphologic and cytochemical reactions. The WHO classification system (Table 2) represents a significant departure from earlier systems in that it classifies certain acute myeloid leukemias on the basis of recurring genetic abnormalities *(21)*. It follows that identification of these abnormalities forms an essential part in the evaluation of patients with AML.

In general, three kinds of genetic abnormality are found in AML *(22)*. First, several recurring chromosomal abnormalities, such as t(8;21), inversion 16 [inv(16)], t(16;16), and t(15;17), are associated with a relatively favorable prognosis. These abnormalities generate fusion proteins that alter the transcription of genes involved in hematopoiesis. Because t(8;21), inv(16), and t(16;16) appear to disrupt the function of a group of transcriptional factors known as core binding factors, they are sometimes called the "core binding factor leukemias." The second kind of genetic abnormality in AML is characterized by recurring chromosomal deletions such as 5-, 5q-, 7-, and 7q-. These generally have a poor prognosis. Finally, approx 45% of cases of AML have no demonstrable cytogenetic abnormality and have an intermediate prognosis. A significant percentage of this group have mutations in the *FLT3* gene, and mutations in this gene represent the most common genetic abnormalities in AML.

Although the presentation here is focused on recurring abnormalities that have been characterized at a molecular level, it should be emphasized that leukemias frequently show highly complex patterns of molecular and cytogenetic abnormalities.

Table 1
The French-American-British (FAB) Classification of AML and Associated Genetic Abnormalities

FAB subtype	Common name (% of cases)	Results of staining			Associated translocations and rearrangements (% of cases)	Genes involved
		Myelo-peroxidase	Sudan Black	Non-specific esterase		
M0	Acute myeloblastic leukemia with minimal differentiation (3%)	−	−	−[a]	inv(3q26) and t(3;3) (1%)	EVI1
M1	Acute myeloblastic leukemia without maturation (15–20%)	+	+	−		
M2	Acute myeloblastic leukemia with maturation	+	+	−	t(8;21) (40%) t(6;9) (1%)	AML1-ETO, DEK-CAN
M3	Acute promyelocytic leukemia (5–10%)	+	+	−	t(15;17) (98%) t(11;17) (1%) t(5;17) (1%)	PML-RARα, PLZF-RARα, NPM RARα
M4	Acute myelomonocytic leukemia (20%)	+	+	+	11q23 (20%), inv(3q26) and t(3;3) (3%) t(6;9) (1%)	MLL, DEK-CAN, EVI1
M4E0	Acute myelomonocytic leukemia with abnormal eosinophils (5–10%)	+	+	+	inv(16), t(16;16) (80%)	CBFβ-MYH11
M5	Acute monocytic leukemia	−	−	+	11q23 (20%) t(8;16) (2%)	MLL, MOZ-CBP
M6	Erythroleukemia (3–5%)	+	+	−		
M7	Acute megakaryocytic leukemia	−	−	+[b]	t(1;22) (5%)	Unknown

[a] Cells are positive for myeloid antigen (e.g., CD13 and CD33).

[b] Cells are positive for α-naphthylacetate and platelet glycoprotein IIb/IIIa or factor VIII-related antigen and negative for naphthylbutyrate.

Table 2
The WHO Classification of Acute Myeloid Leukemias

Acute myeloid leukemia with recurrent genetic abnormalities
    AML with t(8;21)
    AML with abnormal bone marrow eosinophils with inv(16)(p13q22) or
        t(16;16)(p13;q22)
    Acute promyelocytic leukemia [AML with t(15;17)(q22;q12)]
        (PML/RARA) and variants
    AML with 11q23 (MLL) abnormalities
Acute myeloid leukemia with multilineage dysplasia
Acute myeloid leukemia and myelodysplastic syndromes, therapy-related
Acute myeloid leukemia not otherwise categorized
FAB types M0–M7 (but not M4 Eo, which is associated with the recurring
    chromosome 16 abnormalities)
Acute basophilic leukemia
Acute panmyelosis with myelofibrosis
Myeloid sarcoma

RECURRING TRANSLOCATIONS IN AML

t(8;21) (AML1-ETO). The 8;21 translocation is the most common cytogenetic abnormality in AML, being present in 12–15% of all cases of AML, and is strongly associated with the FAB M2 subtype, in which it is present in 40% of cases (23). This translocation is associated with *de novo* AML, younger age (<45 yr), and a relatively favorable prognosis. Laboratory findings that are associated with t(8;21) include the presence of a single Auer rod, abnormal cytoplasmic granules, high levels of expression of the markers CD34 and CD19, and low levels of expression of CD33 (24).

The 8;21 translocation creates a chimeric gene on the der(8) chromosome that is formed by fusion of the *AML1* gene from chromosome 21 and the *ETO* (*e*ight-*t*wenty-*o*ne) gene on chromosome 8. The breakpoint in *AML1* is between exons 5 and 6, and the breakpoint in *ETO* is between the first two alternative exons. Thus, the *AML1-ETO* fusion gene is composed of the first 177 amino acids of *AML1* and most of the *ETO* gene.

The protein product of the normal *AML1* gene forms part of a heterodimeric complex composed of AML1 and core binding factor β (CBFβ) (Fig. 2). This heterodimer binds to DNA via the runt homology domain (RHD) of the AML1 protein. Binding of the het-

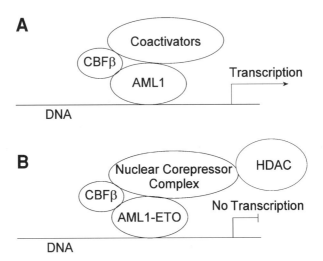

Fig. 2. (A) AML1 and CBFβ proteins form a heterodimer that can bind to DNA and, with other coactivator proteins, stimulate transcription of target genes. **(B)** The AML1-ETO fusion protein binds to DNA but recruits transcriptional repressors and histone deacetylase. These lead to repression of transcription of target genes.

erodimer to regulatory regions of target genes leads to recruitment of other proteins that regulate gene transcription and is essential for normal hematopoiesis. Genes that are known to be regulated by the heterodimer include interleukin-1, interleukin-3, granulocyte-macrophage colony-stimulating factor (CSF), the CSF-1 receptor, myeloperoxidase, *BCL2,* the heavy chain immunoglobulin *(IgH)* gene, T-cell receptor genes, neutrophil elastase, and the multidrug resistance-1 gene encoding the P glycoprotein *(25,26).* Mice in which either *AML1* or *CBFβ* has been experimentally knocked out fail to develop a definitive hematopoietic system and die *in utero.* The protein product of *ETO* can bind to nuclear corepressors and recruit histone deacetylases, thus repressing gene transcription. The protein can also form homodimers and heterodimers with related proteins *(25).*

Because the RHD domain is preserved in the *AML1-ETO* fusion gene, the protein retains the ability to bind to DNA. However, the effect of DNA binding by the fusion protein is dramatically different from the effect that follows DNA binding of normal AML1 protein. Not only does AML1-ETO compete with normal AML1 for binding to target sites in DNA, it actively represses transcription of AML1 target genes by recruiting transcriptional co-repressors and histone deacetylases *(24)*. The *AML1-ETO* fusion gene is therefore a dominant negative mutation that causes inhibition of expression of critical target genes in hematopoietic cells. Loss of expression of these genes appears to cause loss of normal regulation of cell growth. One gene in particular that has been shown to be downregulated by AML1-ETO is the tumor suppressor gene *p14^ARF* *(27)*. p14^ARF stabilizes p53 by antagonizing the effect of the protein mdm2, which is responsible for inactivation of p53 (see Chapt 8). Loss of p14^ARF results in impairment of p53-mediated growth arrest or apoptosis in response to activation of oncogenes and may be an important factor in the development of leukemia.

Point Mutations in AML1. In addition to its involvement in leukemia-associated recurring translocations such as *AML1-ETO* and *TEL-AML1,* the *AML1* gene is inactivated by point mutations in the RHD in approx 27% of patients with the M0 FAB subtype (undifferentiated acute myeloblastic leukemia) *(28,29)*. These point mutations prevent binding of AML1 protein to DNA, thus disrupting normal regulation of transcription of AML1 target genes.

Detection of t(8;21). The 8;21 translocation can be detected by conventional cytogenetic study, FISH, or RT-PCR. Quantification of *AML1-ETO* transcripts by RT-PCR can be used for monitoring minimal residual disease *(30)*.

Clinical Significance of t(8;21). The 8;21 translocation tends to be found in younger patients and portends a relatively favorable prognosis. Qualitative detection of *AML1-ETO* transcripts has limited clinical utility after treatment for leukemia because these transcripts are detectable in many patients in long-term remission *(31,32)*. However, evidence suggests that serial quantitative monitoring of *AML1-ETO* transcripts following treatment is of clinical importance. Increases in the level of these transcripts in bone marrow are predictive of subsequent relapse of leukemia *(30)*.

Inv(16) and t(16;16) (CBFβ-MYH11). The inversion (16) [inv(16)] and t(16;16) abnormalities are present in approx 70–80% of patients with the M4Eo subtype AML, but they are also found occasionally in other subtypes, including M2, M4, and M5 *(26)*. Both inv(16)(p13.1;q22) and t(16;16)(p13.1;q22) involve the *CBFβ* gene, which, as discussed above, is a member of a heterodimeric complex that binds DNA to bring about transcription of genes involved in normal hematopoietic development. In these abnormalities, *CBFβ*, which is located on 16q22, forms a chimeric gene with the myosin heavy chain gene, *MYH11*, located on 16p13. This chimeric gene encodes a fusion protein composed of the N-terminal region of CBFβ fused to the C-terminal region of MYH11 *(33)*. This fusion protein can bind AML1 protein, but at least some of the resulting complex remains in the cytoplasm and cannot function as an activator of gene transcription. In addition, the fusion protein is capable of blocking activation of gene transcription by AML1, an effect similar to that of the AML1-ETO fusion *(34)*.

Although there is variability in the location of breakpoints within *CBFβ* and *MYH11*, in 90% of cases the fusion is between nucleotide 495 of *CBFβ-MYH11* and nucleotide 1921 of *CBFβ-MYH11 (33)*.

Detection of inv(16) and t(16;16). Detection of inv(16) and t(16;16) can be performed by conventional cytogenetics, FISH, or RT- PCR. Because inv(16) may be difficult to demonstrate by conventional cytogenetic evaluation, it has been proposed that all cases with FAB M4 morphology be screened for the presence of the *CBFβ-MYH11* fusion gene or transcripts by FISH or RT-PCR, respectively *(26)*. Following therapy, quantitative assays that measure *CBFβ-MYH11* transcripts may be useful in identifying patients with increasing levels of transcripts who are at increased risk of relapse.

Clinical significance of inv(16) and t(16;16). The presence of inv(16) or t(16;16) is associated with younger age and a relatively favorable prognosis. Limited data are available on the role of monitoring *CBFβ-MYH11* transcripts following treatment. Qualitative RT-PCR appears to have limited clinical utility, whereas quantitative assays appear to predict relapse *(35)*.

11q23 Translocations and MLL. Chromosomal translocations involving 11q23 are found in approx 5% of cases of AML, most commonly in the M4 and M5 subtypes. These translocations are also seen in 10% of cases of ALL *(36)*. 11q23 translocations are notably found in infant and childhood AMLs (up to 80% of cases of infant leukemia) and AMLs, as well as secondary AML, particularly in patients who have been exposed to topoisomerase II inhibitors such as epipodophyllotoxins.

In 95% of 11q23 translocations, the critical gene that is rearranged is the *m*yeloid *l*ymphoid *l*eukemia gene *(MLL)*, which is a member of the homeobox (Hox) family of genes that play roles in development of the soma and in normal hematopoiesis. *MLL* is structurally related to the *Drosophila* gene *trithorax.* Fusions of *MLL* with its partner chromosomes appear to disrupt the ability of Hox to regulate normal hematopoiesis.

A large number of partner chromosomes has been identified, but the most common translocations are t(4;11), t(6;11), t(9;11), and t(11;19) *(37).* As the name indicates, rearrangements of *MLL* can be found in both myeloid and lymphoid leukemias. For example, t(9;11), in which the *AF9* gene is fused to *MLL,* is the most common abnormality in pediatric AML involving 11q23 abnormalities. In contrast, t(4;11), in which the *AF4* gene is fused to *MLL,* is associated with ALL.

Most breakpoints in *MLL* occur in the breakpoint cluster region (BCR), which is an 8.3-kb region encompassing exons 5–11 within the 100-kb gene. The fusion proteins are composed of an N-terminus region derived from *MLL* and a C-terminus region encoded by the partner chromosome in the translocation. Because of the very large number of partner chromosomes, the N-terminal region derived from *MLL* is the only common sequence in these different fusion proteins.

Other 11q23 Abnormalities. In addition to chromosomal translocations, two other kinds of abnormality involving 11q23 have been described: internal tandem duplications within MLL and duplication or amplification of the 11q23 band.

Internal tandem duplication of exons 2–6 (or 2–8) of *MLL* are seen in approx 10% of cases of AML with a normal karyotype, but in up to 90% of cases that have trisomy 11 as a sole cytogenetic abnormality *(38).* In this abnormality, there is a duplication of an internal portion of the gene so that the duplicated sequence is immediately adjacent to the original (i.e., they are in a tandem arrangement). Among patients with AML who do not have a detectable cytogenetic abnormality, the presence of this duplication is associated with a less favorable prognosis *(39).*

Duplication or amplification of 11q23 is also recognized as a recurring abnormality in acute leukemia and in therapy-related myelodysplasia. In this abnormality, a much larger region of DNA is either duplicated or present in larger numbers of copies (amplification) *(40,41)*. These amplified sequences may be contained in chromosomes (including chromosomes other than 11) or present in double minutes (small extrachromosomal particles composed of chromatin).

Detection of 11q23 Abnormalities. Demonstration of 11q23 translocations can be made by routine cytogenetic testing, FISH, Southern blotting, or RT-PCR. Demonstration of the internal duplication is performed by Southern blotting or by PCR. Duplications and amplifications of 11q23 may be demonstrated by FISH.

Clinical Significance of 11q23 Abnormalities. In general, the presence of *MLL* translocations, the *MLL* internal duplication, or 11q23 duplications/amplifications indicate a relatively unfavorable prognosis. An exception to this generalization is that t(9;11) may be a favorable prognostic factor in childhood AML *(42)*.

t(15;17) (PML-RARα). The FAB M3 subtype of AML is strongly associated with t(15;17). This form of leukemia is characterized by the presence in the bone marrow of abnormal promyelocytes that contain many large azurophilic granules and prominent Auer rods. A variant form, M3v, in which granules are not seen by conventional microscopy, is also recognized. The variant form is present in up to 27% of all cases of acute promyelocytic leukemia (APL) *(43)*. Both M3 and M3v commonly present with a severe bleeding diathesis owing to an associated consumptive coagulopathy and fibrinolysis resulting in disseminated intravascular coagulation.

The translocation creates a fusion between the promyelocytic leukemia gene *(PML)* on chromosome 15q22 and the retinoic acid receptor α gene *(RARA)* on 17q21. The normal PML protein appears to play a role in several cellular processes *(44)*. For example, it is essential for formation of the nuclear body, a nuclear structure of largely unknown function. Expression of *PML* is increased in response to interferon I or II through an interferon response element in the promoter region of the *PML* gene, suggesting that *PML* may be involved in immune functions. *PML* is also a proapoptotic factor, and cells from mice in which the *PML* genes have been knocked out show resistance to apoptosis. Finally, *PML* can function as a tumor suppressor.

The *RARA* gene is a member of a superfamily of nuclear receptors that includes the steroid and thyroid hormone receptors. The retinoic acid receptors (RARs) form DNA-binding heterodimers with another class of retinoid receptors called retinoid-X-receptors (RXRs). RARα is also capable of binding retinoic acid (RA). In the absence of RA or in the presence of low concentrations of RA, the RARα/RXR complex binds other proteins including nuclear co-repressors SMRT or N-CoR, the corepressor mSin3A, and histone deacetylases (HDACs). Binding of these leads to repression of transcription of certain target genes needed for differentiation of myeloid cells. In the presence of RA, the RAR/RXR heterodimer dissociates from these other proteins and functions as a transcriptional activator by binding transcriptional coactivators and histone acetyltransferase (HAT). Thus, *RARA* encodes a component of a molecular switch that can activate or repress transcription of certain genes that function in myeloid differentiation. Disruption of this function is critical in the molecular pathology of APL.

The PML-RARα fusion protein binds to transcriptional corepressors and HDACs and leads to decreased gene transcription *(45,46).* Moreover, the fusion protein can bind these other repressors of gene transcription with a stronger affinity than that of normal RARα, so that normal levels of RA are incapable of overcoming the inhibition. In this way, the fusion protein functions as a dominant-negative regulator of transcription of certain genes. Importantly, pharmacological doses of all-*trans* retinoic acid lead to dissociation of the repressors from the fusion protein, allowing expression of critical genes involved in myeloid differentiation (*see* All-*Trans* Retinoic Acid section below).

Breakpoints in PML *and* RARA. The t(15;17) translocation is characterized by three common pairs of breakpoints in *PML* and one common breakpoint in *RARA* (Fig. 3). The breakpoints in *PML* are in intron 3, exon 6, or intron 6. The breakpoint in *RARA* is consistently in intron 2. These combinations give rise to distinct isoforms of the *PML-RARA* transcript from the fusion genes as follows:

PML	*RARA*	Designations
Intron 6	Intron 2	bcr1 or long (L)
Exon 6	Intron 2	bcr2 or variable (V)
Intron 3	Intron 2	bcr3 or short (S)

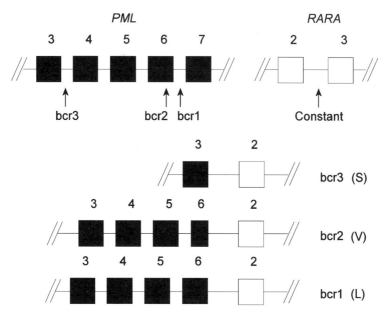

Fig. 3. The breakpoints in *PML* and *RARA* and the resulting proteins.

Patients with the bcr3 isoform of the fusion gene may have a less favorable prognosis than do patients with the bcr1 or bcr2 iso-forms *(47)*.

Variant Translocations in APL. Rarely, patients with APL have other translocations that involve the *RARA* gene. The t(11;17)(q23;q21) translocation fuses the promyelocytic leukemia zinc finger gene with *RARA (PLZF-RARA)*. This fusion differs from the usual *PML-RARA* translocation because PLZF has a domain that is capable of binding co-repressors independently of RA. Patients with this translocation commonly show resistance to treatment with pharmacological doses of RA. Other recognized translocations include t(5;17)(q35;q21), in which the nucleophosmin *(NPM)* gene is fused with *RARA (NPM-RARA);* t(11;17)(q13;q21) (nuclear mitotic apparatus, *NUMA1,* and *RARA*); and t(17;17)(q11;q21) *(STAT5b* and *RARAM) (48)*.

*All-*Trans *Retinoic Acid.* Administration of pharmacological doses of all-*trans* retinoic acid (ATRA) to patients with the *PML-RARA* fusion results in differentiation of the leukemic promyelo-

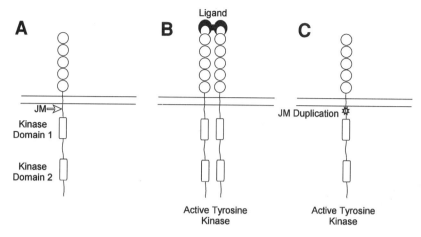

Fig. 4. (A) FLT3 is a transmembrane protein that contains two intracellular tyrosine kinase domains. **(B)** Normally, binding of the ligand, FL, leads to dimerization of FLT3 and activation of tyrosine kinase activity. **(C)** An internal tandem duplication in the juxtamembrane region leads to constitutive activation of the tyrosine kinase.

cytes to more mature myeloid cells. This remarkable therapy does not achieve cure of the patient's leukemia, and treatment with chemotherapy is still required. Nevertheless, the observation that further differentiation of malignant cells is achievable by pharmacological intervention offers the promise that such therapy may be applicable to other kinds of tumors. Patients with the *PML-RARA* fusion can be expected to benefit from ATRA therapy. Patients with the *PLZF-RARA* or the *NPM-RARA* translocations do not respond to ATRA therapy, or have a variable response *(48)*. For this reason, identification of the *PML-RARA* fusion is important in selecting patients for treatment with ATRA *(26)*.

FLT3 Abnormalities in AML. The FEMS-like tyrosine kinase-3 (FLT3) is a membrane-bound receptor that has tyrosine kinase activity (Fig. 4) *(49)*. This protein is normally expressed in primitive hematopoietic cells and is physiologically activated by binding of FLT3 ligand (FL), leading to stimulation of cell proliferation. Importantly, FLT3 has been shown to be activated in most cases of AML and B-cell precursor ALL, and recurring mutations in the *FLT3* gene have been identified. *FLT3* mutations are the most common genetic abnormality in AML.

Mutations in FLT3. The most common mutation in *FLT3* that has been reported is an internal tandem duplication (ITD) in the juxtamembrane domain of the protein *(50)*. This mutation is present in 20–25% of adults with AML (but up to 40% of cases of APL) and in 10–15% of pediatric AML cases *(49)*. The mutation results in an in-frame duplication of several amino acids and appears to block the autoinhibitory effect of the JM domain on the tyrosine kinase domain. This disrupts the normal regulation of tyrosine kinase activity, rendering FLT3 active even in the absence of its ligand.

A second mutation that has been found in a smaller percentage of patients involves a mutation in the activation loop (A-loop) of FLT3 *(51)*. Normally this loop blocks access of ATP and substrate to the tyrosine kinase domain, thereby inhibiting the enzyme activity. Phosphorylation of a tyrosine in this loop alters the configuration of the loop so that the tyrosine kinase domain becomes activated because of accessibility. Missense mutations occur at a specific amino acid, Asp835, and have been found in approx 7% of AML patients and a smaller percentage of patients with myelodysplastic syndrome or ALL. A third reported mutation is a 6-bp insertion in the A-loop that has been seen in a few patients and is also associated with increased tyrosine kinase activity *(52)*.

Detection of FLT3 *Mutations.* The *FLT3* ITD can be detected by PCR, and the Asp835 mutation is detectable by a variety of methods such as PCR-restriction fragment length polymorphism (RFLP) analysis.

Significance of FLT3 *Mutations.* FLT3 mutations are characteristically found in AMLs that do not have visible cytogenetic abnormalities. Of AML cases with a normal karyotype, nearly 40% have the *FLT3* internal duplication *(22)*. Because of this, detection of a *FLT3* mutation may be a useful marker for use in monitoring minimal residual disease in patients in whom a translocation is not present *(22)*. Patients without a visible cytogenetic abnormality generally represent an intermediate prognosis group. The *FLT3* internal tandem duplication is associated with a higher relapse rate but does not appear to have a significant effect on overall survival *(22)*. Like the *BCR-ABL* tyrosine kinase that can be inhibited with imatinib, inhibition of FLT3 tyrosine kinase represents a possible target for pharmaceutical intervention in AML *(53)*.

GENETIC ABNORMALITIES IN LYMPHOID NEOPLASMS

B-Cell Neoplasms

PRECURSOR B-LYMPHOBLASTIC LEUKEMIA/LYMPHOMA

Precursor B lymphoblastic leukemia (B-ALL) is primarily a disease of childhood, with most cases occurring under 6 yr of age *(54)*. A precursor B-cell phenotype is found in up to 85% of cases of ALL. The designation of leukemia versus lymphoma depends on the degree of involvement of lymph nodes and extranodal sites. Precursor B lymphoblastic lymphoma (B-LBL) is relatively uncommon and is primarily a disease of youth, with a median age of 20 yr at presentation. The four common translocations in B-ALL are t(12;21), t(9;22), t(1;19), and t(4;11).

t(12;21) *(TEL-AML1)*. The most common cytogenetic abnormality in children with B-ALL is t(12;21)(p13;q22), which leads to fusion of *TEL* and *AML1*. This translocation is found in 16–32% of cases of childhood B-ALL, but much less commonly in infants or adults with ALL. This translocation is generally associated with a favorable prognosis, although some studies have shown it to be as frequent in patients with relapse as in patients at the time of diagnosis *(55)*.

The *TEL* gene (also called *ETV6*), located on chromosome 12p, forms a fusion with *AML1,* commonly with the breakpoint in intron 5 of *TEL*. The breakpoint in *AML1* is usually in intron 1; thus the fusion includes more of the coding regions from this gene than are seen in the common AML-associated translocation, t(8;21), which also involves *AML1*. Whereas AML1 protein is an activator of gene transcription, the fusion TEL-AML1 protein is a transcriptional repressor *(56)*. This repression appears to be brought about by binding of co-repressors to domains of the fusion protein that are derived from *TEL,* and the subsequent recruitment of HDAC activity.

In leukemias with t(12;21), deletion of the untranslocated 12p is a common finding. This loss, which includes the untranslocated *TEL* gene, is believed to be a secondary event in cells that harbor t(12;21) *(57)*.

Detection of t(12;21). It is important to note that conventional cytogenetic studies using G-banding cannot detect t(12;21) because of the minimal changes in the appearance of the translocated chromosomes. RT-PCR methods that employ primers targeted to exon 5 of *TEL* and exon 2 or 3 of *AML1* will detect most fusions. FISH methods can also be used to detect this translocation. Retrospective studies of blood spots on Guthrie cards collected from newborns have shown that the *TEL-AML1* translocation is detectable at birth in many children who later develop B-ALL *(58)*. This finding implies that the translocation can occur *in utero* and provides important information on the natural history of this disease.

Clinical Significance of t(12;21). The t(12;21) translocation in ALL is generally associated a favorable prognosis.

t(9;22) (BCR-ABL). The t(9;22) translocation is found in approx 30% of adults and 3–5% of children with B-ALL In approx 50% of cases of adult Ph-positive ALL, the breakpoint in the *BCR* gene is in the 5.8-kb M-bcr. In most cases of childhood ALL and the remaining 50% of adult Ph-positive ALL, the breakpoint is in the m-bcr of *BCR*. The location of breakpoints in *BCR* is discussed on page 241.

Detection of t(9;22). Detection of t(9;22) or the *BCR-ABL* transcript is described on page 242.

Clinical Significance of t(9;22) in ALL. In the pediatric population, Ph-positive ALL has a substantially worse prognosis than does Ph-negative ALL. The recent availability of a specific ABL tyrosine kinase inhibitor, imatinib, may improve the prognosis for these patients.

t(1;19) (E2A-PBX1). The t(1;19)(q23;p13.3) translocation results in a fusion of the *E2A* gene on 19p13.3 with the *PBX1* gene on 1q23. The translocation is seen in 5% of all cases of pediatric and adult ALL and is associated with a pre-B-cell phenotype. The cells typically have the following immunophenotype: CD9+, CD10+, CD19+, CD34−, at least partial absence of CD20, cIgμ+, and sIgμ− *(59)*. It is the second most frequent translocation in ALL and is present in approx 25% of pediatric pre-B-cell leukemias.

The *E2A* gene encodes a protein with a basic helix-loop-helix domain. It plays critical roles in directing B-cell lineage commitment, immunoglobulin gene rearrangement, immunoglobulin class switching, and T-cell development *(60)*. It may also function as a tumor suppressor. The *PBX1* gene is the human homolog of the Drosophila gene *extradenticle (exd)*, which, as a cofactor for HOX proteins, plays a role in cell differentiation. Normally, *PBX1* is not expressed in lymphoid cells. Interactions of PBX1 with HOX proteins are through the homeodomain and the HOX cooperativity motif (HCM), both of which are present in the *E2A-PBX1* fusion gene *(60)*.

The *E2A-PBX1* fusion gene is located on the derivative chromosome 19 [der(19)]. The translocation has several effects *(60)*. First, the fusion E2A-PBX protein can function as a strong transcriptional activator of several known HOX/PBX target genes. Second, the encoded E2A protein may function as a tumor suppressor gene, and therefore loss of one allele may impair control of cell division. Third, the fusion protein is constitutively present in the nucleus, whereas normal PBX1 moves between the cytoplasm and the nucleus. The reciprocal product of the translocation, *PBX1-E2A,* which is present on der(1), does not encode a protein.

Detection of t(1;19). The presence of t(1;19) can be demonstrated by conventional cytogenetics, FISH, or RT-PCR.

Clinical Significance of t(1;19). The t(1;19) translocation in pediatric ALL is associated with an unfavorable response to certain chemotherapeutic protocols.

t(4;11) (AF4-MLL). Translocations involving 11q23 are found in up to 80% of infant leukemias. These translocations can be found in myeloid, lymphoid, or mixed myeloid/lymphoid leukemias in this age group. Among patients with B-ALL, t(4;11)(q21;q23) is the most common translocation involving 11q23, followed by t(11;19)(q23;p13). The 4;11 translocation forms a fusion between *AF4* and *MLL* that includes portions of the 5′ region of *MLL* and variable portions of *AF4*. The breakpoints in *MLL* are usually in an 8.3-kb region between exons 5 and 11, the bcr. Leukemic cells with t(4;11) tend to be negative for the marker CD10. 11q23 abnormalities are discussed on page 250.

Detection of t(4;11). The *AF4-MLL* fusion can be detected by RT-PCR, Southern blot, or FISH techniques. Conventional cytogenetics can demonstrate the translocation.

Clinical Significance of t(4;11). The 4;11 translocation is associated with an unfavorable prognosis in childhood leukemia. The complete remission rate tends to be lower, and the relapse rate tends to be very high. For these reasons, allogeneic bone marrow transplantation should be considered as a primary treatment in patients with this translocation *(61)*.

NUMERICAL CHROMOSOMAL ABNORMALITIES IN B-ALL

High hyperdiploidy (51–65 chromosomes) in pediatric B-ALL is a predictor of a favorable response to therapy and is found in 25–30% of pediatric patients with ALL. Hyperdiploidy (47–50 chromosomes), diploidy (46 chromosomes), and pseudodiploidy (46 chromosomes, but with a structural abnormality) are associated with an intermediate prognosis. On the other hand, hypodiploidy (<46 chromosomes), near-haploidy (23 chromosomes), near-triploidy (69 chromosomes), and tetraploidy (92 chromosomes) are associated with an unfavorable prognosis.

Mature B-Cell Neoplasms

CHRONIC LYMPHOCYTIC LEUKEMIA/SMALL
LYMPHOCYTIC LYMPHOMA

B-cell chronic lymphocytic leukemia (B-CLL) is the most common form of adult leukemia. Small lymphocytic lymphoma (SLL) is a closely related disease that presents as a lymphoma without leukemic manifestations. The median age of diagnosis of B-CLL is 65 yr. Symptoms may be related to anemia (often an autoimmune hemolytic anemia), infection, and thrombocytopenia. Commonly the disease is discovered as an incidental finding in asymptomatic patients. There is bone marrow involvement and absolute lymphocytosis with $>10 \times 10^9$ lymphocytes/L, although the disease can be diagnosed with lower lymphocyte counts if typical B-CLL immunophenotyping data and morphology are present (62). The malignant cells are positive for the marker CD5. A small monoclonal gammopathy may be observed on serum protein electrophoresis.

A chromosomal abnormality can be detected in >80% of cases of B-CLL using sensitive techniques such as FISH (63). The most common abnormalities involve deletions of 13q (55% of cases), 11q, 17p, 6q, and trisomy 12q. These have prognostic significance: del(17p) and del(11q) are associated with a worse prognosis, and del(13q) is associated with a better prognosis (63). In addition, molecular genetic analysis of immunoglobulin genes has shown that in approx one-half of cases of B-CLL, the immunoglobulin genes are in the germline (unrearranged) configuration (Ig-unmutated CLL); in the remaining cases, these genes are rearranged and have somatic mutations (Ig-mutated CLL). The former subtype is associated with a more aggressive disease course (64,65).

MULTIPLE MYELOMA

Multiple myeloma is a common disease, accounting for 20% of all hematological malignancies. It is usually seen in middle-aged and elderly patients. In the United States, African Americans have a twofold greater incidence of multiple myeloma than do Caucasians. The disease is characterized by expansion of a clone of malignant plasma cells. Frequently, these produce a monoclonal immunoglobulin (intact or free light chain), and there is associated suppression of production of normal polyclonal immunoglobulins. Clinical features are related to anemia, destruction of bone by osteolytic processes, renal insufficiency, hypercalcemia, and immunological deficiency.

The malignant plasma cells tend to show complex cytogenetic abnormalities that more closely resemble those found in epithelial tumors rather than the simpler translocations that characterize many hematological tumors *(66)*. Gains of chromosome 1q, 3q, 9q, 11q, and 15q are relatively common. Loss of 13q is the most common deletion. It is seen in approximately one-third of cases and is associated with an adverse prognosis. Deletion of 17p13, which eliminates a *TP53* allele, is seen in up to 25% of cases. Translocations involving the immunoglobulin loci, particularly the heavy chain locus *(IGH),* are common. Four recurring partners in these translocations include 11q13 (BCL1/cyclin D1), 6p21 (cyclin D3), 4p16 [multiple myeloma set domain *(MMSET),* which has homology with *MLL* and fibroblast growth factor receptor 3 *(FGR3),*] and 16q23 (c-MAF) *(67).*

FOLLICULAR LYMPHOMA AND T(14;18) (BCL2-IGH)

The t(14;18)(q32;q21) translocation is found in up to 90% of cases of follicular lymphoma and 30% of cases of diffuse large cell lymphoma. The translocation brings the *BCL2* gene on chromosome 18q21 in close proximity to the *IGH* locus with its strong enhancers on chromosome 14q32. This translocation leads to overexpression of the *BCL2* gene. The protein encoded by this gene, Bcl-2, is an important antiapoptotic factor (*see* Chap 6), and the presence of high levels of this protein leads to a survival advantage for cells harboring this translocation.

In approx 70% of cases of follicular lymphoma, the breakpoints in *BCL2* are in the major breakpoint region (MBR), which is in exon 3 of *BCL2*. Most of the remaining *BCL2* breakpoints are in the minor cluster region, which is distal to exon 3. The breakpoint on chromosome 14 is usually 5′ of the joining (J_H) regions of *IGH*.

Detection of t(14;18). t(14;18) can be detected by conventional cytogenetics, Southern blotting, and PCR. With PCR-based detection schemes, the selection of primers and the use of long-range PCR techniques are important to achieve a high rate of identification of the translocation *(68,69)*.

Clinical Significance of t(14;18). Demonstration of t(14;18) is not needed for diagnosis of morphologically typical cases of follicular lymphoma, but it may be useful in unusual cases and for detection of minimal residual disease *(69)*. The translocation is present in some normal individuals, more commonly in the elderly *(70)*.

MANTLE CELL LYMPHOMA AND T(11;14) (BCL1-IGH)

The t(11;14)(q13;q32) is present in up to 95% of cases of mantle cell lymphoma. In this translocation, the *BCL1* region, which contains the cyclin D1 gene, *CCND1* (also known as *PRAD1*), comes in close proximity to the *IGH* locus on chromosome 14. This translocation leads to overexpression of *CCND1*. As discussed in Chapter 6, cyclin D1 is a regulator of the cyclin-dependent kinases cdk4 and cdk6 and is therefore involved in control of the cell cycle at the restriction point between the G_1 and S phases. A major target of cdk4 and cdk6 is the retinoblastoma protein, pRb. Phosphorylation of this protein leads to release of E2F1, which is a transcriptional activator for a set of genes involved in DNA synthesis and cell cycle progression. Elevated levels of cyclin D1 facilitate passage of the cell through the G_1-S restriction point. *CCND1* is not expressed in normal hematopoietic cells, and its presence in mantle cell lymphoma is presumed to be a critical element in oncogenesis.

Detection of t(11;14). Most breakpoints in chromosome 11 occur in the major translocation cluster (MTC) that is located up to 110 kb from *CCND1*. The breakpoints on chromosome 14 are in the J_H region of *IGH*. The translocation does not give rise to a fusion protein, but to aberrant expression of *CCND1*. Because the translocation gives rise to increased levels of cyclin D1, immunohistochemistry can be used to demonstrate the presence of this protein, which is expressed neither in normal lymphoid cells nor in most B-cell lymphomas *(71)*. The typical staining pattern is nuclear.

The translocation can be demonstrated by conventional cytoge-netics, FISH, Southern blotting, and PCR. For PCR, primers are usually selected that anneal to a conserved J_H region and to several sites within the MTC. However, because the chromosome 11 breakpoints can occur over a large distance, PCR is not as sensi-tive as other techniques, particularly FISH, in detecting the translocation *(71)*.

Clinical Significance of t(11;14). The t(11;14) is occasionally found in other lymphoid malignancies including CLL, plasmacy-toma, hairy cell leukemia, splenic marginal zone lymphoma, and B-prolymphocytic leukemia *(71)*. At least 50% of cases of hairy cell leukemia show overexpression of cyclin D1 by immunohistochem-istry, but the underlying mechanism does not involve t(11;14) *(72)*. The strong association with mantle cell lymphoma makes detection of this translocation supporting evidence in favor of a diagnosis of this type of lymphoma.

DIFFUSE LARGE B-CELL LYMPHOMA

Diffuse large B-cell lymphoma (DLBCL) is one of the more common forms of lymphoma, accounting for 30–40% of non-Hodgkin's lymphomas. It has long been recognized that this form of lymphoma has widely variable clinical outcomes and was suspected to represent more than a single disease entity. This impression was confirmed in a landmark study using gene expression arrays to study the patterns of expression of a large number of genes in DLB-CLs *(73)*. This analysis revealed the existence of two principal classes of DLBCL. The first has a pattern of gene expression similar to that of germinal center B-cells and shows an active immunoglob-ulin gene somatic hypermutation machinery that is characteristic of normal germinal B-cells. The second class of DLBCL has a gene expression profile like that of activated peripheral blood B-cells.

This molecular classification generally correlated with clinical outcome: patients with the germinal center B-cell pattern of gene expression tended to have a favorable outcome to therapy, whereas those with the activated B-cell pattern of gene expression tended to have an unfavorable outcome. Moreover, the molecular classifica-tion allowed for further classification of those patients who had been placed in a favorable prognostic group using the International Prognostic Index. Therefore, the pattern of gene expression can provide important prognostic information that is independent of established clinical grading schemes.

Chromosomal Translocations in DLBCL. The most common chromosomal translocations in DLBCL, present in approximately 30–40% of cases, involve the *BCL6* gene on chromosome 3q27. This gene becomes expressed because of placement near a strong promoter in B-cells, such as the promoter of the immunoglobulin heavy chain *(IGH)* locus [t(3;14)] *(74)*. In addition to translocations, deletions and point mutations in the *BCL6* promoter region have been reported in DLBCL. Point mutations appear to be the most common genetic abnormality, being present in 75% of cases; however, these may also be detected in some normal B-cells *(75)*. The role of *BCL6* in oncogenesis remains unclear. Translocations involving this gene are also found in some other types of lymphoma including follicular lymphoma, mucosa-associated lymphoid tissue (MALT) lymphoma, mantle cell lymphoma, chronic lymphocytic leukemia, and Hodgkin's disease *(75)*.

BURKITT'S LYMPHOMA AND *MYC* TRANSLOCATIONS

Translocations involving the *MYC* oncogene on chromosome 8q24.1 and the heavy chain *(IGH)* locus on chromosome 14q32 or light chain loci (κ and λ) on chromosomes 2 and 22, respectively, are associated with L3 morphology B-ALL, or with Burkitt's lymphoma if the disease is characterized predominantly by nodal involvement. In 80% of cases, the translocation involves the *IGH* locus, and the remaining cases are approximately equally divided between the κ and λ light chain loci. These kinds of tumors are aggressive and frequently present with tumor deposits in lymph nodes and in the central nervous system.

Three types of breakpoints are recognized. Class I breakpoints are present in the *MYC* gene, in the region of exon 1 and intron 1, and are often seen in sporadic Burkitt's lymphoma. Class II breakpoints occur 5′ to MYC, and class III breakpoints occur more distantly. MYC protein is a transcriptional regulator that has broad effects on many facets of cell biology including cell cycle progression, differentiation, and apoptosis *(76)*. The translocations that involve the immunoglobulin heavy or light chain loci bring *MYC* under the regulation of these genes, which are active in B-lymphoid tissue, thereby leading to increased expression of *MYC*.

In endemic Burkitt's lymphoma, there is usually evidence of Epstein-Barr virus infection, but the molecular relationship between the infection and the development of the lymphoma remains unclear.

Detection of *MYC.* Translocations The 8;14, 2;8, and 8;22 translocations can be detected by Southern blot, long-range PCR, conventional cytogenetics, and FISH. Because of the large size of the DNA in which breakpoints can occur, PCR is not a preferred method to detect translocations, although technical improvements using long-range PCR have been reported *(77)*.

Clinical Significance of *MYC.* Translocations Translocations involving *MYC* and the immunoglobulin heavy or light chain genes are present in essentially all cases of Burkitt's lymphoma. However, these translocations can be seen in other lymphoid malignancies including DLBCL, T-cell ALL, and multiple myeloma *(78)*.

T-Cell Neoplasms

PRECURSOR T-LYMPHOBLASTIC LEUKEMIA/LYMPHOMA

Precursor T-lymphoblastic leukemia (T-ALL) accounts for approximately 15% of ALL in children. The distinction between the term T-lymphoblastic lymphoma (T-LBL) and T-ALL depends on the relative involvement of the blood and bone marrow versus nodal and extranodal sites.

Approximately 30% of cases of T-cell ALL have translocations that involve the T-cell receptor (TCR) genes. The TCR-α/δ genes are located at 14q11.2, the TCR-β gene is at 7q35, and the TCR-γ gene is at 7p14–15. As in the case of translocations involving the immunoglobulin heavy and light chain genes in B-cell leukemias and lymphomas, fusion of a partner chromosome to a TCR locus brings the partner under the influence of enhancers that upregulate gene expression in T-cells. This leads to overexpression of the partner gene. A number of partner genes have been identified in recurring chromosomal translocations in T-ALL. These include *MYC* (8q24.1), *TAL1* (1p32), *TAL2* (9q31), *RBTN1/LMO2* (11p13), *RBTN2/LMO1* (11p15), *HOX11* (10q24), and *LCK* (1p34). Of these, translocations involving *HOX11* such as t(10;14)(q24;q11) have been associated with a favorable outcome.

ANAPLASTIC LARGE CELL LYMPHOMA
AND T(2;5)(P23;Q35) (ALK-NPM)

Anaplastic large cell lymphoma (ALCL) accounts for 10–30% of childhood lymphomas and 3% of adult lymphomas. Primary systemic ALCL is classified as ALK⁺ or ALK⁻-based on detection of *ALK* expression. ALK⁺ ALCL is most common in the first three decades of life and shows a strong male predominance. ALK⁻ ALCL affects older patients.

The t(2;5)(p23;q35) translocation is found in up to 60% of cases of T cell or null-cell ALCLs. The translocation results in fusion between the anaplastic large cell kinase *(ALK)* gene on chromosome 2p23 and the nucleophosmin *(NPM)* gene on chromosome 5q35, leading to overexpression of ALK protein, which is a membrane receptor tyrosine kinase. Unlike the normal ALK protein, the fusion protein is capable of self-aggregation and activation because of dimerization domains in the nucleophosmin component. In addition, expression of the fusion gene comes under the control of the *NPM* promoter region, which is functional in lymphoid cells. Other translocation partners that activate ALK include 1q21 (tropomyosin 3), 3q21 (TRCK fusion gene), 17q23 (clathrin heavy chain), and Xq11–12 (moesin); it can also be activated by inv(2) (ATIC/Pur H) *(79)*.

Activation of ALK leads to autophosphorylation of the fusion protein and to activation of downstream signaling pathways that include the signal transducer and activation of transcription (STAT) pathways, phosphotidylinositol 3-kinases, phospholipase C-γ, and Ras. There is also evidence of inhibition of apoptosis in ALK⁺ tumors. *(79,80)*.

Detection of t(2;5)(p23;q35). Because ALK is not expressed in normal lymphoid cells, its detection by immunohistochemistry provides evidence of aberrant activation. The immunostaining pattern of ALK in the t(2;5) translocation shows both nuclear and cytoplasmic expression, whereas variant translocations tend to show only cytoplasmic staining *(79)*. The translocation can be demonstrated by cytogenetics, FISH, or RT-PCR. Primers for RT-PCR must be chosen for the specific partner chromosome to be detected.

Clinical Significance of t(2;5)(p23;q35). The t(2;5) translocation is associated with a relatively favorable prognosis in ALCL. Because this and other *ALK* fusions result in overexpression of tyrosine kinase, this enzyme represents a target for future drug development, similar to the development of the tyrosine kinase inhibitor, imatinib, for CML.

MOLECULAR TESTING FOR CLONALITY

Distinction between malignant proliferation of lymphoid cells and reactive processes is not always straightforward by conventional histopathological techniques. Demonstration of monoclonality of cells in a suspicious lesion provides evidence, although not necessarily definitive evidence, that the lesion is malignant. Because B- and T-cells undergo rearrangement of immunoglobulin or T-cell receptor genes during their development, it is possible to demonstrate monoclonality of these cell types by demonstrating a population of cells that share a specific pattern of gene rearrangements.

Clonality detection by molecular methods is a complementary approach to other methods, particularly immunohistochemistry and flow cytometry. Demonstration of κ or λ light chain restriction by these techniques provides evidence of B-cell monoclonality. Because comparable markers are not found on T-cells, assessment of T-cell monoclonality is based on immunophenotypic profiles that are less specific for monoclonality or on molecular techniques *(81)*.

B- and T-Cell Gene Rearrangement Studies

A striking feature of the immune system is the ability to produce a very large number of antigen-binding molecules consisting of immunoglobulins and TCRs. In B- and T-cells, the normal production of this diverse repertoire of immunoglobulin and TCR molecules is accomplished by rearrangement of genes from their germline configuration to a form capable of producing functional mRNAs encoding immunoglobulin heavy or light chains, or subunits of the TCR. These rearrangements are a hallmark of lymphoid tissues. The genes involved in the production of immunoglobulin and TCR molecules are shown in Table 3.

B-CELL REARRANGEMENT EVENTS

The first step in the production of a functional immunoglobulin involves recombination at the heavy chain locus *(IGH)* on chromosome 14q32.2 by joining of a diversity (D) segment with a joining (J) segment to form a DJ fusion (Fig. 5). There are 27 D and 6 J region segments; during the rearrangement DNA between

Table 3
Immunoglobulin and T-Cell Receptor Loci

Gene	Abbreviation	Chromosome
Immunoglobulin heavy chain	IgH	14q32.3
κ light chain	Igκ	2p12
λ light chain	Igλ	22q11.2
T-cell receptor, α-chain	TCR-α	14q11.2
T-cell receptor, β-chain	TCR-β	7q34
T-cell receptor, δ-chain	TCR-δ	14q11.2
T-cell receptor, γ-chain	TCR-γ	7p15

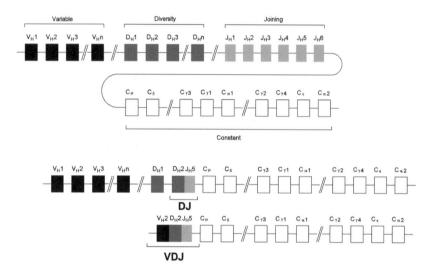

Fig. 5. Rearrangement of immunoglobulin heavy chain genes (IGH). The germline configuration of the variable (V), diversity (D), joining (J), and constant (C) genes is shown at the top. Production of a functional immunoglobulin gene involves joining of a D segment with a J segment to form a DJ fusion. A V segment is then added to form a VDJ fusion. Additional nucleotides are added at the fusion sites that increase sequence diversity among different B-cells (not shown). During rearrangement, DNA sequences between the fused segments are deleted.

the fused D and J segments is removed. In addition to fusion of the D and J segments, additional nucleotides are added randomly between the D and J segments. DJ rearrangement occurs in early pre-B-cells and is the first detectable rearrangement in the immunoglobulin genes.

The second rearrangement in B-cell development involves fusion of one of the *IGH* variable (V) regions to the DJ fusion. Again, additional nucleotides are randomly added at the site of the fusion. With the formation of the VDJ fusion, rearrangement of the immunoglobulin heavy chain locus is complete. During production of immunoglobulin, the unused constant regions (C) are removed from the RNA transcript by splicing. VDJ rearrangement is completed in the late pre-B-cell stage of cell differentiation.

Following rearrangement of *IGH,* the next locus to rearrange is the κ light chain *(IGK)* locus on chromosome 2p12. This locus does not contain D segments, so the rearrangement involves just a VJ recombination with the addition of some random nucleotides at the joining site. Successful rearrangement of *IGK* allows production of a complete immunoglobulin that uses the C_μ segment of the rearranged *IGH* locus and is therefore of the IgM class. If the first attempt to rearrange one of the *IGK* loci fails, the cell will attempt to form an immunoglobulin using the second *IGK* allele. If this also fails, then the cell will attempt to rearrange one of the *IGL* alleles on chromosome 22q11.2. Like the *IGK* genes, the *IGL* genes do not contain D segments.

T-Cell Receptor Rearrangement Events

The TCR exists in two forms, composed of heterodimers of either α and β polypeptides, or γ and δ polypeptides. These types of receptors are termed α/β or γ/δ; of these types, α/β receptors are present on approx 95% of circulating T-cells. Like the rearrangement of immunoglobulin genes in developing B-cells, the TCR genes undergo V(D)J rearrangement in developing T-cells. The order of rearrangement of TCR genes is δ, γ, β, and α. The α and γ genes do not include D segments *(82)*.

Detection of Immunoglobulin and TCR Rearrangements by Southern Blotting

Because the Ig and TCR rearrangements delete large regions of DNA, the distances between restriction sites for several restriction enzymes becomes altered from the germline configuration during rearrangement of these loci. In a pool of polyclonal B- or T-cells, physiologic rearrangements produce a wide variety of alterations in restriction fragment length that are represented in a Southern blot as a smear of bands of different molecular weights. Differences in

M 1   2   3   4   5   6   7 8   9

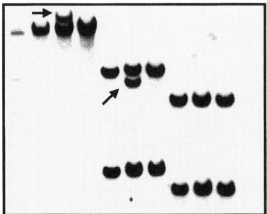

Fig. 6. Evaluation of T-cell clonality with Southern blots using the TCRBC probe (DAKO, Carpenteria, CA) and restriction enzymes *Bam*HI (lanes 1–3), *Eco*RI (lanes 4–6), and *Hind*III (lanes 7–9). Each restriction enzyme has a control lane identifying the germline configuration (lanes 1, 4, and 7). Clonal T-cell gene rearrangements are identified in a case of T-cell non-Hodgkin's lymphoma (lanes 2, 5, and 8) with novel bands present in lanes 2 and 5 (arrows). Only the germline configuration is identified in a lymph node biopsy showing reactive hyperplasia (lanes 3, 6, and 9). M, marker lane. (Reproduced from ref. *85.*)

fragment size arise from the use of different V, D, and J segments and from the addition of extra nucleotides at the joining positions. The only visible discrete band represents the germline pattern. When a clone of cells is present in sufficient abundance, its unique restriction fragment pattern associated with the Ig or TCR loci will be visible as an additional band on a Southern blot (Fig. 6).

Detection of a clonal rearrangement generally requires that at least 5%, and often 10%, of the cells in the sample harbor the rearrangement. Intact DNA, isolated from the tumor sample, is required for a Southern blot analysis, often in large quantities (of 10 μg or more) for each restriction enzyme to be tested. Thus, large amounts of fresh tissue are usually required for detection of B- or T-cell gene rearrangements by Southern blot analysis.

Enzymes and Probes. Detailed laboratory guidelines for the performance of B- and T-cell gene rearrangement assays have been published by the National Committee for Clinical Laboratory

Standards (NCCLS) *(83)*. Restriction enzymes commonly used for gene rearrangement assays are *Eco*RI, *Bam*HI, *Hind*III, and *Bgl*II. The use of multiple enzymes is essential to assess gene rearrangements on Southern blots. Commonly used probes to detect B-cell gene rearrangements are J_H, J_κ, and J_λ. For detection of T-cell gene rearrangements, the TCR β chain probes, C_β and J_β, are commonly used.

DETECTION OF IMMUNOGLOBULIN AND TCR GENE REARRANGEMENTS BY PCR

PCR can be used for immunoglobulin and TCR gene rearrangement studies. Compared with Southern blotting, PCR assays offer the convenience of rapid turnaround time, and relative ease of use and generally do not require the use of radioactive isotopes, unlike many Southern blot procedures.

Because of the large number of possible rearrangements and sequence variations among different genes of the same group (e.g., V genes), it is not possible to use just a single pair of PCR primers to detect Ig or TCR gene rearrangements. The use of multiple primer sets is essential to maximize the likelihood of detection of these rearrangements. Numerous assays using different combinations of primers with varying abilities to detect rearrangements are used in clinical practice *(84)*. In general, amplification of the TCR-β or -γ genes is technically easier than is amplification of the α or δ (which is often deleted) genes *(82)*. A commercially available set of primers has been validated in a large European study (BIOMED-2). In that assay system, detection of rearrangements of the *IGH* locus is performed with several sets of primers that anneal to the framework 1, 2, and 3 regions of the V_H genes, as will as a consensus J_H primer (Fig. 7). Several D_H primers are also used in combination with a J_H consensus primer in parallel reactions. For detection of TCR gene rearrangements, multiple primers are used that anneal to V and J regions or the D and J regions of the TCRβ gene. Optimization and standardization of PCR primer sets and reaction conditions are needed to ensure reliability of these assays between laboratories.

In PCR assays, the presence of clonality is demonstrated by an intense band in a background of a polyclconal PCR products. There may be more than a single band if the development of the clone

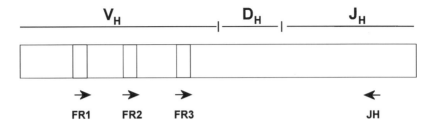

Fig. 7. PCR approach to determining clonality. Primers are used that hybridize to the conserved framework (FR) 1, 2, and 3 regions of the V_H genes, and a consensus J_H region.

involved a failed rearrangement followed by a second, successful rearrangement.

Limitations of Gene Rearrangement Studies

Gene rearrangement studies have several technical and interpretive limitations *(83)*. A clonal population must be sufficiently abundant in a mixed population of cells to be detectable. Incomplete digestion of DNA and crosshybridizing bands on Southern blots can mimic a monoclonal process. Occasionally, B-cell monoclonal processes can demonstrate rearrangement of *TCR* genes, and T-cell monoclonal processes can occasionally demonstrate rearrangement of immunoglobulin genes. Rearrangement of *Ig* and *TCR* genes may be present on occasion even in nonlymphoid lesions. If PCR methods are used to detect gene rearrangement, the possibility of false-negative results arising from failure of assay optimization (e.g., because of failure of primer binding) should be borne in mind. Finally, monoclonality is not always synonymous with malignancy. For these reasons, gene rearrangement studies must be carefully interpreted and placed in the context of other clinical and laboratory findings including morphological and immunophenotyping results.

REFERENCES

1. Kelly LM, Gilliland DG. Genetics of myeloid leukemias. Annu Rev Genomics Hum Genet 2002;3:179–98.
2. Nowell PC, Hungerford DA. A minute chromosome in human chronic granulocytic leukemia. Science 1960;142:1397.
3. Rowley JD. Letter: a new consistent chromosomal abnormality in chronic myelogenous leukaemia identified by quinacrine fluorescence and Giemsa staining. Nature 1973;243:290–3.

 4. Druker BJ, Sawyers CL, Kantarjian H, et al. Activity of a specific inhibitor of the BCR-ABL tyrosine kinase in the blast crisis of chronic myeloid leukemia and acute lymphoblastic leukemia with the Philadelphia chromosome. N Engl J Med 2001;344:1038–42.
 5. Druker BJ, Talpaz M, Resta DJ, et al. Efficacy and safety of a specific inhibitor of the BCR-ABL tyrosine kinase in chronic myeloid leukemia. N Engl J Med 2001;344:1031–7.
 6. Sawyers CL. Chronic myeloid leukemia. N Engl J Med 1999;340:1330–40.
 7. Daley GQ, Van Etten RA, Baltimore D. Induction of chronic myelogenous leukemia in mice by the P210bcr/abl gene of the Philadelphia chromosome. Science 1990;247:824–30.
 8. Baltimore D, Ren R, Cheng G, Alexandropoulos K, Cicchetti P. A nuclear tyrosine kinase becomes a cytoplasmic oncogene. Ann NY Acad Sci 1995;758:339–44.
 9. Ahuja H, Bar-Eli M, Arlin Z, et al. The spectrum of molecular alterations in the evolution of chronic myelocytic leukemia. J Clin Invest 1991;87:2042–7.
10. Bernstein R. Cytogenetics of chronic myelogenous leukemia. Semin Hematol 1988;25:20–34.
11. Advani AS, Pendergast AM. Bcr-Abl variants: biological and clinical aspects. Leuk Res 2002;26:713–20.
12. Melo JV, Myint H, Galton DA, Goldman JM. P190BCR-ABL chronic myeloid leukaemia: the missing link with chronic myelomonocytic leukaemia? Leukemia 1994;8:208–11.
13. Sinclair PB, Nacheva EP, Leversha M, et al. Large deletions at the t(9;22) breakpoint are common and may identify a poor-prognosis subgroup of patients with chronic myeloid leukemia. Blood 2000;95:738–43.
14. Huntly BJ, Reid AG, Bench AJ, et al. Deletions of the derivative chromosome 9 occur at the time of the Philadelphia translocation and provide a powerful and independent prognostic indicator in chronic myeloid leukemia. Blood 2001;98:1732–8.
15. Schoch C, Schnittger S, Bursch S, et al. Comparison of chromosome banding analysis, interphase- and hypermetaphase-FISH, qualitative and quantitative PCR for diagnosis and for follow-up in chronic myeloid leukemia: a study on 350 cases. Leukemia 2002;16:53–9.
16. Hochhaus A, Reiter A, Saussele S, et al. Molecular heterogeneity in complete cytogenetic responders after interferon-alpha therapy for chronic myelogenous leukemia: low levels of minimal residual disease are associated with continuing remission. German CML Study Group and the UK MRC CML Study Group. Blood 2000;95:62–6.
17. Nimmanapalli R, Bhalla K. Mechanisms of resistance to imatinib mesylate in Bcr-Abl-positive leukemias. Curr Opin Oncol 2002;14:616–20.
18. Joensuu H, Roberts PJ, Sarlomo-Rikala M, et al. Effect of the tyrosine kinase inhibitor STI571 in a patient with a metastatic gastrointestinal stromal tumor. N Engl J Med 2001;344:1052–6.
19. Greenberg P, Cox C, LeBeau MM, et al. International scoring system for evaluating prognosis in myelodysplastic syndromes. Blood 1997;89:2079–88.
20. Anonymous. Loss of the Y chromosome from normal and neoplastic bone marrows. United Kingdom Cancer Cytogenetics Group (UKCCG). Genes Chromosomes Cancer 1992;5:83–8.
21. Harris NL, Jaffe ES, Diebold J, et al. The World Health Organization classification of neoplastic diseases of the hematopoietic and lymphoid tissues. Report of the

Clinical Advisory Committee meeting, Airlie House, Virginia, November, 1997. Ann Oncol 1999;10:1419–32.

22. Schnittger S, Schoch C, Dugas M, et al. Analysis of FLT3 length mutations in 1003 patients with acute myeloid leukemia: correlation to cytogenetics, FAB subtype, and prognosis in the AMLCG study and usefulness as a marker for the detection of minimal residual disease. Blood 2002;100:59–66.

23. Lowenberg B, Downing JR, Burnett A. Acute myeloid leukemia. N Engl J Med 1999;341:1051–62.

24. Licht JD. AML1 and the AML1-ETO fusion protein in the pathogenesis of t(8;21) AML. Oncogene 2001;20:5660–79.

25. Downing JR. The AML1-ETO chimaeric transcription factor in acute myeloid leukaemia: biology and clinical significance. Br J Haematol 1999;106:296–308.

26. Willman CL. Molecular evaluation of acute myeloid leukemias. Semin Hematol 1999;36:390–400.

27. Linggi B, Muller-Tidow C, van de Locht L, et al. The t(8;21) fusion protein, AML1 ETO, specifically represses the transcription of the p14(ARF) tumor suppressor in acute myeloid leukemia. Nat Med 2002;8:743–50.

28. Osato M, Asou N, Abdalla E, et al. Biallelic and heterozygous point mutations in the runt domain of the AML1/PEBP2alphaB gene associated with myeloblastic leukemias. Blood 1999;93:1817–24.

29. Roumier C, Eclache V, Imbert M, et al. M0 AML, clinical and biological features of the disease including AML1 gene mutations: a report of 59 cases by the Groupe Français d'Hématologie Cellulaire (GFHC) and the Groupe Français de Cytogénétique Hématologique (GFCH). Blood 2003;101:1277–83.

30. Tobal K, Newton J, Macheta M, et al. Molecular quantitation of minimal residual disease in acute myeloid leukemia with t(8;21) can identify patients in durable remission and predict clinical relapse. Blood 2000;95:815–9.

31. Nucifora G, Larson RA, Rowley JD. Persistence of the 8;21 translocation in patients with acute myeloid leukemia type M2 in long-term remission. Blood 1993;82:712–5.

32. Jurlander J, Caligiuri MA, Ruutu T, et al. Persistence of the AML1/ETO fusion transcript in patients treated with allogeneic bone marrow transplantation for t(8;21) leukemia. Blood 1996;88:2183–91.

33. Liu PP, Hajra A, Wijmenga C, Collins FS. Molecular pathogenesis of the chromosome 16 inversion in the M4Eo subtype of acute myeloid leukemia. Blood 1995;85:2289–302.

34. Lutterbach B, Hou Y, Durst KL, Hiebert SW. The inv(16) encodes an acute myeloid leukemia 1 transcriptional corepressor. Proc Natl Acad Sci USA 1999;96:12822–7.

35. Yin JA, Grimwade D. Minimal residual disease evaluation in acute myeloid leukaemia. Lancet 2002;360:160–2.

36. Kaneko Y, Maseki N, Takasaki N, et al. Clinical and hematologic characteristics in acute leukemia with 11q23 translocations. Blood 1986;67:484–91.

37. Rowley JD. The critical role of chromosome translocations in human leukemias. Annu Rev Genet 1998;32:495–519.

38. Caligiuri MA, Strout MP, Schichman SA, et al. Partial tandem duplication of ALL1 as a recurrent molecular defect in acute myeloid leukemia with trisomy 11. Cancer Res 1996;56:1418–25.

39. Dohner K, Tobis K, Ulrich R, et al. Prognostic significance of partial tandem duplications of the MLL gene in adult patients 16 to 60 years old with acute

myeloid leukemia and normal cytogenetics: a study of the Acute Myeloid Leukemia Study Group Ulm. J Clin Oncol 2002;20:3254–61.

40. Cuthbert G, Thompson K, McCullough S, et al. MLL amplification in acute leukaemia: a United Kingdom Cancer Cytogenetics Group (UKCCG) study. Leukemia 2000;14:1885–91.

41. Andersen MK, Christiansen DH, Kirchhoff M, Pedersen-Bjergaard J. Duplication or amplification of chromosome band 11q23, including the unrearranged MLL gene, is a recurrent abnormality in therapy-related MDS and AML, and is closely related to mutation of the TP53 gene and to previous therapy with alkylating agents. Genes Chromosomes Cancer 2001;31:33–41.

42. Rubnitz JE, Raimondi SC, Tong X, et al. Favorable impact of the t(9;11) in childhood acute myeloid leukemia. J Clin Oncol 2002;20:2302–9.

43. Mattson JC. Acute promyelocytic leukemia. From morphology to molecular lesions. Clin Lab Med 2000;20:83–103.

44. Zhong S, Salomoni P, Pandolfi PP. The transcriptional role of PML and the nuclear body. Nat Cell Biol 2000;2:E85–90.

45. Grignani F, De Matteis S, Nervi C, et al. Fusion proteins of the retinoic acid receptor-alpha recruit histone deacetylase in promyelocytic leukaemia. Nature 1998;391:815–8.

46. Lin RJ, Nagy L, Inoue S, Shao W, Miller WH Jr, Evans RM. Role of the histone deacetylase complex in acute promyelocytic leukaemia. Nature 1998;391:811–4.

47. Weil SC. Minimal residual disease in acute promyelocytic leukemia. Clin Lab Med 2000;20:105–17.

48. Zelent A, Guidez F, Melnick A, Waxman S, Licht JD. Translocations of the RAR-alpha gene in acute promyelocytic leukemia. Oncogene 2001;20:7186–203.

49. Gilliland DG, Griffin JD. The roles of FLT3 in hematopoiesis and leukemia. Blood 2002;100:1532–42.

50. Nakao M, Yokota S, Iwai T, et al. Internal tandem duplication of the flt3 gene found in acute myeloid leukemia. Leukemia 1996;10:1911–8.

51. Yamamoto Y, Kiyoi H, Nakano Y, et al. Activating mutation of D835 within the activation loop of FLT3 in human hematologic malignancies. Blood 2001;97:2434–9.

52. Spiekermann K, Bagrintseva K, Schoch C, Haferlach T, Hiddemann W, Schnittger S. A new and recurrent activating length mutation in exon 20 of the FLT3 gene in acute myeloid leukemia. Blood 2002;100:3423–5.

53. Sawyers CL. Finding the next Gleevec: FLT3 targeted kinase inhibitor therapy for acute myeloid leukemia. Cancer Cell 2002;1:413–5.

54. Brunning RD, Borowitz M, Matutes E, et al. Precursor B lymphoblastic leukaemia/lymphoblastic lymphoma (precursor B-cell acute lymphoblastic leukaemia). In: Jaffe ES, Lee Harris N, Stein H, Vardiman JW, eds. Pathology and Genetics of Tumours of Haematopoietic and Lymphoid Tissues. Lyon: IARC, 2001;111–114.

55. Kelly L, Clark J, Gilliland DG. Comprehensive genotypic analysis of leukemia: clinical and therapeutic implications. Curr Opin Oncol 2002;14:10–8.

56. Loh ML, Rubnitz JE. TEL/AML1-positive pediatric leukemia: prognostic significance and therapeutic approaches. Curr Opin Hematol 2002;9:345–52.

57. Kempski HM, Sturt NT. The TEL-AML1 fusion accompanied by loss of the untranslocated TEL allele in B-precursor acute lymphoblastic leukaemia of childhood. Leuk Lymphoma 2000;40:39–47.

58. Gale KB, Ford AM, Repp R, et al. Backtracking leukemia to birth: identification of clonotypic gene fusion sequences in neonatal blood spots. Proc Natl Acad Sci USA 1997;94:13950–4.

59. Borowitz MJ, Hunger SP, Carroll AJ, et al. Predictability of the t(1;19)(q23;p13) from surface antigen phenotype: implications for screening cases of childhood acute lymphoblastic leukemia for molecular analysis: a Pediatric Oncology Group study. Blood 1993;82:1086–91.

60. Aspland SE, Bendall HH, Murre C. The role of E2A-PBX1 in leukemogenesis. Oncogene 2001;20:5708–17.

61. McKenna RW. Multifaceted approach to the diagnosis and classification of acute leukemias. Clin Chem 2000;46:1252–9.

62. Müller-Hermelink HK , Montserrat E, Catovsky D, Harris NL. Chronic lympho-cytic leukemia/small lymphocytic lymphoma. In: Jaffe ES, Harris NL, Stein H, Vardiman JW, eds. World Health Organization Classification of Tumors. Pathology and Genetics of Tumors of the Hematopoietic and Lymphoid Tissues. Lyon: IARC, 2001:127–130.

63. Dohner H, Stilgenbauer S, Benner A, et al. Genomic aberrations and survival in chronic lymphocytic leukemia. N Engl J Med 2000;343:1910–6.

64. Hamblin TJ, Davis Z, Gardiner A, Oscier DG, Stevenson FK. Unmutated Ig V(H) genes are associated with a more aggressive form of chronic lymphocytic leukemia. Blood 1999;94:1848–54.

65. Damle RN, Wasil T, Fais F, et al. Ig V gene mutation status and CD38 expression as novel prognostic indicators in chronic lymphocytic leukemia. Blood 1999;94:1840–7.

66. Kuehl WM, Bergsagel PL. Multiple myeloma: evolving genetic events and host interactions. Nature Rev Cancer 2002;2:175–87.

67. Bergsagel PL, Kuehl WM. Chromosome translocations in multiple myeloma. Oncogene 2001;20:5611–22.

68. Albinger-Hegyi A, Hochreutener B, Abdou MT, et al. High frequency of t(14;18)-translocation breakpoints outside of major breakpoint and minor cluster regions in follicular lymphomas: improved polymerase chain reaction protocols for their detection. Am J Pathol 2002;160:823–32.

69. Aster JC, Longtine JA. Detection of BCL2 rearrangements in follicular lym-phoma. Am J Pathol 2002;160:759–63.

70. Liu Y, Hernandez AM, Shibata D, Cortopassi GA. BCL2 translocation frequency rises with age in humans. Proc Natl Acad Sci USA 1994;91:8910–4.

71. Hankin RC, Hunter SV. Mantle cell lymphoma. Arch Pathol Lab Med 1999;123:1182–8.

72. Foucar K, Catovsky D. Hairy cell leukemia. In: Jaffe ES, Lee Harris N, Stein H., Vardiman JW, eds. Pathology and Genetics of Tumours of Haematopoietic and Lymphoid Tissues. Lyon: IARC, 2001:138–141.

73. Alizadeh AA, Eisen MB, Davis RE, et al. Distinct types of diffuse large B-cell lymphoma identified by gene expression profiling. Nature 2000;403:503–11.

74. Ye BH, Chaganti S, Chang CC, et al. Chromosomal translocations cause deregu-lated BCL6 expression by promoter substitution in B cell lymphoma. EMBO J 1995;14:6209–17.

75. Dent AL, Vasanwala FH, Toney LM. Regulation of gene expression by the proto-oncogene BCL-6. Crit Rev Oncol Hematol 2002;41:1–9.

76. Napoli C, Lerman LO, de Nigris F, Sica V. c-Myc oncoprotein: a dual pathogenic role in neoplasia and cardiovascular diseases? Neoplasia 2002;4:185–90.

77. Basso K, Frascella E, Zanesco L, Rosolen A. Improved long-distance polymerase chain reaction for the detection of t(8;14)(q24;q32) in Burkitt's lymphomas. Am J Pathol 1999;155:1479–85.
78. Boxer LM, Dang CV. Translocations involving c-myc and c-myc function. Oncogene 2001;20:5595–610.
79. Kutok JL, Aster JC. Molecular biology of anaplastic lymphoma kinase-positive anaplastic large-cell lymphoma. J Clin Oncol 2002;20:3691–702.
80. Scheijen B, Griffin JD. Tyrosine kinase oncogenes in normal hematopoiesis and hematological disease. Oncogene 2002;21:3314–33.
81. Gorczyca W, Weisberger J, Liu Z, et al. An approach to diagnosis of T-cell lymphoproliferative disorders by flow cytometry. Cytometry 2002;50:177–90.
82. Rezuke WN, Abernathy EC, Tsongalis GJ. Molecular diagnosis of B- and T-cell lymphomas: fundamental principles and clinical applications. Clin Chem 1997;43:1814–23.
83. NCCLS. Immunoglobulin and T-Cell Receptor Gene Rearrangment Assays; Approved Guideline, 2nd ed. Wayne, PA: NCCLS, 2002.
84. Bagg A, Braziel RM, Arber DA, Bijwaard KE, Chu AY. Immunoglobulin heavy chain gene analysis in lymphomas: a multi-center study demonstrating the heterogeneity of performance of polymerase chain reaction assays. J Mol Diagn 2002;4:81–9.
85. Tsongalis GJ, Rezuke WN. Molecular genetic applications to the diagnosis of non-Hodgkin's lymphoma. In: Coleman WB, Tsongalis GJ, eds. The Molecular Basis of Human Cancer. Totowa, NJ: Humana, 2002:461–74.

9   Pharmacogenetics

Pharmacogenetics is a branch of human genetics that relates genetic variation to interindividual differences in pharmacokinetics or pharmacodynamics of drug action. Within most populations, and certainly between ethnic groups, there are important, heritable differences that determine the rate of drug metabolism or the efficacy of certain drugs. Usually these differences are discovered when a drug is administered to a large number of subjects among whom some proportion demonstrates a distinctive drug toxicity, altered effectiveness, or pharmacokinetic difference from the rest of the population. Commonly, such variation is manifested as a bimodal or trimodal distribution of the phenotype within the population.

Ideally, recognition of important genetic determinants of drug action would be made before a drug is administered, so as to allow for an informed decision regarding the best drug or dosage for a given patient. For example, a physician would not prescribe a particular drug for a patient if it were known that the patient had a genetic defect that would lead to toxicity. Similarly, awareness that a patient had a genetic predisposition to slow or rapid metabolism of a drug could be used to influence the choice of dosage and thereby achieve the desired therapeutic effect.

PHARMACOKINETICS AND PHARMACODYNAMICS

Following administration of an oral dose, a drug is absorbed, distributed throughout the body, undergoes metabolism, and is finally eliminated. Pharmacokinetics deals with these properties of drugs. The metabolism of most drugs takes place primarily in the liver and produces metabolites that may be inactive or may have different biological effects than the parent drug. Enzymes that are responsible for drug metabolism are conventionally grouped into phase I and phase II drug-metabolizing enzymes (DMEs). Phase I DMEs catalyze what are commonly called functionalization reactions. These

From: *Principles of Molecular Pathology*
Edited by: A. A. Killeen © Humana Press Inc., Totowa, NJ

include oxidation, reduction, or hydrolysis reactions that render the drug more soluble or provide chemical groups for further metabolic reactions. Phase I reactions are catalyzed by a variety of enzymes, notably cytochrome P450s. Phase II enzymes include conjugating enzymes that produce more water-soluble compounds by conjugation of the drug with hydrophilic groups such as glucuronide or sulfate. Some pharmacological agents undergo metabolism to form the biologically active drug. The administered forms of these drugs are often called prodrugs.

Pharmacodynamics deals with factors that regulate the pharmacological effect of drugs. Most drugs interact with a biological receptor to exert their pharmacologic effect. Genetically determined variation in the structure of drug-binding receptor molecules can also influence the pharmacological effect of the drug.

EXAMPLES OF GENES DEMONSTRATING PHARMACOKINETIC VARIATION
Cytochrome P450s

The cytochrome P450s (CYPs) are a group of enzymes that are responsible for phase I metabolism of most drugs. At least 40 CYPs are present in humans, and several display polymorphisms that influence the pharmacokinetics or pharmacodynamics of certain drugs. These polymorphic CYPs include 1A1, 2A6, 2C9, 2C19, 2D6, 3A4, and 3A5. Examples of clinically important polymorphisms in several of these enzymes are discussed here.

CYP2D6

CYP2D6 is responsible for metabolism of several dozen drugs (Table 1). These include tricyclic antidepressants, neuroleptics, antiarrhythmics, and β-blockers. This enzyme is also known as debrisoquine 4-hydroxylase. Based on the rate of metabolism of debrisoquine, the population can be divided into three groups: extensive metabolizer (EM), poor metabolizer (PM), and ultraextensive metabolizer (UEM). Among Caucasian populations, most subjects are EM; however, approx 5–10% are PM, and a similar percentage are UEM. By contrast, PMs are infrequent among African and most Asian populations, but up to 29% of Ethiopians are UEM.

Table 1
Examples of Drugs That Are Substrates of Cytochrome P450 CYP2D6

Drugs for treating psychiatric and neurological disease
Amitriptyline, clomipramine, clozapine, desipramine, desmethylcitalo-
pram, fluvoxamine, fluoxetine, haloperidol, imipramine, levomepromazine,
maprotiline, mianserin, nortriptyline, olanzepine, paroxetine, perphenazine,
risperidone, thioridazine, tranylcypromine, venlafaxine, zuclopenthixol
Drugs for treating cardiovascular disease
Alprenolol, amiodarone, flecainide, indoramin, mexiletine, nimodipine,
oxprenolol, propanolol, timolol.

From Wolf CR, et al., BMJ 2000;320:987–90. Published with permission of BMJ
Publishing Group.

Subjects with the PM phenotype metabolize a number of drugs at a greatly reduced rate compared with EMs. This can lead to a reduced rate of elimination of the drug or, in the case of drugs that are converted to their active form by the enzyme, failure to achieve a therapeutic level of the active drug despite administration of an adequate dose.

The molecular bases of the PM phenotype are inactivating mutations in the *CYP2D6* gene on chromosome 22. A list of mutations with their corresponding allele designation is maintained at www.imm.ki.se/cypalleles/cyp2d6.htm. The most common of these mutations is a single nucleotide mutation, G1934A, at the intron 3/exon 4 splice junction. This disrupts the normal splicing of the mRNA and results in an inactive enzyme. This variant allele is termed *CYP2D6*4,* or the B allele, and accounts for approximately 75% of *CYP2D6* mutations in Caucasians. Other mutations include deletion of *CYP2D6 (CYP2D6*5),* present in approx 26% of PM alleles, and a single nucleotide deletion, A2637 *(CYP2D6*3),* which causes a frame shift mutation, present in approx 3% of PM alleles *(1)*. Most subjects with the PM phenotype are homozygous or compound heterozygous for these inactivating mutations, i.e., the phenotype is inherited as an autosomal recessive trait.

Subjects with the UEM phenotype have increases in copy number of *CYP2D6*. This leads to increased levels of the enzyme activity in the liver and thus to increased metabolism of substrate drugs. Genotypes associated with the UEM may contain from 2 to 13 copies of a functional gene. The UEM is transmitted as an autosomal dominant trait.

PHENOTYPING

The CYP2D6 phenotype of a subject can be determined by administration of debrisoquine or dextromethorphan followed by measurement of the ratio in urine of parent drug to metabolite (4-hydroxydebrisoquine or dextrorphan, respectively). This approach has several disadvantages including inconvenience and potential adverse effects for the subject, the possible confounding effects of other drugs that might induce or inhibit the enzyme, and instability of the sample *(2)*. Alternatively, and more conveniently, the phenotype can be inferred by determination of the presence of mutations in a subject's DNA.

CLINICAL SIGNIFICANCE OF CYP2D6 POLYMORPHISMS

Subjects with the PM phenotype achieve higher blood levels for a given dose of a drug that is metabolized by CYP2D6 than do EM or UEM subjects. Another effect of the PM phenotype is that certain prodrugs are converted to their active forms at a slower rate than occurs in EM or UEM phenotypes. Drugs in this category include codeine, which is metabolized by CYP2D6 to the more potent analgesic agent, morphine. This means that PM subjects given codeine may fail to achieve the desired analgesic effect of a standard dose *(3)*.

CYP2C9

CYP2C9 is responsible for the metabolism of several drugs including warfarin, tolubutamide, phenytoin, and nonsteroidal anti-inflammatory agents. Based on frequencies of deficiency alleles, a PM phenotype with respect to warfarin is found in 4% of Caucasians and 0.2% of Japanese *(4)*.

The wild-type or most common allele is *CYP2C9*1,* which contains Arg144 and Ile359. The most common deficiency alleles, *CYP2C9*2* and *CYP2C9*3,* both contain missense mutations: *CYP2C9*2* contains Cys144/Ile359, whereas *CYP2C9*3* contains Arg144/Leu359 *(5)*. *CYP2C9*2* is present in approx 10% of Caucasians and 3% of African Americans, whereas *CYP2C9*3* is present in approx 8% of Caucasians, 1% of African Americans, and 1–2% of Asians *(5)*. *CYP2C9*2* has approx 12% of the activity of *CYP2C9*1,* whereas *CYP2C9*3* has approx 5% of the activity *(4)*. *CYP2C9*5* is found in approx 3% of African Americans and is associated with impaired enzyme activity *(6)*. Other deficiency alleles have also been reported. A list of genetic variants is maintained at www.imm.ki.se/CYPalleles/cyp2c9.htm.

PHENOTYPING

Tolbutamide can be used for in vivo CYP2C9 phenotyping. The ratio of parent drug to the metabolite, 4-hydroxytolbutamide (measured in urine), is predictive of the genotype. DNA analysis can be performed to determine the presence of known deficiency alleles.

CLINICAL SIGNIFICANCE OF CYP2C9 POLYMORPHISMS

Among the various drugs that are metabolized by CYP2C9, much clinical interest has focused on the effect of genetic variations on metabolism of warfarin. The required dose of warfarin to achieve a desired international normalized ratio (INR) in prothrombin time can vary significantly between subjects, and much of the difference is attributable to genetic variation in CYP2C9. Pharmacological preparations of warfarin are racemic mixtures of *R*- and *S*-enantiomers of the drug. *(S)*-warfarin is the more active enantiomer and is metabolized principally by *CYP2C9*. Subjects with *CYP2C9* deficiency alleles tend to require lower doses of warfarin because of the longer half-life of the drug in these subjects. This suggests that there may be utility in determining a patient's genotype prior to administration of warfarin; however, this remains to be proved in clinical trials *(7)*. Other factors are also implicated in determining the response to warfarin. A warfarin-resistant phenotype is recognized that is characterized by a need for very high doses of drug to achieve a pharmacological response. A possible mechanism of this may involve alterations in vitamin K1 2,3-epoxide reductase, the enzyme that is inhibited by warfarin-like compounds *(4)*.

The response to phenytoin is known to be partly dependent on the *CYP2C9* genotype; because of the narrow therapeutic range of this drug, determination of the genotype may be useful prior to dosage selection. However, this remains to be demonstrated in prospective trials *(7)*.

CYP2C19

CYP2C19 is responsible for the metabolism of a variety of drugs including imipramine, omperazole, diazepam, propanolol, and chloroguanide. As in the case of *CYP2D6,* polymorphisms in

CYP2C19 alter the activity of the enzyme, with resulting alterations in the rate of metabolism of substrate drugs. A PM phenotype is present in up to 5% of Caucasians, but up to almost 25% of Asians. The normal allele is termed *CYP2C19*1*. The common mutant alleles are *CYP2C19*2* and *CYP2C19*3*. These are caused by a splice mutation and a nonsense mutation, respectively.

PHENOTYPING

Oral administration of mephenytoin is commonly used for CYP2C19 phenotyping. The ratio of *(S)*-mephenytoin to *(R)*-mephenytoin in urine predicts the phenotype. Subjects with the PM phenotype have higher *S/R* ratios.

CLINICAL SIGNIFICANCE OF CYP2C19 POLYMORPHISMS

CYP2C19 is required for activation of the antimalarial drugs proguanil and chloroproguanil. Subjects with deficiency of this enzyme have reduced efficacy of these drugs. By contrast, subjects with deficiency of this enzyme show increased activity of omeprazole, a gastric proton pump inhibitor (PPI) used in the treatment of *Helicobacter pylori* infections. The effect on the metabolism of omeprazole has been related to different cure rates in subjects with *H. pylori* infections and seems to vary among different PPI drugs *(8–10)*.

Thiopurine S-Methyltransferase

Thiopurine *S*-methyltransferase (TPMT) is involved in the metabolism of azathioprine, 6-mercaptopurine (MP), and 6-thioguanine (TG). The enzyme catalyzes methylation of sulfur atoms using *S*-adenosylmethionine as a methyl donor. The physiological function of this enzyme, which is expressed primarily in the liver and kidney, is unknown. The genetic locus, *TPMT,* which is on chromosome 6p22.3, encodes a protein comprised of 245 amino acids with a molecular weight of 28 kDa.

Three TPMT phenotypes are associated with high (i.e., normal), intermediate, and low enzyme activity levels. Approximate frequencies of these phenotypes are 90%, 10%, and 1 in 300 in Caucasian and African populations *(11)*. Under normal circumstances, none of these is associated with any adverse consequences. However, administration of MP, TG, or azathioprine (which is metabolized in vivo to MP) to subjects with low TPMT activity is associated with bone marrow suppression, which can be fatal. Subjects with inter-

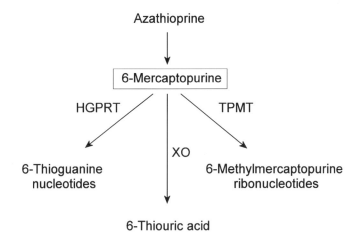

Fig. 1. Metabolism of azathioprine and 6-mercaptopurine (6MP). Azathioprine is converted to 6-mercaptopurine by a nonenzymatic reaction. 6MP can be metabolized to 6-methylmercaptopurine ribonucleotides by thiopurine methyltransferase (TPMT), to 6-thiouric acid by xanthine oxidase (XO), or to 6-thioguanine ribonucleotides (6TGNs). The first reaction in the 6TGN pathway is catalyzed by hypoxanthine guanine phosphoribosyl transferase (HGRPT). 6TGNs are the principal agents responsible for the action of azathioprine and 6MP and are also responsible for bone marrow toxicity. If TMPT activity is reduced, relatively more 6MP is converted to 6TGN.

mediate levels of enzyme activity are at intermediate risk of toxicity from these drugs. In subjects with deficiency of TPMT activity, metabolism of MP to 6-methylmercaptopurine is decreased, and more MP is converted to cytotoxic 6-thioguanine nucleotides (TGNs) (Fig. 1). An inverse relationship exists between TPMT activity and red cell TGN levels *(12)*.

The most active (i.e., normal) allele is termed *TPMT*1*. Common deficiency alleles are *TPMT*2* (G238C), *TPMT*3A,* which has two missense mutations (G460A and A719G), and *TPMT*3B,* which has one missense mutation (G460A). In Ghana, *TPMT*3C* (A719G) accounts for 15% of mutations. Other rare deficiency alleles also exist. Individuals with deficiency alleles have intermediate enzyme activities.

PHENOTYPING

TPMT enzyme activity can be measured in red cells, although there is little standardization of methods. These measurements are unreliable in patients who have been transfused with red cells in the preceding 2–3 mo *(12)*. DNA analysis to detect mutant alleles can also be performed. Depending on the number of mutations tested, this technique may miss rare deficiency alleles. Testing for *TPMT*2,-*3A,* and *-*3B* will detect most deficiency alleles in Caucasians. The value of genotyping *TPMT* prior to administration of azathioprine has been reported in a few studies that have concluded that genotyping is a convenient method to identify patients at risk of drug toxicity *(13,14)*.

CLINICAL SIGNIFICANCE OF GENETIC VARIANTS OF THIOPURINE S-METHYLTRANSFERASE

Subjects with extremely low or undetectable TPMT activity are at risk of serious, potentially fatal, bone marrow suppression when they are given azathioprine, MP, or TG. This particularly applies to patients receiving high doses of these drugs as chemotherapy for malignancies. Recommendations advocating administration of just 10% of the usual dose of azathioprine for treating inflammatory bowel disease in subjects with low activity have been made *(15)*. These recommendations also call for a 50% dose reduction in subjects with an intermediate phenotype.

N-*Acetyltransferase*

Arylamide *N*-acetyl transferase (NAT) is responsible for the "acetylator" phenotype shown in the 1950s to be associated with the development of isoniazid-induced neuropathy. The recognized phenotypes are slow, intermediate, or rapid. Frequently, the latter two are grouped as rapid. Among Caucasians, approx 40–60% are slow acetylators. In some Middle Eastern countries, 80% of the population has the slow-acetylator phenotype, whereas among Japanese and certain Eskimo populations, only 10% are slow acetylators. The reason for these marked differences in frequency of the phenotypes among different ethnic groups is unknown, but it is of interest that the global frequency of the slow-acetylator phenotype in populations generally decreases with increasing distance from the equator.

Two *NAT* genes are found on chromosome 8p: *NAT1* and *NAT2*. Both genes encode proteins with 290 amino acids and have extensive homology. *NAT2* encodes the enzyme responsible for the slow/fast acetylator phenotype associated with isoniazid toxicity.

Whereas *NAT1* has wide tissue distribution, *NAT2* is found predominantly in the liver.

As with many drug metabolizing enzymes, the physiologic substrates for NAT1 and NAT2 are essentially unknown. A folate metabolite is produced by the action of NAT1, suggesting that this enzyme may play a role in folate metabolism. The enzymes are capable of N- and O-acetylation of substrates using acetyl-CoA as a provider of the acetyl group.

The rapid acetylator allele (i.e., the wild type in Caucasians) is termed *NAT2*4*. The common slow acetylator alleles are *NAT2*5* and *NAT2*6*. These have single nucleotide substitutions giving rise to missense mutations: Ile114Thr and Arg197Gln, respectively. A database of *NAT* alleles is maintained at www.louisville.edu/medschool/pharmacology/NAT2.html.

PHENOTYPING

NAT2 phenotyping can be performed by administering caffeine and measuring the ratio of the metabolites, 5-acetylamino-6-formylamino-3-methyluracil (AFMU) and 1-methylxanthine (1X). DNA testing for the presence of mutations can also be performed.

CLINICAL SIGNIFICANCE OF *N*-ACETYLTRANSFERASE VARIANTS

Several drugs show a prolonged half-life in subjects who have the slow acetylator phenotype. These include isoniazid, some sulfonamides, dapsone, phenelzine, hydralazine, procainamide, and caffeine *(16)*. In cancer epidemiology, interest in *NAT1* mutations has increased following evidence that variants of this gene may increase or decrease risk for certain tumors *(17)*.

Cholesteryl Ester Transfer Protein

Cholesteryl ester transfer protein (CETP) is a plasma protein that is involved in exchange of cholesteryl esters and triglycerides between lipoprotein particles. There is an inverse correlation between plasma CETP and high-density lipoprotein (HDL) levels. The gene, which is located on chromosome 16q21, contains a single nucleotide polymorphism within intron 1 that destroys a restriction site for the enzyme, *Taq*I. This *Taq*I site is termed *Taq*IB. Alleles with the restriction site are termed B1; alleles in which the site is destroyed are termed B2.

The B1 allele is present at a frequency of 0.56 among Caucasians. Relative to the B2 allele, the B1 allele is associated with lower blood levels of HDL cholesterol and increased activity of CETP. These differences are associated with a 30% reduction in coronary heart disease risk among subjects with the B2 allele. The mechanism of the effect of this intronic polymorphism is unknown.

Pharmacogenetic interest in this enzyme arises because of the association between the polymorphism and efficacy of the 3-hydroxy-3-methylglutaryl coenzyme A (HMG-CoA) reductase inhibitor, pravastatin (Pravachol). By comparison with subjects who are homozygous for the B1 allele, subjects with the B2 allele have been shown to have a decreased response to pravastatin in terms of progression of coronary heart disease (18). This suggests that B2 homozygotes, who account for approx 16% of the Caucasian population, will have reduced benefit from treatment designed to slow or halt the progression of coronary heart disease using this drug.

Apolipoprotein E

The association between the ε4 allele of apolipoprotein E (APOE) and Alzheimer disease is discussed in Chapter 2. Pharmacogenetic interest in the APOE gene in Alzheimer disease stems from the observation that patients administered tacrine, an inhibitor of acetylcholinesterase, show a variable response to the drug that depends on the APOE genotype (patients with ε4 respond less favorably) (19). A similar trend was observed with metrifonate, which is also a cholinesterase inhibitor, and with a cholinergic agonist, Xanomeline. By contrast, administration of an experimental compound, S12024, which is a noradrenergic/vasopressinergic agent, was found to give the best results, in terms of cognitive performance, in subjects with ε4. Similarly, the beneficial effects of deprenyl, a monoamine oxidase inhibitor, were most pronounced in subjects with an ε4 allele.

These results lend support to the concept that the choice of drug for treatment of Alzheimer disease may depend on the APOE genotype of the subject and that subjects with one or two ε4 alleles might obtain benefit from a different group of drugs than subjects without an ε4 allele (20).

Butyrylcholinesterase (Pseudocholinesterase)

Two distinct enzymes show cholinesterase activity. True acetyl-cholinesterase is present in neurological tissues and in red cells. This enzyme is responsible for the hydrolysis of acetylcholine after its release at a cholinergic synapse. Butyrylcholinesterase (BChE), which is also called pseudocholinesterase or plasma cholinesterase, is found in plasma and other tissues such as liver. The physiological function of plasma BChE is unknown, but it hydrolyzes a number of substrates, including succinylcholine, a muscle relaxant that acts by inhibiting true cholinesterase and thus preventing repolarization of muscle. The locus of *BCHE* is on chromosome 3q26.

The normal or usual allele of *BCHE* is termed U. The enzyme encoded by the K allele has about 70% of the activity of U and is present in 9% of Caucasians but is nearly twice as frequent in Japanese *(21,22)*. This allele has a missense mutation, Ala539Thr, caused by a point mutation, G1615A. Approximately 1 in 100 Caucasians is homozygous for this mutation. Subjects with the U/U, U/K, or K/K genotypes cannot be distinguished from each other based on plasma BChE activity because of the wide range of enzyme activity in plasma. U/K or K/K subjects generally do not have a clinically important impairment in their ability to hydrolyze succinylcholine. The K allele has been associated with late-onset Alzheimer's disease *(21)*.

A variety of rare silent (S) alleles exist that are associated with minimal or no enzyme activity. Approximately 1 in 100,000 Caucasians is homozygous for S. Rare fluoride-resistant (F) alleles that encode enzymes with reduced, but not absent, activity also exist. The homozygote frequency of F alleles is approx 1 in 150,000.

The atypical (A) allele contains a single missense mutation (Asp70Gly) resulting in decreased affinity for the substrate. This manifests as in vitro resistance to inactivation by dibucaine. The great majority (approx 90%) of alleles that harbor the A mutation also contain the K mutation and can be described as AK rather than A. Approximately 1 in 3000 Caucasians is homozygous or compound heterozygous for AK and A and shows prolonged apnea after administration of succinylcholine. The most commonly seen genotypes in subjects with reduced ability to hydrolyze succinylcholine are therefore (in order of decreasing frequency) AK/AK, AK/A, and A/A. Genotypes with the S and F alleles are rarely seen.

PHENOTYPING

Total butyrylcholinesterase activity in plasma or serum is determined using butyrylcholine as a substrate. In addition to genetic deficiencies, low levels of enzyme activity can be seen following exposure to organophosphate insecticides, during pregnancy, and in patients with liver disease. Incubation of the sample with dibucaine or fluoride is useful for characterizing genetic variants and is used for screening. The percentage inhibition of enzyme activity in the presence of standardized concentrations of these agents is reported as the dibucaine number or the fluoride number. Atypical alleles are less inhibited by dibucaine (i.e., they are associated with a lower than normal dibucaine number). Reference ranges vary among laboratories, but typical dibucaine numbers and their associations are as follows: <35 is indicative of homozygosity for an atypical allele, 35–75 indicates heterozygosity, and >75 is normal. DNA analysis can be used to identify specific alleles.

CLINICAL SIGNIFICANCE OF BCHE MUTATIONS

The most important clinical significance of *BCHE* mutations is prolonged action of the muscle relaxant succinylcholine in subjects harboring mutations who undergo surgical procedures during which this drug is administered. Any genotype composed of a homozygous or compound heterozygous combination of atypical or silent alleles (i.e., AK, A, and S) can be expected to have prolonged apnea following administration of succinylcholine. These genotypes are found in approx 1 in 3000 Caucasians. Because the genotype is recessive, a single U or K allele is generally sufficient to provide enough enzyme activity to avoid the marked apnea seen in patients who lack at least one of these alleles.

Deficiencies of Conjugation Enzymes

Uridine diphosphate glucuronosyltransferase (UGT) catalyzes a conjugation step (phase II drug metabolism) that increases the solubility of drug metabolites and facilitates their excretion. In humans, at least 15 UGT transcripts exist, which derive from two loci: *UGT1A* on chromosome 2q37 and *UGT2A* on chromosome 4q13. The *UGT1A* locus encodes 12 alternative exons, which can serve as exon 1 of the mRNA, and a common set of exons, 2–5 *(23)*. The functional mRNA is encoded by one of the alternative first exons and by exons 2–5. The presence of alternative first exons gives rise to isoforms of this enzyme.

The most important disease-associated allele is *UGT1A1,* which is responsible for glucuronidation of bilirubin. Mutations in exon 1 of this variant are associated with Gilbert's syndrome and Crigler-Najjar syndromes (types 1 and 2). These are autosomal recessive disorders characterized by deficiencies in UGT1A activity and associated increases in bilirubin, particularly unconjugated bilirubin. Gilbert's syndrome is a common disorder found in up to 7% of Caucasians; it is characterized by episodic jaundice, particularly following stress. More severe enzyme deficiencies cause the rare Crigler-Najjar syndrome type 1 (complete deficiency) or type 2 (partial deficiency). Of these, Crigler-Najjar type 1 is the most severe disease and presents with severe neonatal hyperbilirubinemia in the newborn period. These diseases are therefore allelic and are caused by homozygosity or compound heterozygosity for mutations in the *UGT1A1* allele.

The allele usually associated with Gilbert's syndrome is characterized by the presence of an additional (TA) repeat in the promoter region of the gene, i.e., $(TA)_7TAA$ instead of the usual $(TA)_6TAA$ in the TATA box *(24).* The molecular etiology of this disease is therefore an expanded nucleotide repeat *(25).* Patients with Crigler-Najjar syndrome, types 1 or 2, have been shown to have any of about three dozen other mutations involving missense, deletion, frameshift, and nonsense mutations that abolish hepatic UGT1A1 activity.

PHENOTYPING

No established method of phenotyping *UGT1A1* exists. The promoter mutation can be identified by molecular methods.

CLINICAL SIGNIFICANCE OF POLYMORPHISMS IN UGT1A

Mutations in *UGT1A1* have been associated with a pharmacokinetic variation in the population. Subjects with reduced activity of UGT1A1 because of the presence of the $(TA)_7$ allele in the homozygous form have diminished ability to conjugate and eliminate SN-38, the active metabolite of the chemotherapeutic drug irinotecan (CPT-11) *(26).* Subjects with this deficiency experience increased toxicity, including myelosuppression, but particularly diarrhea, when they are given irinotecan. This is believed to be a toxic effect of SN-38 on the gastrointestinal epithelium. Other mutations in UGT1A1 that also decrease glucuronosyltransferase activity have been shown to be associated with increased side effects of irinotecan *(27)*.

Glucose-6-Phosphate Dehydrogenase Deficiency

Glucose-6-phosphate dehydrogenase (G6PD) is involved in the pentose phosphate pathway for producing NADPH, which is required for maintenance of glutathione in a reduced state. A deficiency of G6PD affects 10% of the world's population. Subjects with this deficiency have an increased risk of developing hemolytic anemia following oxidative stress to red cells. It is believed that subjects with deficiency of G6PD have increased resistance to infection by *Plasmodium falciparum (28)*.

The G6PD locus is on the X chromosome. Males are therefore more frequently affected by deficiency of this enzyme. In heterozygous females carrying a deleterious mutation, red cells express one of the two alleles (because of lyonization); therefore two populations of red cells exist, one of which is G6PD-deficient. The usual allele in most populations is the B allele. Another allele with normal activity, termed the A+ allele, is commonly found in Africans. Numerous mutations have been described. The most common among subjects of African origin is the A– allele, which is associated with decreased stability of the enzyme. Among subjects of Mediterranean origin, a large number of mutations with decreased activity have been described.

PHENOTYPING

G6PD deficiency can be detected by determining activity of the enzyme in red cells by an in vitro assay.

CLINICAL SIGNIFICANCE OF G6PD MUTATIONS

Mutations in G6PD affect not only metabolism of certain drugs, but are also associated with neonatal hyperbilirubinemia. Infection, ingestion of some foods, notably fava beans, and certain drugs can lead to hemolysis characterized by the presence of Heinz bodies in affected red cells *(29)*. Drugs that have been associated with hemolysis in subjects with G6PD deficiency include chloramphenicol, primaquine, phenacetin, vitamin K, sulfonamides, acetanilide, and nitrofurans.

EXAMPLES OF GENES DEMONSTRATING PHARMACODYNAMIC VARIATION

β_2-Adrenergic Receptor

The β-adrenoceptors are G protein-coupled, cell membrane receptors that bind catecholamines and are responsible for signal transduction to the cell interior through generation of the second messenger, cAMP, by activation of adenylate cyclase.

Three types of β-adrenergic receptors exist: β_1, β_2, and β_3. Within the respiratory tract, β_2 is the predominant receptor type. This receptor, which is encoded by the *ADRB2* gene, shows polymorphism at several positions. A missense mutation, Arg16Gly, is found in 63% of alleles in Caucasians and 39% of alleles in Hispanics. Gly16 is associated, in a dose-dependent manner, with resistance to the pharmacological effects of certain β_2 agonists, including albuterol, which is commonly used to treat asthma *(30)*. This suggests that testing for this allele may be used to guide therapy.

Mitochondrial 12S Ribosomal Subunit and Aminoglycoside Ototoxicity

A mutation, A1555G, in the gene encoding the ribosomal 12S subunit in mitochondria has been shown to be associated with an increased risk of aminoglycoside-induced ototoxicity and with non-syndromic deafness (OMIM 561000) *(31)*.

Aminoglycosides exert their antibiotic effect by inhibiting bacterial ribosomes, which are structurally similar to mitochondrial ribosomes. It is believed that this drug-induced ototoxicity is caused by damage to cochlear mitochondria. In some regions of the world, up to 25% of deafness is aminoglycoside-induced *(32)*. Aminoglycoside-induced deafness is irreversible, and pretreatment identification of the mutation in members of families with a history of aminoglycoside toxicity may be of benefit in avoiding the use of this class of antibiotic with its associated toxicity *(32)*.

REFERENCES

1. Bertilsson L, Dahl ML, Dalen P, Al-Shurbaji A. Molecular genetics of CYP2D6: clinical relevance with focus on psychotropic drugs. Br J Clin Pharmacol 2002;53:111–22.
2. Shi MM, Bleavins MR, de la Iglesia FA. Technologies for detecting genetic polymorphisms in pharmacogenomics. Mol Diagn 1999;4:343–51.

3. Williams DG, Patel A, Howard RF. Pharmacogenetics of codeine metabolism in an urban population of children and its implications for analgesic reliability. Br J Anaesth 2002;89:839–45.

4. Linder MW. Genetic mechanisms for hypersensitivity and resistance to the anticoagulant Warfarin. Clin Chim Acta 2001;308:9–15.

5. Xie HG, Kim RB, Wood AJ, Stein CM. Molecular basis of ethnic differences in drug disposition and response. Annu Rev Pharmacol Toxicol 2001;41:815–50.

6. Dickmann LJ, Rettie AE, Kneller MB, et al. Identification and functional characterization of a new CYP2C9 variant (CYP2C9*5) expressed among African Americans. Mol Pharmacol 2001;60:382–7.

7. Lee CR, Goldstein JA, Pieper JA. Cytochrome P450 2C9 polymorphisms: a comprehensive review of the in vitro and human data. Pharmacogenetics 2002;12:251–63.

8. Furuta T, Ohashi K, Kamata T, et al. Effect of genetic differences in omeprazole metabolism on cure rates for *Helicobacter pylori* infection and peptic ulcer. Ann Intern Med 1998;129:1027–30.

9. Furuta T, Shirai N, Takashima M, et al. Effect of genotypic differences in CYP2C19 on cure rates for *Helicobacter pylori* infection by triple therapy with a proton pump inhibitor, amoxicillin, and clarithromycin. Clin Pharmacol Ther 2001;69:158–68.

10. Inaba T, Mizuno M, Kawai K, et al. Randomized open trial for comparison of proton pump inhibitors in triple therapy for *Helicobacter pylori* infection in relation to CYP2C19 genotype. J Gastroenterol Hepatol 2002;17:748–53.

11. Weinshilboum RM, Sladek SL. Mercaptopurine pharmacogenetics: monogenic inheritance of erythrocyte thiopurine methyltransferase activity. Am J Hum Genet 1980;32:651–62.

12. Krynetski EY, Evans WE. Genetic polymorphism of thiopurine S-methyltransferase: molecular mechanisms and clinical importance. Pharmacology 2000;61:136–46.

13. Black AJ, McLeod HL, Capell HA, et al. Thiopurine methyltransferase genotype predicts therapy-limiting severe toxicity from azathioprine. Ann Intern Med 1998;129:716–8.

14. Colombel JF, Ferrari N, Debuysere H, et al. Genotypic analysis of thiopurine S-methyltransferase in patients with Crohn's disease and severe myelosuppression during azathioprine therapy. Gastroenterology 2000;118:1025–30.

15. Sandborn WJ. Rational dosing of azathioprine and 6-mercaptopurine. Gut 2001;48:591–2.

16. Grant DM, Goodfellow GH, Sugamori K, Durette K. Pharmacogenetics of the human arylamine N-acetyltransferases. Pharmacology 2000;61:204–11.

17. Hein DW. Molecular genetics and function of NAT1 and NAT2: role in aromatic amine metabolism and carcinogenesis. Mutat Res 2002;506–507:65–77.

18. Kuivenhoven JA, Jukema JW, Zwinderman AH, et al. The role of a common variant of the cholesteryl ester transfer protein gene in the progression of coronary atherosclerosis. The Regression Growth Evaluation Statin Study Group. N Engl J Med 1998;338:86–93.

19. Poirier J, Delisle MC, Quirion R, et al. Apolipoprotein E4 allele as a predictor of cholinergic deficits and treatment outcome in Alzheimer disease. Proc Natl Acad Sci USA 1995;92:12260–4.

20. Poirier J. Apolipoprotein E: a pharmacogenetic target for the treatment of Alzheimer's disease. Mol Diagn 1999;4:335–41.

21. Lehmann DJ, Johnston C, Smith AD. Synergy between the genes for butyryl-cholinesterase K variant and apolipoprotein E4 in late-onset confirmed Alzheimer's disease. Hum Mol Genet 1997;6:1933–6.
22. Maekawa M, Sudo K, Dey DC, et al. Genetic mutations of butyrylcholine esterase identified from phenotypic abnormalities in Japan. Clin Chem 1997;43:924–9.
23. Tukey RH, Strassburg CP. Human UDP-glucuronosyltransferases: metabolism, expression, and disease. Annu Rev Pharmacol Toxicol 2000;40:581–616.
24. Bosma PJ, Chowdhury JR, Bakker C, et al. The genetic basis of the reduced expression of bilirubin UDP-glucuronosyltransferase 1 in Gilbert's syndrome. N Engl J Med 1995;333:1171–5.
25. Schmid R. Gilbert's syndrome—a legitimate genetic anomaly? N Engl J Med 1995;333:1217–8.
26. Ratain MJ. Irinotecan dosing: does the CPT in CPT-11 stand for "Can't Predict Toxicity"? J Clin Oncol 2002;20:7–8.
27. Ando Y, Saka H, Ando M, et al. Polymorphisms of UDP-glucuronosyltransferase gene and irinotecan toxicity: a pharmacogenetic analysis. Cancer Res 2000;60:6921–6.
28. Tishkoff SA, Varkonyi R, Cahinhinan N, et al. Haplotype diversity and linkage dis-equilibrium at human G6PD: recent origin of alleles that confer malarial resis-tance. Science 2001;293:455–62.
29. Mehta A, Mason PJ, Vulliamy TJ. Glucose-6-phosphate dehydrogenase deficiency. Baillieres Best Pract Res Clin Haematol 2000;13:21–38.
30. Martinez FD, Graves PE, Baldini M, Solomon S, Erickson R. Association between genetic polymorphisms of the beta2-adrenoceptor and response to albuterol in children with and without a history of wheezing. J Clin Invest 1997;100:3184–8.
31. Prezant TR, Agapian JV, Bohlman MC, et al. Mitochondrial ribosomal RNA muta-tion associated with both antibiotic- induced and non-syndromic deafness. Nat Genet 1993;4:289–94.
32. Pandya A, Xia X, Radnaabazar J, et al. Mutation in the mitochondrial 12S rRNA gene in two families from Mongolia with matrilineal aminoglycoside ototoxicity. J Med Genet 1997;34:169–72.

10 Identity Testing

Identity testing by DNA analysis has acquired an important role in areas such as paternity testing, forensic sample identification, and bone marrow engraftment monitoring. The large number of DNA polymorphisms that exist in humans, the feasibility of extracting DNA from small specimens that are obtained from crime scenes, and the analytical sensitivity of techniques such as polymerase chain reaction (PCR) make DNA an ideal molecule for identity testing.

Until the 1980s, laboratory identity testing for forensics and paternity determination was performed primarily by analysis of polymorphisms in red blood cell antigens, certain serum proteins and enzymes, and HLA markers. In the 1980s, the discovery of variable number tandem repeat markers led many laboratories to add DNA analysis for these applications. These assays were generally performed using Southern blotting. In the 1990s, numerous laboratories adopted techniques based on analysis of short tandem repeats (STRs) that are suitable for PCR-based amplification. DNA analysis has now become the dominant technology for identity testing in most laboratories that perform parentage or forensic testing or bone marrow engraftment monitoring.

SAMPLES

In all cases of identity testing that are performed for legal reasons, e.g., paternity testing or forensic analysis, it is essential that chain-of-custody procedures be maintained and that the identity of sample donors be carefully recorded. Blood is the most common source of DNA for identity testing; however, many sources of DNA can be used including buccal scrapings, hair roots, semen, saliva, and bone. In sexual assault investigations, vaginal epithelial cells and leukocytes from the victim can be separated from sperm cells, and DNA can be extracted from each.

From: *Principles of Molecular Pathology*
Edited by: A. A. Killeen © Humana Press Inc., Totowa, NJ

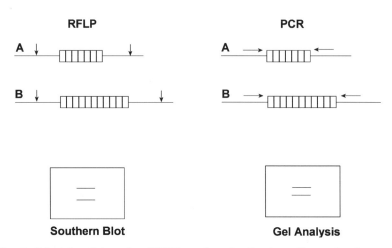

Fig. 1. Principle of detecting VNTR markers by Southern blot and polymerase chain reaction (PCR). Two alleles that differ in length can be detected by performing a Southern analysis or by PCR amplification. The latter method offers a much faster analysis. RFLP, restriction fragment length polymorphism.

VARIABLE NUMBER TANDEM REPEATS

Tandem repeats are a class of satellite DNA in which a specific sequence is repeated multiple times, generally in a head-to-tail fashion (Fig. 1). When there is variation between chromosomes in the number of copies of the repeating unit, it is termed a variable number tandem repeat (VNTR). Some VNTR loci are highly polymorphic with regard to the number of repeating units present on different chromosomes in the population. These markers are very useful for applications involving identity testing because unrelated individuals commonly have different alleles at these loci. If a sufficiently large panel of VNTR markers is examined from different people, it may be possible to identify a set of markers that is essentially unique to each person (Fig. 2).

Analysis of VNTRs involves determination of the size of the whole segment of DNA at the locus. The more copies of the repeating unit that are present, the larger the segment. The analysis therefore involves size determination, and this can be performed by Southern analysis or on PCR products. Southern analysis is based on determining the size of fragments generated when genomic DNA is cut on both sides of the VNTR by a restriction enzyme (Fig. 1).

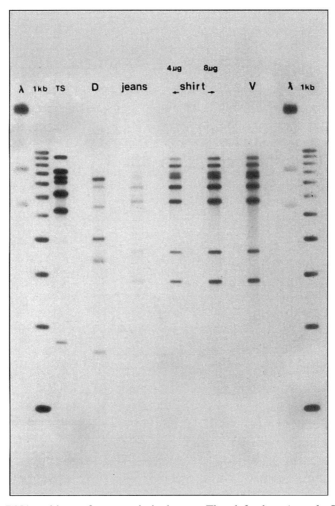

Fig. 2. DNA evidence from a criminal case. The defendant (sample D) was charged with fatally stabbing a young woman. Blood on the defendant's clothing (jeans and shirt) matched the DNA pattern from the victim (sample V) and did not match his own DNA pattern. This provides evidence of his close contact with the (bleeding) victim. (Courtesy of Orchid Cellmark, Germantown, MD.)

PCR involves amplification of DNA across the VNTR followed by determination of the size of the PCR product using a suitable sizing system, for example, gel or capillary electrophoresis. The choice of which method is used depends partly on the overall sizes of VNTRs that are found at the locus. If the overall size is relatively large (for example, >1 kb), it may be difficult to amplify the VNTR by PCR, in which case Southern analysis may be a more suitable approach.

SHORT TANDEM REPEATS

STRs, also known as microsatellites, are a type of VNTR composed of repeating units of 2–6 bp in length. Segments of DNA containing STRs can often be amplified by PCR because the total length of these markers is commonly <500 bp. This makes STRs useful markers for analysis of samples that contain degraded DNA that is unsuitable for analysis by Southern blots. In addition, because of the use of PCR to amplify STRs, smaller amounts of starting material are needed for analysis than are required for Southern blotting. In a PCR analysis, primers are selected that flank the STR. Size analysis of the PCR products is performed by gel analysis, capillary electrophoresis, or another suitable technique *(1)*.

PATERNITY TESTING

Probability of Exclusion

The mean probability of exclusion is a measure of the ability of a test, with its specific panel of genetic markers, to exclude correctly a random man in the population as being the father of a child. The probability of exclusion is therefore a function of the power of the method being used for paternity testing. The higher the value, the more likely a random man will be excluded by the test. The probability of exclusion depends on the number of alleles at a marker locus, the frequency distribution of alleles, and the ethnic population. For example, a value of 0.95 (95%) for the mean probability of exclusion of a specific set of genetic markers means that, on average, of 100 random men, 95 would be excluded as being the father of a child. With blood group typing, the mean probability of exclusion is relatively low: using ABO, MNSs, and Rhesus blood group markers, for example, the probability of excluding a falsely accused Caucasian man is only 53% *(2)*. With panels of DNA markers used in paternity testing laboratories, the probability of exclusion is often over 99.9%.

Obligatory Genes and the Paternity Index

Examination of genetic markers in a mother-child pair will reveal which markers in the child are not present in the mother and therefore must have been transmitted from the father to the child. The markers that must have been contributed by a father are known as paternal obligatory genes (OGs). For example, if a child has alleles A and C at a locus, and the mother has alleles A and B, then the father must have contributed allele C to the child. The likelihood that an alleged father might contribute allele C depends on his genotype. If he is homozygous C, then the probability of his transmitting this allele is essentially 1.0. If he is heterozygous for markers C and D, then the probability of his transmitting C is 0.5. Within a population, the chance of a random man transmitting marker C is the frequency of the allele in that population.

The paternity index (PI) is the ratio of the probability *(X)* of an alleged father transmitting an obligatory gene to the probability *(Y)* that a random man might transmit that gene i.e., *X/Y.* For example, if the father is heterozygous for *C,* and the frequency of *C* in the population is 0.01, then the PI for this locus is 0.5/0.01, which is 50. The paternity indices from several loci can be multiplied to give a cumulative paternity index (CPI). Current AABB standards require that the CPI be at least 99 to demonstrate paternity.

New Mutations

It is possible for a father to transmit an allele with a new mutation, and the more loci are tested, the more likely it is that one locus in the child will have a new mutation. This could lead to erroneous exclusion of an alleged father if he does not have an obligatory gene that, in reality, is a new mutation in the child. Because of this possibility, exclusion generally is not based on only one marker, especially if the remaining markers indicate a very high value for the PI.

Direct and Indirect Exclusion

If an alleged father does not have an obligatory gene, he is excluded using that marker; however, he can be excluded directly or indirectly depending on the genotypes in the family. As an illustration of the difference between these, consider a trio with the following genetic markers at a given locus:

Mother	Child	Alleged father
A, B	A, C	D, E

The OG is C; however, the alleged father does not have this allele but has two other identifiable alleles and is therefore excluded using this system. This type of exclusion is known as a *direct exclusion.* Now consider the following trio:

Mother	Child	Alleged Father
A, B	B	D

In this case, the child and alleged father are both apparently homozygous for markers B and D. Using these markers, the alleged father would be excluded, but this type of exclusion is known as an *indirect exclusion,* which does carry the same weight of evidence as a direct exclusion. If it could be demonstrated by some other method that the alleged father was actually homozygous for D, then this system would provide a direct exclusion. However, the genotypes shown could be found if a father had a null allele at this locus (i.e., if his genotype were D/null). A null allele is undetectable using routine laboratory procedures. In that case, the observed genotypes could be found if he had transmitted the null allele to the child, whose correct genotype is therefore B/null.

In practice, DNA markers that are used in paternity testing occasionally exhibit null alleles. This leads to mistyping of the homologous allele as being homozygous and potentially to false exclusion of an alleged father, as shown in the above example. Explanations for a null allele include a deletion of the marker locus on one chromosome, or a mutation that prevents a PCR primer from annealing to, or priming, one of the alleles to be amplified *(3).* Testing of markers in a child with maternal uniparental disomy also has the potential to lead to erroneous exclusion of an alleged father *(4).*

Probability of Paternity

The probability of paternity is calculated by bayesian analysis. This uses an estimate of the *a priori* probability of paternity and the observed CPI. The *a priori* probability of paternity is normally assigned a value of 0.5, which means that the alleged father and a random man are considered equally likely to have fathered the child. This is considered a neutral value because it does not bias the bayesian calculation in favor of either the alleged father or the party seeking to establish paternity. However, as a criticism of this approach, there are situations in which setting the *a priori* probability at 0.5 can be unrealistic, for example, if the alleged father were infertile, or if he were the only sexual partner of the child's mother.

With a prior probability of 0.5, the bayesian formula to calculate the probability of paternity, W, can be simplified as:

$$W = CPI/CPI + 1$$

If the CPI is 500, W is 99.8%. This expression of the probability of paternity may be more readily understood by a jury than the corresponding CPI value. Various states have assigned a value of W that is needed to support an allegation of paternity, commonly this is >99%.

FORENSIC APPLICATIONS OF IDENTITY TESTING

DNA analyses are commonly used in forensic applications, and aspects of this work have been standardized by the Federal Bureau of Investigation (FBI) in a DNA identification system known as CODIS (*c*ombined *D*NA *i*ndex *s*ystem). This system is authorized by the federal DNA Identification Act of 1994. CODIS uses information on DNA profiles from two sources. The Convicted Offender Index contains results of DNA profiles of criminals convicted of certain offences. The Forensics Index contains results of DNA profiles from unsolved crimes. The latter can be used to establish evidence of a common perpetrator of multiple crimes. DNA profiles can be searched using the CODIS system to determine whether a sample matches that in either index. This system has been successfully used to identify perpetrators of hundreds of crimes by finding profile matches with those from samples previously entered in the database.

CODIS operates at three levels, each with its legal requirements that govern the circumstances under which profiles may be entered into a DNA database and under which a database may be searched for a possible match. The Local DNA Identification System operates at a local level. The State DNA Identification System operates on a state-wide basis in each state. The National DNA Index System is maintained by the FBI.

To establish uniformity of reporting of DNA profiles from different jurisdictions, the FBI in 1997 adopted a panel of 13 STR markers for use in CODIS. These are shown in Table 1. In 2001, most

Table 1
CODIS Core STR Markers

STR Name	Chromosome	Locus	Core sequence in STR
TPOX	2p23-2pter	Thyroid peroxidase, intron 10	[AATG]
D3S1358	3p	[TCTA]	
D5S818	5q21-q31	[AGAT]	
CSF1PO	5q33.3-q34	CSF1 receptor	[AGAT]
D7S820	7q	[GATA]	
D8S1179	8	[TCTA]	
THO1	11p15-p15.5	Tyrosine hydroxylase, intron 1	[AATG]
vWF	12p12-pter	von Willebrand factor	[TCTA]
D13S317	13q22-q31	[TATC]	
D16S539	16q22-q24	[GATA]	
D18S51	18q21.3	[AGAA]	
D21S11	21q11-21	[TCTA]	
AMEL	X, Y	Amelogenin	

crime laboratories used two commercially available kits for STR typing, the Profiler Plus and COFiler, both produced by Applied Biosystems. These kits can be used to amplify the 13 CODIS STR markers in two separate PCR reactions. Some markers are included in both reactions to confirm that the same sample was used for both analyses. The success of DNA profiling is attested to by the thousands of successful identifications of perpetrators of serious crimes and the exclusion of falsely accused individuals.

In forensic applications, the objective is to match a DNA sample from a known individual with evidence related to a crime. The utility of DNA-based tests depends on the number of loci tested, their allele numbers, and the frequency distributions of the alleles. The power of discrimination [(also known as the matching probability (pM)] is the average number of people (in theory) one would have to genotype to find a profile that matches that of a random individual. When several STR markers are used to generate a profile, extremely large numbers of people would have to be screened to find a match, or, in other words, the likelihood of two random people having the same profile is extremely small.

Mitochondrial DNA

Mitochondrial DNA (mtDNA) has several distinctive features that make it useful for identity testing. DNA is present in multiple copies in each mitochondrion, and most cells have up to 1,000 mitochondria. By contrast, there only two copies of most genes in the diploid nucleus and a single copy of most genes on the X and Y chromosomes in males. For this reason, mtDNA can often be amplified from samples in which nuclear DNA is too degraded to be amplifiable, or is present in only tiny amounts, e.g., hair and bone fragments. Mitochondria are transmitted from mother to child. All individuals in a family who share a matrilineal relationship therefore share a common mitochondrial genome. This imposes the limitation that a sample cannot be determined with certainty to belong to a specific individual within a family based on mtDNA alone. On the other hand, it is not necessary to have a reference sample from a putative mother to compare with a forensic sample for identification. Any person in the maternal lineage of the family can provide a reference sample.

As discussed in Chapter 5, mitochondria from a single individual may have different sequences—a phenomenon known as heteroplasmy. In mitochondrial testing, this can be manifest as either length heteroplasmy or as site heteroplasmy *(5)*. In length heteroplasmy, a variation in the length of a homopolymeric run of a particular nucleotide can obscure sequencing results downstream from the polymorphic site. Site heteroplasmy manifests as two nucleotide peaks appearing coincidentally in a sequencing reaction. Recognition of the existence of mitochondrial heteroplasmy is important in not excluding otherwise matching samples as originating from the same source.

The mitochondrial genome is polymorphic, particularly in two parts of the control region in the D loop known as hypervariable regions 1 and 2 (HV1 and HV2). However, relative to markers in nuclear DNA such as STRs, the power of discrimination of mitochondrial polymorphisms is low. Moreover, because all polymorphisms are on the same piece of DNA, one cannot treat the probabilities of finding individual polymorphic markers as independent events for statistical purposes. A few common mitochondrial genotypes at HV1 and HV2 exist, as well as a large number of rare genotypes. In the United States, the FBI has organized a database of mitochondrial sequences that can be searched by law enforcement agencies for identification of human specimens.

Sex Determination

Detection of Y chromosomal DNA indicates that the sample is of male origin. Both the *SRY* (testis-determining factor) gene and a variety of other Y chromosome markers can be used for this purpose. Amelogenin is commonly used to determine the sex of the person of origin of a human sample. Amelogenin is encoded by loci on both the X and Y chromosomes *(6)*. The X chromosome gene is known as *AMELX,* and the Y chromosome gene is known as *AMELY.* These two genes differ in that *AMELX* has a 6-bp deletion in intron 1. PCR amplification across this region therefore leads to fragments of differing sizes depending on the sex chromosome complement of the subject. The presence of a single fragment of the expected size indicates that the sample is from a female. The presence of both fragments indicates that the sample is from a male.

STRs encoded on the Y chromosome are useful for identification of male cells *(7)*. In sexual assault cases, these markers provide increased detection sensitivity and so are useful in samples containing low numbers of sperm, or for identification in cases where there are cells from more than one male. Because all males who share a patrillineal relationship have the same pattern of Y chromosome STRs, these markers are of use in forensic analysis in an analogous fashion to the use of mitochondrial markers described above.

BONE MARROW ENGRAFTMENT MONITORING

Bone marrow transplantation is used to treat a variety of disorders, primarily hematological malignancies. Before a bone marrow transplant, a patient's marrow is eliminated by radiation and/or chemotherapy, and then the patient is rescued by infusion of marrow or stem cells from a donor. Following bone marrow transplantation, a comparison is made between polymorphisms in the post-transplant marrow and those identified in the donor and recipient prior to the transplant. The purpose of the analysis is to identify markers unique to both recipient and donor and, using these, to determine whether donor engraftment has occurred *(1)*.

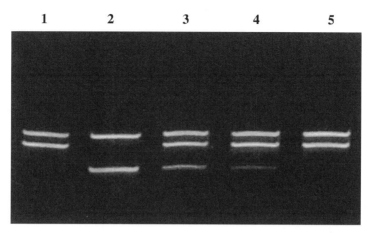

Fig. 3. Polyacrylamide gel stained with ethidium bromide showing PCR products from a bone marrow engraftment analysis. The polymorphic marker used is Col-IIA1. Lane 1, donor DNA; lane 2, bone marrow recipient DNA (obtained prior to transplant); lane 3, artificial mixture (75% donor DNA, 25% recipient DNA); lane 4, artifical mixture (90% donor DNA, 10% recipient DNA); lane 5, post-transplantation sample showing only the donor pattern. This result indicates complete engraftment of the donor marrow in the recipient. Note that the mixing studies are run as laboratory controls to ensure that a relatively minor amount of recipient DNA is detectable in the assay in a case of mixed chimerism. (Reproduced from ref. *1.*)

For this analysis, PCR amplification of STRs is commonly used. In situations of mixed chimerism in which both recipient and donor cells are present, PCR becomes competitive (e.g., if there is a preponderance of donor cells, the signal from these will be stronger than the signal from recipient cells). This enables the laboratory to provide information on the relative abundance of donor and recipient cells. In situations of mixed chimerism, the lesser population of cells can usually be detected by this analysis if it accounts for at least 1% of the total population of cells in the sample. The clinical significance of finding recipient cells following transplantation needs careful consideration and depends on the relative abundance of recipient cells, the clinical context, the bone marrow morphology, and other clinical and laboratory information. Correlation of data from different laboratory studies with clinical data is essential for interpretation of bone marrow engraftment studies. An example of bone marrow engraftment assessment by VNTR analysis is shown in Fig. 3.

REFERENCES

1. Woronzoff-Dashkoff KP, McGlennen RC. Monitoring of bone marrow transplant engraftment. In: Killeen AA, ed. Molecular Pathology Protocols. Totowa, NJ: Humana, 2001;211–25.
2. Dykes DD, Polesky HF. The usefulness of serum protein and erythrocyte enzyme polymorphisms in paternity testing. Am J Clin Pathol 1976;65:982–6.
3. Alves C, Amorim A, Gusmao L, Pereira L. VWA STR genotyping: further inconsistencies between Perkin-Elmer and Promega kits. Int J Legal Med 2001;115:97–9.
4. Bein G, Driller B, Schurmann M, Schneider PM, Kirchner H. Pseudo-exclusion from paternity due to maternal uniparental disomy 16. Int J Legal Med 1998;111:328–30.
5. Patel PI, Roa BB, Welcher AA, et al. The gene for the peripheral myelin protein PMP-22 is a candidate for Charcot-Marie-Tooth disease type 1A. Nat Genet 1992;1:159–65.
6. Nakahori Y, Takenaka O, Nakagome Y. A human X-Y homologous region encodes "amelogenin." Genomics 1991;9:264–9.
7. Carey, L, Mitnik L. Trends in DNA forensic analysis. *Electrophoresis* 2002;23:1386–97.

11 Molecular Diagnoses of Human Immunodeficiency Virus and Hepatitis C Virus

Molecular diagnostic applications promise to revolutionize the practice of medical microbiology. Identification of many microorganisms can be made more rapidly using molecular techniques than can be achieved by traditional culture methods. Molecular techniques are particularly useful for rapid detection of slow-growing organisms such as *Mycobacterium tuberculosis,* or organisms that cannot be conveniently grown such as viruses. Detection of microbial virulence or antibiotic resistance factors is also an area that is amenable to molecular approaches.

Some of the most common examples of applications of molecular techniques in medical microbiology are in the area of viral infections. These illustrate the larger themes of molecular diagnostic applications in microbiology: organism identification and quantification, identification of microbial genetic resistance factors to antimicrobial drugs, and the role of host genetic factors in susceptibility or resistance to infection.

In this chapter, the molecular principles related to diagnosis and monitoring of two common viral infections are reviewed. Human immunodeficiency virus (HIV) is responsible for the epidemic of acquired immune deficiency syndrome (AIDS). Hepatitis C virus (HCV) is a leading cause of chronic hepatitis, with severe and often fatal outcomes in a large number of patients.

HUMAN IMMUNODEFICIENCY VIRUS

HIV is the agent of a epidemic that is responsible for over 2 million deaths worldwide. It is estimated that over 40 million people worldwide were infected with HIV at the end of 2001; most infected people live in sub-Saharan Africa *(1).* The HIV-1 virus was identi-

From: *Principles of Molecular Pathology*
Edited by: A. A. Killeen © Humana Press Inc., Totowa, NJ

fied as the responsible agent for AIDS in the early 1980s *(2,3)*. A second, structurally related virus, HIV-2, which can also cause AIDS, is found predominantly in west Africa *(4)*.

Clinical Description

Both HIV-1 and HIV-2 infections are contracted through exposure to body fluids of an infected patient. The viruses are usually transmitted by sexual spread or by blood exchange associated with intravenous drug use. Prior to screening of blood donors for infection, transmission by blood products was a common route of infection and remains frequent in developing countries in which there is inadequate screening of blood donors. HIV can also be transmitted from an infected mother to her child before or during delivery, or by breast feeding, but maternal transmission of HIV-2 to children appears to be less efficient than is that of HIV-1.

Acute infection is characterized by a flu-like illness with lymphadenopathy that presents within a few months of exposure. Following the acute infection, a chronic infection is established that lasts for many years, leading to gradual destruction of the patient's CD4+ T-helper cells. This destruction of T-cells compromises the immune system, leading to the eventual appearance of opportunistic infections, neurological diseases, malignancies, and wasting, which are the usual causes of death.

Genomic Structure

HIV-1 is a RNA retrovirus that has a genome of 9.5 kb in length. The genome encodes a single protein that is subsequently cleaved by a viral protease to generate functional viral proteins. The structure of the HIV-1 genome is shown in Fig. 1.

Viral Life Cycle

Following initial infection through sexual contact, the gp120 protein of HIV-1 binds to tissue macrophages that express CD4. The presence of a cell membrane co-receptor is also required for successful infection. The great majority of HIV infections are initiated by macrophage-tropic (M-tropic) strains of HIV-1, which require the presence of the CCR5 receptor on the surface of the target cell for infection. Other, T-cell-tropic (T-tropic), strains require the co-presence of the CXCR4 receptor on the membrane of the target cell for infection.

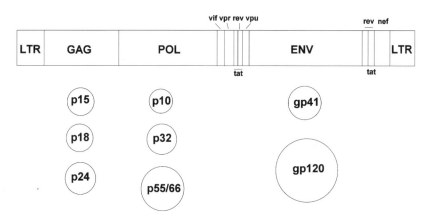

Fig. 1. Organization of the HIV-1 RNA viral genome. Long terminal repeats (LTRs) flank the coding region. Proteins encoded by viral genes are shown below these genes. The GAG gene encodes core proteins. The POL gene encodes the reverse transcriptase, integrase, and protease. The ENV gene encodes envelope proteins.

Following binding, the virus enters the cell and the RNA is reverse transcribed using the viral reverse transcriptase to form a cDNA that, in turn, is copied to form a double-stranded DNA molecule that is integrated into the host genome. Integration is accomplished by a viral integrase. Transcription of the integrated viral genome leads to the formation of a messenger RNA that is translated into a viral protein. This undergoes cleavage by a viral protease to generate the viral proteins needed to form mature virus particles. The mature virus is assembled in the membrane of the infected T-cell and is liberated to attack another CD^{4+} T-cell, causing destruction of the host cell. This leads to eventual depletion of CD4+ T-cells, resulting in impaired immunity and susceptibility to a variety of infections and malignancies.

Detection of HIV

SEROLOGICAL TESTS

Enzyme Immunoassay. Routine testing for the presence of HIV-1 and HIV-2 in blood is performed by detecting antibodies against specific viral proteins. In a popular format for this analysis, the HIVAB HIV-1/HIV-2 enzyme immunoassay (Abbott Laboratories, Abbott Park, IL, recombinant viral proteins (*gag* and *env* proteins for HIV-1 and *env* for HIV-2) are immobilized on the surface of polystyrene beads. The patient sample (plasma or serum) is added. If the sample contains antibodies to the bound proteins, these antibodies become attached to the immobilized proteins and are detected using a colorimetric signal generation system The change in color is detected and quantified by a spectrophotometer. Known positive and negative controls are run in parallel with patient samples and are used to determine the cutoff point of optical absorbances that indicate sample positive reactivity. Other assay formats are reviewed in ref. 5.

False-positive and false-negative results are uncommon in serological assays. Causes for false-negative results include the presence of very low levels of antibody, as might be seen in the window period—the time between infection and the development of a detectable immune response. This window period can last for up to 6 mo. During the window period, patients can have very high levels of HIV-1 virus in the circulation and can transmit the virus. False-positive results can be seen in several situations. Newborns may have acquired maternal antibodies by placental transfer and therefore may have antibody reactivity to HIV-1 but not be infected with the virus. False-positive results have also been described in multi-parous women *(6)*. This is believed to be owing to the development of antibodies to fetal HLA antigens to which they have been exposed to during pregnancy. These may crossreact with viral proteins in some assay systems. False-positive results have also been associated with autoimmune disease and may be seen in persons who have received multiple blood transfusions and in persons vaccinated against influenza and hepatitis B *(7)*.

Western Blots. Because of the presence of occasional false-positive results obtained by enzyme-linked immunosorbent assay (ELISA) screening, it is usual practice to confirm all positive results with a Western blot test. In this procedure, purified HIV-1 proteins are immobilized onto a solid phase. Patient sample (plasma or serum) is applied to the membrane. If the sample contains antibodies against viral proteins, as would be expected in an infected patient who has mounted an immune response to the virus, these antibodies will bind to the viral proteins. Detection of bound antibodies is achieved using a labeled anti-human immunoglobulin system that produces visible bands. The demonstration of antibodies

Table 1
Criteria for Determination of Western Blot Reactivity[a]

Pattern observed	Interpretation
No HIV-1 bands positive	Negative
Any two or more of the following positive: p24, gp41, gp120/160	Positive
Other pattern	Indeterminate

[a] Criteria defined by U.S. Centers for Disease Control and Prevention/Association of Public Health Laboratories *(40)*. Interpretive guidelines of other organizations may differ.

against the HIV-1 proteins confirms infection by the virus. Criteria for confirmation of a Western blot result are specified by various organizations. The criteria defined by the Centers for Disease Control and Prevention and the Association of Public Health Laboratories in the United States are shown in Table 1.

MOLECULAR TESTS

Molecular tests for HIV-1 include qualitative and quantitative assays and detection of mutations associated with viral drug resistance. Qualitative tests are used to identify the presence of virus in patient samples. This is of value in evaluating patients with indeterminate Western blots and newborns of infected mothers, and for testing blood donations in an effort to identify units collected during the serological window period. Quantitative tests are used to assess the viral load and to monitor response to therapy. Assays to identify viral drug resistance are of rapidly growing importance in patient care.

Quantification. Quantification of HIV viral load is commonly performed to monitor the response to anti-retroviral drug treatment. The goal of treatment is to suppress viral replication to the maximal achievable extent, as evidenced by undetectable HIV in sensitive assays *(8)*. This goal therefore places a large emphasis on the lower limit of detection of HIV quantitative assays. Quantification of HIV-1 is achieved through a variety of quantitative techniques including PCR, NASBA, TMA, and bDNA (*see* Chap. 4). The lower limit of quantification for current assays is 50 viral copies/mL.

Assay Calibration. A longstanding problem with quantitative HIV-1 assays is lack of agreement between methods. Because of this, patient results depend, in part, on the analytical method used, and so consecutive samples from an individual patient should be monitored using a single method to ensure that variation over time is biological and not a result of different analytical techniques. In part, this problem has been owing to lack of an agreed standard reference material that assay manufacturers could use to calibrate assays. Different manufacturers developed and used their own assay calibrators based on such diverse techniques as viral particle counting by electron microscopy and ultraviolet absorption of viral nucleic acid content. In 2001, the World Health Organization (WHO) approved a reference material as the First International Standard for HIV-1 RNA *(9)*. Adoption of this material should lead to improved harmonization of assay calibration and closer agreement of patient results between different analytical methods.

HIV-1 Groups. Three major groups of HIV-1 exist: M (major), O (outlier), and N (non-M, non-O). Group M is responsible for most infections in the United States and Europe. This group is composed of subtypes A–J, also known as clades. Most infections are caused by subtype B. Group O is primarily found in parts of west Africa and in France. Evidence indicates that each of these groups represents a separate cross-species transfer of simian retroviruses to humans *(10)*. In addition to being of epidemiological interest, the existence of different groups and clades of HIV-1 is of importance in the clinical laboratory. Various molecular assays have different sensitivities for different groups and subtypes *(11),* which can affect the ability of these assays to detect and quantify diverse viral groups and subtypes.

Mutations in HIV-1. HIV-1 replication is extremely error-prone because of the lack of proof reading capability of the viral reverse transcriptase. Given the extraordinarily large number of new viruses produced each day in an infected person, estimated to be 10^9–10^{10}, viral mutations are continually arising. HIV-1 viruses in an infected patient therefore contain genetically related, but different genomes, forming quasispecies. In the presence of anti-retroviral drug therapy, quasispecies that have resistance to the drug(s) administered may have a growth advantage over drug-sensitive quasispecies and become relatively more abundant in an infected patient. This leads to the emergence of drug-resistant strains in patients being treated with anti-retroviral agents.

HIV Mutation and Drug Resistance Monitoring. Currently, three classes of anti-retroviral drugs are used to treat HIV-1 infections. These are nucleoside analog reverse transcriptase (RT) inhibitors (NRTIs), non-nucleoside analog RT inhibitors (NNRTIs), and protease inhibitors (PIs). Testing, or consideration of testing, for anti-retroviral drug resistance has been recommended by a international panel in the following situations *(12):*

1. Patients with newly acquired HIV-1 infections. Many patients who acquire HIV-1 infection in countries in which anti-retroviral drugs are in use may acquire a strain of virus that has been selected for drug resistance in a previously infected patient. In addition, some strains of virus may naturally harbor polymorphisms that confer low-level resistance to NNRTIs. In these patients, testing should be considered prior to commencing drug therapy.
2. Patients with established HIV-1 infection who have not been previously treated with anti-retroviral drugs. In these patients, testing should also be considered because of the possibility that a drug-resistant strain may be present.
3. Patients whose drug therapy is being changed because of failure of viral response. In these patients, several issues are relevant. First, the patient may not be adhering to therapy, or there may be pharmacokinetic abnormalities that limit a drug's effectiveness. In these cases, demonstration of the presence of wild-type HIV-1 would be evidence that viral drug resistance is not the reason for therapeutic failure. Second, HIV-1 in patients on a multidrug regimen may develop resistance to only one or two of the drugs being used. Resistance testing will indicate which drug(s) may still be used. The sample for testing should be collected while the patient is still on the regimen.
4. Patients who have had multiple drug regimen failures. Testing for drug resistance in these patients will indicate what therapeutic options remain.
5. Pregnant patients with HIV-1 infection.

Resistance Monitoring. Three principal methods are in use to determine whether a patient's HIV-1 strain is resistant to anti-retroviral therapy. These methods are HIV-1 genotyping, phenotyping, and virtual phenotyping.

Genotyping. Genotyping of HIV-1 involves examining portions of the viral sequence for the presence of mutations that are associated with anti-retroviral drug resistance. Because most drugs in current use are targeted against the viral reverse transcriptase or the protease, these genes are examined for mutations. Methods in use to detect mutations are performed on RT-PCR-amplified regions of the HIV-1 genome followed by mutation detection. The mutation detection schemes in use include sequencing, using either standard sequencing technology or microarrays, and oligonucleotide probes directed against common mutations. Compared with the use of oligonucleotide probe sets, sequencing has the advantage that novel mutations can be discovered. In samples with mixtures of two or more different populations of virus, sequencing methods can usually detect the minor population if it accounts for at least 10–20% of the total viral population. Below this level, viral variants that contain drug-resistance mutations may not be detectable in a background of wild-type viruses.

Genotyping approaches to determining drug resistance are limited by the difficulties associated with interpretation of the effects of multiple mutations and benign polymorphisms on drug sensitivity. The combined effects of different mutations are not easily predicted. For example, T215Y confers resistance to azidothymidine (AZT); however, if both T215Y and M184V are present, the latter increases sensitivity to AZT and at the same time confers resistance to lamivudine (3TC) *(13)*. Other mutations are only of significance if a second mutation is also present. Computer programs are available to assist in interpretation of genotype data *(14)*.

Phenotyping. Viral phenotyping assays are similar in concept to conventional bacterial antibiotic susceptibility tests. The growth of the virus in the presence of different concentrations of anti-retroviral drugs is determined in vitro. In the more common formats of this assay, regions of the viral genome isolated from a patient's blood sample are cloned into a modified virus, and the growth of the resulting recombinant virus in a standard culture system is monitored. Typically, concentrations of drug needed to inhibit growth by 50% or 90% (IC_{50} or IC_{90}) are reported.

Phenotyping assays have the advantage that interpretation of results is much more straightforward than is interpretation of genotyping results. The complexities of extrapolating from mutation identification to a predicted phenotype do not arise. However, like assays based on genotype determination, phenotyping assays may not detect quasispecies that account for <10–20% of the total viral population. The techniques required to perform phenotypic assays are beyond the current capabilities of most clinical laboratories, and these assays are therefore performed only in specialized reference laboratories. The cost of these assays is also generally greater than the cost of genotyping assays.

Virtual Phenotyping. Analysis of drug-resistance mutations in viral isolates from a patient can be used to predict the phenotype based on knowledge from previous experience of the genotype-phenotype relationship in samples from other patients. In this approach, which has been commercialized, mutations identified in a patient sample are compared with a large database of information about phenotypes that have been previously associated with different mutations. Samples with a mutation profile that has previously been associated with a particular phenotype will be expected to have the same phenotype. This approach is known as virtual phenotyping. A limitation of this approach is the number of mutations tested and the quality of the information of the database against which a particular strain is compared.

Clinical Evidence of Benefit of Resistance Testing. Both retrospective and prospective clinical trials have demonstrated the benefits of adjusting anti-retroviral drug regimens based on HIV-1 genotyping to determine resistance *(15)*. For example, among prospective trials, the Viradapt study demonstrated a mean reduction of 1.04 $\log_{10}$ in viral loads over a 3-mo period in patients given treatment based on HIV-1 genotype versus a reduction of 0.46 $\log_{10}$ in patients treated without this knowledge. At 6 mo, the reductions were 1.15 $\log_{10}$ and 0.67 $\log_{10}$ *(16)*. The Community Programs for Clinical Research on AIDS (CPCRA) study revealed that for patients failing while on existing drug regimens, expert drug selection based on knowledge of HIV-1 mutation status was superior, as evidenced by decreases in viral load, to drug regimens selected by experts without knowledge of mutations *(17)*. Drug resistance monitoring is becoming a routine component of care for HIV-1-infected patients.

Host Factors Implicated in Resistance to Infection

Chemokine Receptors. HIV-1 infects cells that express the CD4 protein. Binding of the virus to CD4$^+$ cells involves the viral protein gp120. However, other receptors, identified as chemokine receptors, are also required for infection of a cell (Fig. 2). T-cell tropic HIV-1 (also known as X4) infects T-cells that coexpress the chemokine

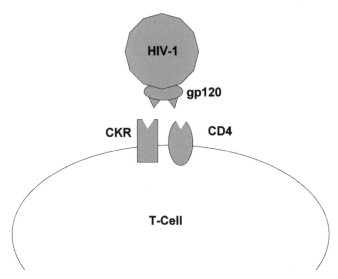

Fig. 2. Infection of a cell by HIV-1. The virus binds to both the CD4 molecule and to a chemokine receptor (CKR) through the viral gp120 protein.

receptor CXCR4. M-tropic HIV-1 (also known as R5) infects macrophages, monocytes, and some T-cells that coexpress another chemokine receptor, CCR5. R5 strains tend to predominate during early infection, whereas X4 strains tend to be associated with later, more aggressive disease *(18)*. Some strains of HIV-1 can utilize other chemokine receptors to effect entry into a target cell. Binding of the virus through gp120 to CD4 is followed by binding to the chemokine receptor and entry of the virus into the cell.

The chemokine receptor genes are polymorphic, and certain variants, including nonfunctional mutant forms, have been shown to influence host susceptibility to HIV-1 infection. The best characterized polymorphism of clinical importance is a deletion of 32 bp in the *CCR5* gene, generating a frameshift mutation and leading to premature protein truncation that inactivates the receptor *(19,20)*. The frequency of this mutant gene, which is designated *CCR5-2,* is approx 10% among Europeans, 2–5% among Middle-Eastern and Indian populations, and very rare in West Africans *(21,22)*. Subjects who are homozygous for the mutant gene have significant resistance to infection by HIV-1 following exposure to the virus *(23)*. Heterozygous subjects show delayed progression of disease.

HEPATITIS C

Clinical Description

Hepatitis C is a frequent infection, with an estimated 170 million people infected worldwide. In the United States, an estimated 4 million people have hepatitis C, many of whom are unaware that they are infected. The disease is caused by HCV, which is transmitted by blood exchange, commonly in connection with intravenous drug use. Vertical transmission (i.e., mother to fetus) can occur but is not a major route of infection. Transmission during sexual intercourse is also not a major mechanism of spread of the virus.

HCV causes hepatitis and leads to chronic hepatitis in approximately 80% of infected patients. The factors that lead to successful clearing of the viral infection in the remaining 20% may include host factors such as the immune response as well as viral factors such as genotype *(24)*. The presence of the HLA allele, DRB1*01, or a recognized episode of acute icteric hepatitis may be associated with a higher rate of viral clearance *(25)*. However, most patients do not experience an acute hepatitis, and many patients are asymptomatic when HCV infection is discovered during evaluation for another medical condition or a routine examination reveals unexpected abnormalities in liver function tests. Approximately 20% of chronically infected patients develop cirrhosis, and of these, the annual risk of developing hepatocellular carcinoma has been estimated to be 1–4%. In the United States, HCV infection is the most common indication for liver transplantation.

Genomic Structure

HCV is a single-stranded 9.5-kb RNA virus. It is related to hepatitis G virus, dengue virus, and yellow fever virus *(26)*. The genome has two untranslated regions and encodes a single polypeptide, which undergoes proteolytic cleavage to form 10 distinct proteins (Fig. 3).

Detection

SEROLOGICAL TESTS

Enzyme Immunoassay. Antibodies against HCV antigens develop in response to infection. Detection of these antibodies forms the basis of the usual method for screening for HCV infec-

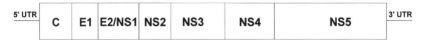

Fig. 3. Organization of the HCV RNA viral genome. C, E, and NS indicate core, envelope, and nonstructural genes, respectively.

tion, namely, enzyme immunoassay (EIA). In a popular commercial version of this assay, the Abbott HCV EIA 2.0 (Abbott Laboratories), HCV proteins are immobilized on the surface of microparticles. The patient sample (serum or plasma) is added, and if anti-HCV antibodies are present in the sample, these bind to their immobilized targets. Detection of bound antibodies is performed using a colorimetric procedure that is quantified using a spectrophotometer. Other serological methods are reviewed in ref. 5.

The current generation of EIA tests has excellent sensitivity and specificity and for most practical purposes a positive test is sufficient to diagnose exposure to the virus, particularly in a patient with known risk factors. The EIA cannot distinguish between past infection that has been cleared, and current, active infection, either acute or chronic. A positive EIA does not provide any information on the extent of liver damage. False-negative test results have been reported in patients with HIV-1 infection (presumably owing to immune suppression) and in patients with essential mixed cryoglobulinemia.

Recombinant Immunoblot Assay. The recombinant immunoblot assay (RIBA) is a serologic test, similar to a Western blot, in which individual, recombinant HCV proteins are applied to a membrane in known locations. This allows detection and identification of patient antibodies against specific antigens. Like the EIA test, a positive RIBA test cannot be used to confirm the presence of active disease or to assess the extent of liver damage. A RIBA assay is used to provide a confirmation of a positive result from EIA screening, particularly in patients who have no known risk factors for HCV infection.

In a popular format for the RIBA assay (HCV 3.0 Strip Immunoblot Assay, Chiron, Emeryville, CA), the test uses two recombinant antigens (c33c and NS5) and three synthetic peptides, c100p, 5-1-1, and c22p. Data indicate that the most common pattern found in positive samples involves detection of antibodies to c33c and c22p *(27)*.

RIBA results are reported as positive, negative, or indeterminate. The status of patients with an indeterminate RIBA result may be clarified by performing a nucleic acid test for HCV RNA or by repeating the workup on a new sample collected at a later time.

LIVER BIOPSY

Liver biopsy is considered the gold standard for assessment of the degree of liver damage, the presence of cirrhosis, and the prognosis. A biopsy that shows absent or only minimal fibrosis implies a good prognosis and may be used in deciding whether to begin antiviral treatment.

MOLECULAR TESTS

Molecular testing can be performed for the following purposes: qualitative detection of the virus, quantification of the viral load, and identification of viral genotypes.

Qualitative Assays. Detection of HCV by RT-PCR is useful in diagnosing suspected acute infections following a known exposure. The time to develop an antibody response in a subject after a known exposure varies from a few weeks to several months. During this period, serological tests are negative, and RT-PCR is the standard method for demonstrating the virus. Conversely, newborns of infected mothers may have passively acquired maternal antibodies to HCV but may not be infected. In this situation, RT-PCR is useful in determining whether the newborn is infected with HCV. RT-PCR may also be useful for evaluating patients with an indeterminate RIBA assay result. A positive RT-PCR result implies the presence of replicating virus.

In addition to PCR-based detection of HCV RNA, nucleic acid amplification tests that can be used include transcription-mediated amplification (TMA) and nucleic acid sequence-based amplification (NASBA) (*see* Chap. 4).

Quantification. Quantification of the baseline HCV viral load before initiation of therapy provides important predictive information regarding response to therapy. Patients with viral loads $>2 \times 10^6$ viral genomes/mL respond less well to drug therapy than do patients with lower levels of viral load. Viral quantification is also used to monitor the response to therapy. In general, patients who do not show a response within 24 wk of therapy are unlikely to benefit from further therapy. An important caveat of quantitative studies is that there is no correlation between the degree of liver damage and the HCV viral load.

Methods commonly used in clinical practice include RT-PCR and branch DNA (bDNA). Different analytical methods give different results on the same sample. This means that periodic samples from patients who are being monitored during therapy should be analyzed using the same method so that changes in viral load can be attributed to biological effects and not to analytical variation. An important reason for lack of agreement between different methods for HCV quantification was lack of availability of an accepted calibration material. Different manufacturers and laboratories used different standards to calibrate HCV assays. This problem has been addressed by the production of the WHO First International Standard for HCV RNA *(28,29)*. After reconstitution of the lyophilized material, the standard contains 10^5 IU/mL of genotype 1 HCV. The availability of this material should lead to improved harmonization of results of quantitative assays.

Genotyping. HCV exists in 6 major subtypes and over 50 subtypes. These differ from each other by up to 50% of their RNA sequence. These subtypes are found with varying frequencies in different parts of the world. In the United States, 70% of infections are associated with subtypes 1a and 1b, and most of the non-genotype 1 cases are caused by genotypes 2 and 3 *(30)*. Genotype 1 is also frequent in Europe. Subtypes 2a and 2b are found widely throughout North America, Europe, and Japan. Additional geographical associations of subtypes are as follows: subtype 4, North Africa and the Middle East (4a is particularly common in Egypt); subtype 5, South Africa; subtype 6, Asia.

In addition to their geographical associations, subtypes are of interest because they may indicate different severity of liver disease, although this remains controversial. Studies on the association between the severity of liver disease in patients with HCV infection and the genotype of the virus have yielded conflicting results, but several studies have tended to associate genotype 1b infections with a worse prognosis than is seen with other genotypes *(24)*. A possible explanation for the discrepancies among studies is that patients identified to date with 1b infections may have been infected for a longer period and thus have more severe disease because of chronicity *(31)*. Prospective studies that have examined the factors influencing disease progression have implicated male gender, age, alcohol consumption, and the hepatitis activity index (but not genotype) as adverse factors *(32–34)*. Currently, the weight of evidence does not support a strong association between genotype and the rate of disease progression in chronic HCV infection.

A study of the association between acute (post-transfusion) hepatitis C infection and the development of chronic infection indicated that infection with genotype 1b was more likely to lead to chronic infection than was infection with non-1b genotypes *(35)*. This observation also needs to be confirmed.

Response to Therapy. The association between genotype and response to therapy has been more clearly defined. It is generally accepted that the genotype influences the response to therapy, with evidence indicating that genotype 1 infections respond less favorably to current therapeutic regimens. Treatment of chronic HCV infection involves therapy with interferon-α (IFN-α) and ribavarin *(36,37)*. Linkage of interferon to polyethylene glycol (Peginterferon) increases the half-life of the drug, reduces the dosing schedule to once weekly, and is associated with improved viral response *(38)*. The initial response to IFN-α is important. Patients who have an early favorable response to therapy are more likely to achieve a long-term response. Among the factors that are associated with long-term response are the dose and duration of IFN-α treatment, the viral load, the degree of liver damage, and the viral genotype *(24)*. Sustained virologic response, which is defined as absence of detectable HCV RNA 24 wk after the cessation of therapy, has been shown to be achieved more commonly in patients with non-1 genotypes than in patients infected with genotype 1 (particularly genotype 1b) *(37,38)*. For patients with genotype 1 infections, high-dose IFN-α induction therapy is associated with a significantly higher rate of achieving long-term response than is conventional therapy *(39)*. For these reasons, genotyping of HCV is of value in deciding the duration and dosage of therapy that are most likely to lead to a sustained viral response.

REFERENCES

1. UNAIDS. Aids Epidemic Update, December, 2001 (www.unaids.org).
2. Gelmann EP, Popovic M, Blayney D, et al. Proviral DNA of a retrovirus, human T-cell leukemia virus, in two patients with AIDS. Science 1983;220:862–5.

3. Laurence J, Brun-Vezinet F, Schutzer SE, et al. Lymphadenopathy-associated viral antibody in AIDS. Immune correlations and definition of a carrier state. N Engl J Med 1984;311:1269–73.

4. Bock PJ, Markovitz DM. Infection with HIV-2. AIDS 2001;15(suppl 5):S35–45.

5. Dow BC. 'Noise' in microbiological screening assays. Transfus Med 2000;10:97–106.

6. Celum CL, Coombs RW, Jones M, et al. Risk factors for repeatedly reactive HIV-1 EIA and indeterminate western blots. A population-based case-control study. Arch Intern Med 1994;154:1129–37.

7. Wai CT, Tambyah PA. False-positive HIV-1 ELISA in patients with hepatitis B. Am J Med 2002;112:737.

8. Anonymous. Report of the NIH Panel to Define Principles of Therapy of HIV Infection. Ann Intern Med 1998;128:1057–78.

9. Holmes H, Davis C, Heath A, Hewlett I, Lelie N. An international collaborative study to establish the 1st international standard for HIV-1 RNA for use in nucleic acid-based techniques. J Virol Methods 2001;92:141–50.

10. Hahn BH, Shaw GM, De Cock KM, Sharp PM. AIDS as a zoonosis: scientific and public health implications. Science 2000;287:607–14.

11. Burgisser P, Vernazza P, Flepp M, et al. Performance of five different assays for the quantification of viral load in persons infected with various subtypes of HIV-1. Swiss HIV Cohort Study. J Acquir Immune Defic Syndr 2000;23:138–44.

12. Hirsch MS, Brun-Vezinet F, D'Aquila RT, et al. Antiretroviral drug resistance testing in adult HIV-1 infection: recommendations of an International AIDS Society-USA Panel. JAMA 2000;283:2417–26.

13. Tisdale M, Kemp SD, Parry NR, Larder BA. Rapid in vitro selection of human immunodeficiency virus type 1 resistant to 3'-thiacytidine inhibitors due to a mutation in the YMDD region of reverse transcriptase. Proc Natl Acad Sci USA 1993;90:5653–6.

14. Shafer RW, Jung DR, Betts BJ, Xi Y, Gonzales MJ. Human immunodeficiency virus reverse transcriptase and protease sequence database. Nucleic Acids Res 2000;28:346–8.

15. Hanna GJ, Caliendo AM. Testing for HIV-1 drug resistance. Mol Diagn 2001;6:253–63.

16. Durant J, Clevenbergh P, Halfon P, et al. Drug-resistance genotyping in HIV-1 therapy: the VIRADAPT randomised controlled trial. Lancet 1999;353:2195–9.

17. Baxter JD, Mayers DL, Wentworth DN, et al. A randomized study of antiretroviral management based on plasma genotypic antiretroviral resistance testing in patients failing therapy. CPCRA 046 Study Team for the Terry Beirn Community Programs for Clinical Research on AIDS. AIDS 2000;14:F83–93.

18. Davenport MP, Zaunders JJ, Hazenberg MD, Schuitemaker H, van Rij RP. Cell turnover and cell tropism in HIV-1 infection. Trends Microbiol 2002;10:275–8.

19. Samson M, Libert F, Doranz BJ, et al. Resistance to HIV-1 infection in Caucasian individuals bearing mutant alleles of the CCR-5 chemokine receptor gene. Nature 1996;382:722–5.

20. Liu R, Paxton WA, Choe S, et al. Homozygous defect in HIV-1 coreceptor accounts for resistance of some multiply-exposed individuals to HIV-1 infection. Cell 1996;86:367–77.

21. Martinson JJ, Chapman NH, Rees DC, Liu YT, Clegg JB. Global distribution of the CCR5 gene 32-basepair deletion. Nat Genet 1997;16:100–3.

22. Zimmerman PA, Buckler-White A, Alkhatib G, et al. Inherited resistance to HIV-1 conferred by an inactivating mutation in CC chemokine receptor 5: studies in pop-

ulations with contrasting clinical phenotypes, defined racial background, and quantified risk. Mol Med 1997;3:23–36.

23. Berger EA, Murphy PM, Farber JM. Chemokine receptors as HIV-1 coreceptors: roles in viral entry, tropism, and disease. Annu Rev Immunol 1999;17:657–700.

24. Zein NN. Clinical significance of hepatitis C virus genotypes. Clin Microbiol Rev 2000;13:223–35.

25. Barrett S, Goh J, Coughlan B, et al. The natural course of hepatitis C virus infection after 22 years in a unique homogenous cohort: spontaneous viral clearance and chronic HCV infection. Gut 2001;49:423–30.

26. Robertson B, Myers G, Howard C, et al. Classification, nomenclature, and database development for hepatitis C virus (HCV) and related viruses: proposals for standardization. International Committee on Virus Taxonomy. Arch Virol 1998;143:2493–503.

27. Tobler LH, Lee SR, Stramer SL, et al. Performance of second- and third-generation RIBAs for confirmation of third-generation HCV EIA-reactive blood donations. Retrovirus Epidemiology Donor Study. Transfusion 2000;40:917–23.

28. Saldanha J, Lelie N, Heath A. Establishment of the first international standard for nucleic acid amplification technology (NAT) assays for HCV RNA. WHO Collaborative Study Group. Vox Sang 1999;76:149–58.

29. Jorgensen PA, Neuwald PD. Standardized hepatitis C virus RNA panels for nucleic acid testing assays. J Clin Virol 2001;20:35–40.

30. Bukh J, Miller RH, Purcell RH. Genetic heterogeneity of hepatitis C virus: quasispecies and genotypes. Semin Liver Dis 1995;15:41–63.

31. Zein NN, Rakela J, Krawitt EL, Reddy KR, Tominaga T, Persing DH. Hepatitis C virus genotypes in the United States: epidemiology, pathogenicity, and response to interferon therapy. Collaborative Study Group. Ann Intern Med 1996;125:634–9.

32. Benvegnu L, Pontisso P, Cavalletto D, Noventa F, Chemello L, Alberti A. Lack of correlation between hepatitis C virus genotypes and clinical course of hepatitis C virus-related cirrhosis. Hepatology 1997;25:211–5.

33. Poynard T, Bedossa P, Opolon P. Natural history of liver fibrosis progression in patients with chronic hepatitis C. The OBSVIRC, METAVIR, CLINIVIR, and DOSVIRC groups. Lancet 1997;349:825–32.

34. Fontaine H, Nalpas B, Poulet B, et al. Hepatitis activity index is a key factor in determining the natural history of chronic hepatitis C. Hum Pathol 2001;32:904–9.

35. Hwang SJ, Lee SD, Lu RH, et al. Hepatitis C viral genotype influences the clinical outcome of patients with acute posttransfusion hepatitis C. J Med Virol 2001;65:505–9.

36. McHutchison JG, Gordon SC, Schiff ER, et al. Interferon alfa-2b alone or in combination with ribavirin as initial treatment for chronic hepatitis C. Hepatitis Interventional Therapy Group. N Engl J Med 1998;339:1485–92.

37. Davis GL, Esteban-Mur R, Rustgi V, et al. Interferon alfa-2b alone or in combination with ribavirin for the treatment of relapse of chronic hepatitis C. International Hepatitis Interventional Therapy Group. N Engl J Med 1998;339:1493–9.

38. Manns MP, McHutchison JG, Gordon SC, et al. Peginterferon alfa-2b plus ribavirin compared with interferon alfa-2b plus ribavirin for initial treatment of chronic hepatitis C: a randomised trial. Lancet 2001;358:958–65.

39. Ferenci P, Brunner H, Nachbaur K, et al. Combination of interferon induction therapy and ribavirin in chronic hepatitis C. Hepatology 2001;34:1006–11.

40. Anonymous. Interpretation and use of the western blot assay for serodiagnosis of human immunodeficiency virus type 1 infections. MMWR 1989;38:1–7.

INDEX